AMYLOIDOSIS

Amyloidosis

Edited by
JAN MARRINK, Ph. D. & MARTIN H. VAN RIJSWIJK, M.D.
Department of Internal Medicine, University Hospital
Groningen, The Netherlands

1986
MARTINUS NIJHOFF PUBLISHERS
A MEMBER OF THE KLUWER ACADEMIC PUBLISHERS GROUP
DORDRECHT - BOSTON - LANCASTER

Distributors

for the United States and Canada: Kluwer Academic Publishers, 101 Philip Drive, Assinippi
Park, Norwell MA 02061, USA.
for the UK and Ireland: Kluwer Academic Publishers, MTP Press Limited, Falcon House,
Queen Square, Lancaster LA1 1RN, England
for all other countries: Kluwer Academic Publishers Group, Distribution Center, P.O. Box
322, 3300 AH Dordrecht, The Netherlands

ISBN-13:978-94-010-8415-4   e-ISBN-13:978-94-009-4309-4
DOI:10.1007/978-94-009-4309-4

PREFACE

This book is a gift from the international community of amyloid friends, presented to Professor Dr. Enno Mandema on the occasion of his retirement from the University of Groningen, the Netherlands. It is the "precipitation" of up to date knowledge of amyloidosis, as presented at the International Course on Amyloidosis in Groningen, on the 10th and 11th of October 1986.

Twenty years ago, Professor Mandema invited a group of scientists, who were studying the various aspects of amyloidosis from different points of view, to discuss their mutual interest in the subject. This "First International Symposium" was held for five days in September 1967. It was a wonderful experience for the participants, as most of them had until then only read each others work in the literature. The proceedings of that symposium, which contained the "lively" discussions, became a text-book for the following years.

Research continued, and while the book was still in preparation, the revolutionary method of "water-soluble amyloid" was published. In the following years, different amyloid proteins were discovered and the molecular basis of the different amyloid syndromes was elucidated. The increase in knowledge parallelled the availability of modern, ingenious and also rapid methods in the biomedical sciences.

The progress of the investigations was reported at international symposia in Helsinki (1974), Povoa de Varzim (1979), Bristol (1981) and New York (1984), as well as in workshops at other large scale congresses. New groups of scientists emerged, and so the "family" of amyloid friends increased. In 1986 they are meeting again in Groningen, but nowadays things move faster and the book is ready at the same time.....

Drs. Jan Marrink and Martin H. van Rijswijk are to be complimented on their enormous effort in the organization of this "state-of-the-art" course and in the editing of the book.

By their presence the participants of this course, have demonstrated that these efforts for organizing such a meeting, have been of great value.

On behalf of all our amyloid friends, I thank Enno Mandema for his continuous stimulation of these international contacts and for the friendly way in which he did it. Last, but not least, I would also like to thank Mrs. Atie Mandema-Polman, whose charm and hospitality is well known to the many amyloid friends who have either visited Groningen or have met her elsewhere during the past 20 years.

Lucas Ruinen

INTRODUCTION

Amyloidosis is the common denominator for a disease complex caused by the extra-cellular deposition of a protein substance with a characteristic tertiary molecular structure, namely, the beta-pleated sheet conformation. This molecular structure is responsible for the insolubility of amyloid under physiological circumstances and for its resistance to proteolytic digestion. As a result of this particular stable structure, amyloid deposition causes progressive replacement and destruction of vital organ tissues. Significant progress has been made in the elucidation of the pathogenesis of the different forms of amyloidosis within the last decade.

Although all types of amyloid display the same conformational characteristics, fundamental differences have been found in the primary structure of the amyloid protein, which appear to be related to differences in the clinical picture of the amyloid syndromes. Different amyloid proteins have been characterized in the amyloid deposits associated with:

* chronic inflammatory diseases,
* plasma cell dyscrasia,
* familial Mediterranean fever,
* the urticaria-deafness-nephropathy syndrome,
* familial amyloidotic polyneuropathy,
* hereditary cerebral hemorrhage (Icelandic type)
* Alzheimer's disease,
* chronic hemodialysis,
* hormone producing tumors.

Circulating precursors have been identified for most of these different amyloid proteins. The practical consequences of these developments are rapidly emerging.

It is incredible to realize that minor substitutions in the amino acid sequence of common proteins may result in a devastating disease such as familial amyloidotic polyneuropathy. It is fascinating that the genetic basis of this substitution is a single base substitution in chromosomal DNA. Nowadays antenatal determination of such a defect has been shown to be possible, thus providing the means for genetic counselling in this troublesome disease.

The awareness of the precursor-product relationship between the acute phase protein SAA and AA amyloidosis has triggered the attention of clinicians to a more vigorous treatment of chronic inflammatory conditions. The question as to whether the amyloid-prone constitution relies on an amino acid substitution of the precursor protein in this type of amyloidosis (e.g. indicated by the heterogeneity of SAA), or on a defect in the degrading system, is as yet unanswered.

The characterization of amyloid in the central nervous system types of amyloidosis, has broadened the scope of amyloid research. The most recent characterization of the amyloid protein in chronic hemodialysis associated amyloidosis as beta-2-microglobulin, demonstrates the rate at which knowledge is increasing in this field.

Amyloid research bears a close relationship to the fundamental biological mechanisms like protein synthesis and processing, as well as to the pathophysiology of inflammation and degeneration.

The acceleration of amyloid research has been greatly stimulated by the regular international symposia on amyloidosis. Ever since Professor Mandema initiated this series of scientific encounters, in 1967, progress has been so rapid, that a "state of the art" anno 1986 seems an appropriate theme for a book covering the present achievements in amyloid research. It was, therefore, decided to organize an International Course on Amyloidosis on the 10th and 11th of October 1986, and at the same time to publish a book reviewing the history, the state of the art, and the perspectives of amyloid research. A team of authors, representative of all those active in the field of amyloid research have dedicated their time and energy to the completion of this volume, which is published in honour of Enno Mandema on the occasion of his retirement from a multifaceted clinical, educational and scientific career. It is hoped that this book - as Professor Mandema himself wrote in his preface of the 1967 symposium book - "may inspire new invest-igations, so that, in the end, we can hope to solve all problems concerned with the amyloid diseases".

The entire area of amyloid syndromes and their pathophysiological aspects is covered in 40 chapters written by the international experts in the field of amyloidosis research. It should be noted that all the chapters were indeed written in 1986!
A book such as "Amyloidosis" is a must for every specialist working in the fields of internal medicine, nephrology, rheumatology, neurology, paediatrics, pathology, clinical biochemistry etcetera.

Acknowledgements

The work of the sub-editors of the different sections, Alan S. Cohen, Gunnar Husby, Mark B. Pepys, Mordechai Pras, George G. Glenner and Keith P.W.J. McAdam, was highly appreciated, as were the contri-butions of the authors of the respective chapters.

We are also indebted to Mrs. Lineke van der Wijk-Stahl for her transformation of all the manuscripts into uniform chapters.

The critical and constructive advice and expert proof-reading of Lucas Ruinen, has been greatly appreciated.

The Assistant Publisher of Martinus Nijhoff Publishers, Ms Drs. A.D.E. Greeven, has devoted her energy to the accomplishment of this tightly scheduled publishing adventure.

Finally we would like to acknowledge the financial and moral support of:

* The Royal Dutch Academy of Sciences
* The State University of Groningen
* The Department of Internal Medicine
* ABBOTT, Diagnostics Division
* BECKMAN Instruments (Nederland) b.v.
* BEHRING Diagnostica
* BOEHRINGER Mannheim b.v.
* CIBA-GEIGY b.v.
* LAMEPRO b.v.
* PFIZER b.v.
* SMITH, KLINE & FRENCH b.v.

Groningen,   Jan Marrink
October 11th, 1986   Martin H. van Rijswijk

CONTENTS

SECTION I

SECTION II

CHEMICAL AND ULTRASTRUCTURAL ASPECTS
sub-editor: Gunnar Husby

SECTION III

CLINICAL ASPECTS
sub-editor: Alan S. Cohen

Contents

SECTION IV

PATHOGENESIS
sub-editor: Mark B. Pepys

Contents

SECTION V

FAMILIAL AMYLOIDOSIS
sub-editor: Mordechai Pras

XIII

Contents

SECTION VI

SENILE AMYLOIDOSIS
sub-editor: George G. Glenner

Contents

XV

Contents

SECTION I

I.1 GENERAL INTRODUCTION AND A BRIEF HISTORY OF AMYLOIDOSIS

and Background of the Groningen, Helsinki, Oporto and Harriman Amyloid Symposia

Alan S. Cohen

Boston University School of Medicine,
Thorndike Memorial Laboratory,
Boston City Hospital,
Arthritis Center of Boston University School of Medicine,
Boston, MA 02118, U.S.A.

1.Amyloid: a historical perspective

Literary research into the history of amyloid is fascinating, and underscores the complexity of scientific discoveries, the blending of different ideas and concepts, the overlap of new and old information and the ultimate evolution of scientific truths. It also underscores the importance of nomenclature as a unifying force in delineating to scientists whether or not they are talking about the same disease, the same syndrome, the same phenomenon. This is particularly important in dealing with ill-defined entities.

Just as there are milestones and key treatises in the elucidation of scientific events, there are milestone reviews, which in the past quarter century have inabled us to trace with reasonable accuracy, the early history of amyloidosis. The treatise of Schwartz (1970) (1) and the papers of Puchtler and Sweat (1966) (2), of Letterer (1969) (3), of Aterman (1976) (4,5) and several other papers (6-8) are major guideposts to the study of early data.

Since there was no terminology by which amyloid was uniquely described until its name was popularized by Virchow in 1854 (9-12), it is difficult to be sure of its true origins. Was the lardaceous liver or the waxy liver always amyloid? Was the spongy and "white stone" containing spleen always an amyloid spleen? While we shall never know precisely, clearly entities consistent with amyloid were described in autopsies carried out as early as 1639 (by Nicolous Fontanus), in 1657 (by Thomas Bartholin), in works by Theophile B. Bonet (1620-1689), Malpighi (1628-1694), Morgagni (1682-1770) and others (1). Portal in 1813 was felt by Dr. Schwartz to be the first to compare what was probably amyloid to "lard" and to "tallow". Rokitansky in 1842 (13) described the "waxy" liver variety of the lardaceous liver and splenomegaly consistent with amyloid, as did Budd in 1845 (14). An Edinburgh group (15) apparently without knowledge of Virchow's work described cases in which liver, spleen and kidney were affected with waxy substances, certainly consistent with amyloid.

Rokitansky and Budd are often given credit for the first descriptions of amyloid although clearly the earlier pathologists had encountered this substance. The key to progress, however, lay in Virchow's assigning to this substance a name, and the fascinating prevailing philosophy and medical knowledge of that era. The name ultimately has its root in the Latin-Amylum and Greek-Amylon. When Virchow discovered that the corpora amylacea stained pale blue on treatment with iodine, and violet on the addition of sulfuric acid, he had no doubt that these bodies were composed of cellulose and at age 32 sent his report to the French Academy (1). His successor as prosector at a Berlin hospital, H. Meckel (1821-1856), however, was considered by Schwartz as "truly the author who inaugurated the exploration of the disease we presently call amyloidosis" (Schwartz, p. 296). Meckel's interest was in the application of the iodine-sulfuric acid test to other organs, and he was able to demonstrate the "lardaceous" material in liver, spleen, kidney, aorta, arteries and intestinal wall. He preferred the name cholesterin and a lively debate with Virchow ensued (16). Virchow himself disagreed with Rokitansky in that the latter's "waxy" liver appeared "lardaceous" to him. He seemed to believe that there was a difference between the two, and that the waxy spleen derived from the degeneration of tissue compounds. The universal use of the term amyloid for tissues or organs staining positively with iodine-sulfuric acid was, however, established and the debate about the similarity or lack of similarity of cerebral corpora amylacea to the tissue lesions and Virchow's views as to the nature of amyloid degeneration were less in vogue.

Aterman (4,5) has nicely reviewed the historical, translational and indeed modern confusion that arose in the seventies based on the usage of the term amyloid, its derivation, original use and historical meaning. Clearly, as noted above, what we now accept as amyloid was known to pathologists as "waxy" or "lardaceous" abnormalities for centuries before Virchow; what we accept as having been coined by Virchow, (i.e. the term amyloid) was used by Schleiden (17) and by Harting (18) before him. Indeed, the modern confusion over Virchow's use of the term amyloid (i.e. starch vs. cellulose) has been clearly shown by Puchtler and Sweat (2) as having been used to indicate cellulose in paper after paper. Interestingly, the improper attribution, i.e., that Virchow regarded amyloid as starch rather than cellulose, took place as early as 1854 through the work and translations of Busk (19). The argument of starch vs. cellulose was far more poignant in the 1850's than it is today, for then scientific debates about the separation of the plant and animal kingdoms were prominent, -and to find so called "cellulose" in the brain of the human body was truly remarkable. Indeed Harting (18,4), who helped develop the iodine-sulfuric acid method in 1847 (and whom Virchow quoted) used the term amyloid as meaning cellulose.

Thus, the major method of diagnozing amyloid was the use of the iodine-sulfuric acid stain, when in 1875 Cornil (20), Heschl (21) and Jurgens (22,5) independently discovered that amyloid deposits stained with methyl violet. Although the term metachromasia was not in use then, by common usage and according to early usage (metachromasia first being used to indicate color change) these analine dyes have been regarded as metachromatic (for discussion see Cohen (6), Aterman (4)) and their impact in the precise in diagnosis of amyloid should not be underestimated. Curiously, Virchow, even 10 years after its introduction, disavowed the dye as a test for amyloid, despite a number of publications demonstrating its clearcut superiority to iodine-sulfuric acid methodology.

It is remarkable how soon after nosology was defined, more precise definition was possible. In 1859, Friedreich and Kekule (23) demonstrated the absence of carbohydrate in a "mass" of amyloid and literally discredited Virchow's concept of amyloid as cellulose or cellulose-like. Attention was then and subsequently has been focused on amyloid as a protein and in recent years as different classes of proteins with common biophysical configuration and properties.

Before we dismiss carbohydrates completely, we must realize that although several complete amino acid sequences of isolated amyloid proteins reveal them to be without carbohydrate moieties the possible linkage of certain proteoglycans or glycosaminoglycans to amyloid in situ or amyloid in its cross-β configuration remains a possibility. Tantalizing data on their presence may have begun with Virchow, but were picked up in 1894 by Oddi (24) and amplified by Krawkow (25). Indeed studies in the 1980's still suggest that this relationship has not yet been completely elucidated.

Another major advance in our understanding of amyloid came with the introduction of Congo red, first as a diagnostic test, then as a histological stain by Bennhold in 1922 (26). When combined with polarization microscopy it becomes the simplest and most useful histologic test for the presence of amyloid (27).

Until the introduction of electron microscopy, polarization microscopy played a major role in the delineation of the submicroscopic structure of tissues and cells. Indeed, the first hint that amyloid might have an organized submicroscopic structure was obtained by Divry working on the central nervous system in 1927 (28). His studies demonstrating the double refraction of the senile plaque was also a landmark in establishing the amyloid nature of these lesions. He also examined experimental murine amyloid, stained it with Congo red, observed the same phenomenon and attributed it to the crystalline structure of the amyloid lesion. This work was sporadically confirmed (Romhanyi, 1949 (29); Ladewig, 1945 (30); Pfeiffer, 1953 (31) but was largely neglected as amyloid was regarded pathologically as composed of a variety of nonspecific proteins.

In 1953, Missmahl (32) started reporting on his extensive series of studies on the birefringence of amyloid, found that both primary and secondary amyloid exhibited positive form birefringence and that Congo red imparted a marked anisotropy to the tissues with a green coloration. After I confirmed the studies of Missmahl in 1956-7 (33), I undertook electron microscopic studies of human primary, secondary, then heredofamilial (familial Mediterranean fever) associated amyloid (34) as well as experimental amyloid, with the hypothesis that an organized ultrastructure should be apparent (35,36). It was clearly demonstrated that all forms of amyloid studied had a comparable fibrillar ultrastructure both in fixed tissue and in isolation of the fibrils, although minor differences concerning their precise dimensions exist. It was subsequently demonstrated that the other protein AP (or SAP when isolated from serum), an almost invariate associate of amyloid fibrils, has a unique pentagonal fine structure of 5 globular subunits and unique amino acid sequence (37-40). Indeed, it has amino acid homologies and a similar appearance to AP (41) and extensions of these studies have led to the identification of a new class of substances, the pentraxins.

Many other landmarks exist if we were to trace the history of significant advances in our knowledge of amyloid. Several of these have been listed on the accompanying table (Table I[a,b]).

TABLE I[a]: MILESTONES IN THE HISTORY OF AMYLOID STUDIES

Early descriptions of <u>a</u>. waxy and lardaceous liver and spleen
<u>b</u>. studies with iodine-sulfuric acid and cellulose
Rokitansky-Budd-others

Year	Author	Description
1854	Virchow	- corpora amylacea and the name amyloid
1855	Meckel; Virchow	- systemic nature
1859	Friedreich & Kekule	- amyloid as a protein, demonstrated probable absence of CHO
1875	Cornil; Heschl; Jurgens	- methyl violet stain for amyloid
1876	Soyka	- amyloid increased in heart of older patients and amyloid in absence of predisposing disease (also probably Wilks, 1856; Wild, 1886)
1894	Krawkow	- systemic experimental amyloid with infection
1922	Bennhold	- Congo red and amyloid; use as diagnostic test and stain
1922	Kuczynski	- casein induction of experimental amyloid
1924	Domagk	- role of reticuloendothelial system
1925	Letterer	- globulins and immune mechanisms
1927	Divry	- first description of birefringence and amyloid in aged
1932	Ostertag	- first description of hereditary amyloid
1952	Teilum	- two-phase theory of pathogenesis

Clearly, the discovery by Soyka (42) in 1876 and by Wild (43) in 1886 and possibly by Wilks (44) in 1856 that amyloid could exist in the absence of predisposing disease ultimately led to our understanding of primary amyloid as opposed to the disorder that characteristically followed chronic infectious and inflammatory disorders. From the early years on, it was always assumed that amyloid existed in conjunction with or as a complication of tuberculosis, osteomyelitis and similar chronic infections. In 1872, Adams and Dowse (45) reported the association of multiple myeloma and amyloid without recognizing the amyloid for what it was. It is probable that Askanazy-Koenigsberg wrote the first clear description of amyloid in multiple myeloma (46). It was Magnus-Levy (47) in 1931 who deduced that the occurrence of amyloid in multiple myeloma was somehow connected to Bence-Jones protein formation, and Apitz (48) in 1940 who noted increased bone marrow plasma cells in primary amyloid.

Our understanding of the whole area of the heredofamilial amyloidoses began with Ostertag's 1932 (49) description of renal disease caused by amyloid in several generations and Andrade's landmark observation starting in 1939 and culminating in his 1952 (50) description of familial amyloid polyneuropathy. The early description by Siegal in 1945 (51) of benign paroxysmal peritonitis and the 1955 studies of Heller and associates (52) clearly defining familial Mediterranean fever and amyloid have been exciting chapters in the development of our understanding of amyloid disease. A multiplicity of genetically determined amyloidoses from Japan, Sweden, Portugal, Italy, Iceland, Denmark, Germany, and elsewhere have emphasized the importance of these genetic disorders.

One should also note the pioneer studies of Krawkow (53) in 1894-5, of Bennhold (1922) (54), Kuczynski (1922) (55), Letterer (1925) (56) and Teilum (1952) (57) in experimentally induced amyloidosis, whose models advanced rapidly our understanding of its pathogenesis.

Arguably, the modern era began when we all came to understand that amyloid was a specific entity, i.e., a fibrillar protein, that could be visualized, isolated and ultimately characterized. I was fortunate, as a Fellow in Rheumatology at the Massachusetts General Hospital in 1956 to be asked to run Dr. Evan Calkins' Laboratory and to see if I could find out anything further about this strange substance amyloid. Together with Giles, Calkins had undertaken a study of whole amyloid tissue and started to characterize its overall biochemical nature (58). Clearly, isolation of a specific component or components would make this a more possible undertaking.

As a clinical investigator, I utilized several approaches to the problem. First, an incidence analysis of amyloid in rheumatoid arthritis to reevaluate the significance of this problem to rheumatology (and I found a 26% incidence in patients with RA who came to postmortem examination at the MGH (59)) and the induction of amyloid experimentally with an attempt to determine physiochemically if there was an organized subunit structure to amyloid (33). As a novice, I was unaware at that time of the studies of Divry, Hartwig, Missmahl and was delighted when I re-

7

discovered the birefringence of amyloid. I quickly hypothesized that amyloid had an organized submolecular structure and undertook to become an electron microscopist to prove or disprove this hypothesis. The laboratory down the corridor housed a collagen chemist who possessed an electron microscope, but I had to go to the Department of Anatomy where I learned tissue techniques from Dr. Leon Weiss, who fortunately was an expert on the spleen. Studies on experimental animal spleens and livers in 1957-1959 led to an abstract in 1958 on the fibrous structure of splenic amyloid (35), then renal amyloid (36) - and the parallel breakthrough came in that same period when we examined human primary, myeloma related and secondary amyloid tissues obtained at biopsy and found them to be clearly fibrous (34). After these studies had been completed and extended to renal biopsies, we split one tissue with a pathologist who verified our finding in this tissue.

TABLE I[b]: MILESTONES IN THE HISTORY OF AMYLOID STUDIES

Modern Era

1959	Cohen[*]	- electron microscopic identification of amyloid as a fibril
1964	Schwartz	- amyloid in senile and presenile dementias
1967	Ranløv	- accelerated induction leading to AEF
		(also Janigan, 1967; Kisilevsky & Axelrad, 1975)
1967	Shirahama[*]	- high resolution EM of fibril
1968	Eanes	- cross-β X-ray diffraction pattern
		(also Bonar[*], 1969)
1971	Glenner	- light chain fragments as component of primary and myeloma amyloid
		(also Natvig; Skinner[*], subsequently)
1972	Benditt	- amyloid A (AA) as the new protein in secondary amyloid
		(also Franklin; Husby; Natvig; Skinner[*])
1972	Goldfinger	- treatment of familial Mediterranean fever with colchicine
1973	Franklin	- serum amyloid A related component (SAA)
	Levin	
1975	Benson[*]	- SAA isolation and identification
1978	Costa	- prealbumin nature of familial amyloidotic polyneuropathy
		(biochemical identification: Skinner[*] & Benson, 1981)
1979	Sipe	- SAA inducer i.e. later interleukin-1
1983	Tawara	- single amino acid substitution (Met for Val) in Japanese familial amyloidotic polyneuropathy
		(1984, Portuguese, Saraiva; 1984, Swedish, Dwulet; Whitehead)
1983	Cohen, D.	- gamma-trace protein (cystatin C) nature of hereditary cerebral amyloid angiopathy
1985	Gejyo[*]	- β_2-microglobulin nature of chronic hemodialysis associated amyloid
	Shirahama[*]	

[*: our laboratory]

8

New information followed rapidly and I was privileged to be in communication in the 1960's with Dr. Philip Schwartz (60) whose career devotion to the study of amyloid, before the ubiquitous nature of amyloid was widely accepted, had highlighted the significance of amyloid in aging. I have preserved correspondence recording his indignation when I suggested that he redo his "nonspecific" thioflavin stained slides. Before responding he sent a selection to a colleague in Germany, and had proof of their green birefringence after Congo red staining! Dr. Earl Benditt was actively at work in the early 60's developing his isolation techniques for what was to be AA amyloid, Dr. Teilum had developed his two phase theory of amyloid formation, - how astutely he had interpreted his histologic data. I was later privileged to be visited on a number of occasions by Dr. Glenner as he was developing his interest in amyloid that led to such significant breakthroughs, and by Drs. Ed Franklin and Dr. Zucker-Franklin as they tooled up for their studies.

It would seem appropriate at this point to mention (at the risk of slighting my friends whom I might not mention) several other critical discoveries. The finding of cross-β X-ray diffraction pattern of amyloid by Eanes and Glenner (61), and our subsequent publication (Bonar, Cohen and Skinner (62)) clarified the definition of amyloid as a substance defined by 3 major parameters (a) green birefringence after Congo red staining, (b) 70-90 Å fibrils on electron microscopy, and (c) cross-β pattern on X-ray diffraction. These have stood the test of time and are the litmus test for all known amyloid(s).

The discovery of the light chain nature of primary and myeloma related amyloid by the amino acid sequencing technique by Glenner and colleagues (63,64) and the subsequent sequence studies from his lab, those in Scandinavia (65) and in Boston (66) clearly delineated this fascinating form of amyloid.

This was closely followed by the description of AA amyloid in animals and in man by Benditt's group (67), by Franklin's group (68), by Husby and Natvig (69), by Skinner (70) so that the second major class was defined. Studies on the pathogenesis of amyloid identified a major acute phase reactant, SAA, the putative precursor of AA protein of secondary amyloid (71,72) and soon thereafter a mediator produced by macrophages, SAA activator (73), which stimulated the production of SAA by hepatocytes (74). SAA activator itself was soon proven to be synonymous with interleukin-1 (75) and SAA was shown to be an apolipoprotein (76). Another fascinating facet of amyloid research has had to do with the accelerated induction of amyloid and the finding of amyloid enhancing factor (AEF) by Ranløv (77), Janigan (78) in 1966-1967 and its pursuit by Kisilevsky and Axelrad (79).

The important observation that the Portuguese familial amyloid neuropathy fibrils were immunologically identical to prealbumin was made by Costa in 1978 (80) and was verified chemically soon thereafter (81,82). Work progressed rapidly in Japan, Portugal and the United States and it was reported by Araki's group (Tarawa) in 1984 that Japanese FAP on sequence analysis had a single amino acid substitution

9

of methionine for valine at position 30 (83). This was found to be the case in Portuguese FAP (84) by Saraiva in 1984 and in two separate Swedish kinships by Dwulet (85) and by Whitehead (86) who also localized the gene to chromosome 18. Other amino acid substitutions have subsequently been recognized and it is clear that amyloid research has entered the era of molecular biology. DNA hybridization techniques and other methodologies now allow for the predictive diagnosis of FAP amyloidosis in family members at risk.

Another fascinating hereditary amyloid was found in 1983 to be identical to another circulating protein, gamma trace (Cystatin C), by Jensson's group in Iceland who were studying hereditary amyloid cerebral angiopathy (87). Even more recent was our laboratory's observation in 1985 in collaboration with Gejyo's group in Japan that the amyloid protein found in the carpal tunnel syndrome and elsewhere in chronic hemodialysis is β_2-microglobulin (88,89).

Starting with the early pathologists there has been an awareness of the role of amyloid in the brain and in association with aging. These concepts, particularly regarding the brain, were stressed by Schwartz (1) and brought to the forefront again by Divry (28). Soyka (42), as early as 1876, noted the association of aging and increased amyloid of the heart. In the modern era, Westermark in 1977 (90) isolated fibrils from the amyloid of the heart associated with aging and showed them to be prealbumin. The literature on the association of amyloid and Alzheimer's disease, senile plaques and tangles has developed rapidly since the electron microscopic confirmation of the nature of these lesions in 1963 by Terry (91). Since this is a rapidly evolving area, I shall leave further discussion of these lesions and the new proteins just being isolated and characterized to another section of this volume.

Other forms of amyloid exist. Some relate to local lesions in the skin, some to endocrine organs where studies since 1975 (92) have suggested that these forms of amyloid relate to polypeptide hormones or their precursors. Finally, as a clinician one must stress the clearcut importance of all these studies leading to better treatment. While it is known that clearing an infection such as osteomyelitis can reverse the disease, the treatment of all forms of established amyloid, i.e. AA (secondary or acquired), AL (primary or myeloma related) or A prealbumin (FAP or that of the aged heart) is not very successful with one exception. The latter is the clearcut evidence based on the 1972 observation of Goldfinger (93), that colchicine used over long term, clearly prevents and may reverse the AA amyloid associated with the hereditary recessive disorder, familial Mediterranean fever, -as shown by the investigators in Israel (94). Animal models also suggest that it may have a broader role in inhibiting amyloidogenesis (95,96).

2. International Amyloid Symposia

Now that I have dealt with these many landmark historical aspects, let me turn to the other topic I have been asked to address. The history of the 4 major Amyloid Symposia leading to the current course honoring Professor Enno Mandema. Sporadically, small international amyloid meetings have taken place, and while none had the participation of virtually all amyloid research scientists who have been present at the major 1967, 1974, 1977 and 1984 meetings, they did represent milestones in their own right (Table II). Several of these meetings were identified by Dr. Mandema in 1967, i.e. (a) the paramyloidosis symposium in Antwerp in 1960, held by the World Federation of Neurology's Problem Commission of Neurochemistry (97); (b) the reports on the geographic distribution of amyloid developed at the 1963, VIII Conference of the International Society of Geographical Pathology in Milan (98); and (c) the Amyloid Research Colloquium in 1964 in Halle, sponsored by the Deutsche Akademie der Naturforscher (99).

TABLE II: MISCELLANEOUS AMYLOID MEETINGS WITH INTERNATIONAL PARTICIPANTS

	Meeting	Publication
1960	World Federation of Neurology's Problem Commission of Neurochemistry - Antwerp	(97)
1963	VIIIth World Conference of the International Society of Geographical Pathology - Milan	(98)
1964	Deutsche Akademie der Naturforscher Leopoldina. Fortschritte der Amyloidforschung - Halle (Saale)	(99)
1969	International Symposium on Hereditary Amyloidosis - Indiana	(100)
1972	Extension Meeting at the IXth International Congress of the International Academy of Pathology - Jerusalem	(101)
1973	XXth Colloquium Protides of the Biological Fluids - Brugge	(102)
1981	European Amyloid Research Symposium - Bristol	(103)
1982	New York Academy of Sciences Conference on CRP and the Plasma Protein Response to Tissue Injury - New York	(104)
1985	First Symposium on Hereditary Central Nervous System Amyloid Angiopathy - Reykjavik	(105)

In addition, the Caylor-Nickel Research Foundation in Indiana on September 29, 1969 held possibly the first international conference on heredofamilial amyloidosis, hosted by Dr. Jackson and which I and several others identified with the study of heredofamilial amyloid in the United States (i.e. Dr. Van Allen) plus investigators from Japan (Dr. Araki), Portugal (Dr. Andrade) and Israel (Dr. Sohar) attended as well (100). Several years later, in 1972 a small international symposium on amyloid was held in conjunction with the International Academy of Pathology's 9th meeting in Jerusalem (101). The annual colloquium of the

Protides of the Biological Fluids had a small symposium on amyloid in 1972 as well (102). Our European colleagues instituted the European Amyloidosis Research Symposium (EARS) in Bristol, England in 1981 (103), and in 1982 there was a symposium sponsored by the New York Academy of Science on CRP and the plasma protein response to tissue injury that included substantial numbers of papers on SAA, AP (SAP) and AEF (104). Very recently, our colleagues in Iceland, Drs. Jensson and Gudmundsson, hosted the first International Symposium on Hereditary Central Nervous System Amyloid Angiopathy, whose responsible protein has been shown to be cystatin C (gamma trace) (105).

TABLE III: INTERNATIONAL AMYLOID SYMPOSIA

Date	Place	Publication	Participants listed	Pages No.	Papers No.
1967 Sept. 24-28	Groningen The Netherlands	Amyloidosis, Proc. International Symposium on Amyloidosis, 1968	46	462	41
		Eds. Mandema, Ruinen, Scholten & Cohen, Excerpta Medica, Amsterdam			
1974 Aug. 26-28	Helsinki Finland	Amyloidosis, Proc. 5th Sigrid Juselius Foundation Symposium, 1976	89	605	49
		Eds. Wegelius & Pasternack, Academic Press, London			
1979 Sept. 23-28	Povoa de Varzim Portugal	Amyloid and Amyloidosis, Proc. 3rd International Symposium on Amyloidosis, 1980	89	629	86
		Eds. Glenner, Costa & Freitas Excerpta Medica, Amsterdam			
1984 Nov. 9-12	Harriman, NY U.S.A.	Amyloidosis, Proc. 4th International Symposium on Amyloidosis: The Disease Complex, 1986	130	857	103
		Eds. Glenner, Osserman, Benditt, Calkins, Cohen & Zucker-Franklin, Plenum Press, New York			

We now turn to the 4 major International Amyloid Symposia (Table III). The first was organized in Groningen, September 24-28, 1967 by my colleague Professor Enno Mandema and his colleagues Drs. Ruinen and Scholten (106). It was very important at that time, for it allowed the investigators from all over the world not only the opportunity to exchange the latest scientific ideas, but also to develop certain generalizations which were clinically as well as investigatively useful. In my discussions of these 4 Symposia, I shall not reference each article, but will refer to the text as a whole. This meeting was truly a working one. It was held at a small rural inn, discussions about amyloid continued at breakfast, lunch and dinner, and various experts made their special contributions. Dr. Missmahl brought along his polarizing microscope and demonstrated green birefringence of Congo red stained amyloid to all who needed such instruction and Dr. Schwartz prepared extensive demonstrations of amyloid in the central nervous system. There were 46 participants, the publication wisely included details of the discussions and 41 papers were presented. It is interesting to note in the last symposium in 1984, we had almost a threefold increase in contributors, $2\frac{1}{2}$ fold increase in the number of papers and twofold increase in the number of pages in the publication. Amyloid research has grown from a cozy cottage industry to a modern science now driven by molecular biologic technology! While we are sad to see the loss of the close exchanges of the 5-10 major groups in the world studying amyloid, we are excited by the multiple advances made now in so many laboratories throughout the world. There is scarcely a "Current Contents" without 2-4 or more citations of amyloid literature per week.

To return to our first Groningen meeting. What were the general outcomes? First, it was again agreed that the use of an appropriate biopsy (probably rectal) and Congo red stain followed by polarization microscopy to demonstrate green birefringence was the best diagnostic method available. Clinical symptoms and signs were stressed and the electron microscopic appearance of fibrils as well. The discovery of the immunoglobulin nature of primary and myeloma related amyloid had not yet been made and the same confusion about the biochemical nature of amyloid persisted, - in retrospect not surprising since multiple biochemical forms of amyloid have been found to exist.

This was the meeting where a number of investigators reported on the isolation of a unique component from amyloid, i.e. amyloid component AP. It was here also that its pentameric electron microscopic configuration was stressed. There were also a significant number of papers on the experimental amyloid model, the role of the reticuloendothelial system in the pathogenesis and various transfer experiments, the latter the precursor of the AEF studies that are still somewhat mysterious.

A considerable amount of time was spent on the ultrastructure of amyloid and its genesis, - leading to one of the more memorable statements after a prolonged discussion as to whether the rigid long amyloid fibrils were intra- or extracellular and whether the nearby cells produced them or not. Dr. Bywaters at that time noted that these comments "reminded me of the pictures of San Sebastian transfixed with arrows: he looked a bit sick too, but nobody has suggested he was secreting them". (p. 80). This, quite eloquently, closed the discussion and led to Dr. Mandema's use of the San Sebastian (Matteo di Giovanni di Bartolo; 1430(?)-1495) painting as the core illustration of the Symposium!

The biochemistry stressed the role of isolation techniques, need for more painting, and the role of carbohydrates i.e. linked or not to the amyloid protein. Histochemical techniques were often used to help to determine the composition of the amyloid deposit.

While familial amyloid polyneuropathy was included (1 paper) and amyloid in the aged was noted in several clinical papers, they clearly did not play a prominent role in this symposium. I personally had the opportunity of summing up the meeting, getting to know Enno Mandema better and wish now, 19 years later, again to thank him for having originated these symposia and having set such an excellent standard.

Finally, it should be noted that among the participants in that meeting were individuals with a long history of study of amyloid i.e. Professors Schwartz, Andrade, Letterer, Teilum, Missmahl plus the new groups of investigators such as those from Groningen (Mandema), Boston (Cohen), Washington, D.C (Glenner), Seattle (Benditt), Tel-Aviv (Gafni) as well as others from Canada, Denmark, Spain, Great-Britain, Italy and Germany.

Seven years later, August 26-28, 1974, the second International Amyloid Symposium took place in Helsinki, Finland (107). It was ably organized by Drs. Otto Wegelius and Amos Pasternack and was as successful as the first. Sponsored by the Sigrid Juselius Foundation, the meeting took place in Hotel Haaga and was charmed each evening by dinners at Hvittrask (Eliel Saarinen's atelier home), then Walhalla restaurant in the Suomenlinna Fortress and finally at Kalastajatorppa. Perhaps the most exciting highlight of the meeting came on the motor launch return from the Walhalla restaurant, when in a deep fog, the launch containing about ½ of the world's "amyloidologists" struck a rock in the Bay of Helsinki, which led to a helicopter and fireboat rescue which made the local headlines. No one was injured, our hosts were wonderful and the meeting went on uneventfully.

Our size had grown significantly in the intervening years, for the biochemical breakthroughs attracted many new investigators. The participants virtually doubled to 89, the number of papers rose to 49 and the text length to 605 pages. In this Symposium some of the discussion was also included. The shift in material presented is interesting for the largest section now had to do with the biochemistry of amyloid. Osserman appropriately in his summation stressed the immunoglobulin nature of primary and myeloma amyloid that was so clearly reconfirmed here, after the initial Glenner discovery in 1971. The presence of the nonimmunoglobulin protein A was also reported on and discussed extensively, as well as P-component. Pathogenetic studies in experimental amyloid evolved to studies of cellular immunity and of the transfer of amyloid, while for the first time there was a small component devoted to several forms of hereditary amyloidosis.

Clinical studies stressed diagnosis, pathology, amyloid in various organs and in association with a number of diseases, and several possible modes of treatment were discussed. One of the milestones of this meeting was the establishment for the first time of internationally accepted criteria (p. ix, Nomenclature) by a Committee consisting of Benditt, Cohen, Franklin, Glenner, Natvig, Osserman and Wegelius. The P-component was officially termed AP, amyloid protein A was termed AA and their serum counterparts SAP and SAA respectively. The immunoglobulin type of amyloid utilized the established immunoglobulin chain nomenclature i.e. AκI etc. Dr. Wegelius and associates had a most successful meeting.

Five years later, September 23-28, 1979, the 3rd International Symposium was held at the Hotel Vermar Dom Pedro, Povoa de Varzim, Portugal. It was hosted by Drs. Andrade and Costa and their colleagues and again was an immense success. The listed participants were again 89, but the number of papers almost doubled to 86 and the book length increased to 629 pages (108). Discussion was still included, but due to the increasing length of the book, was summarized by the chairman of each section.

It was now clear that the new emphasis was on the hereditary amyloid syndromes, particularly the Portuguese familial amyloid neuropathy (FAP) and the Japanese as well as Swedish form. The first detailed discussion of the biochemical nature of the FAP amyloid as prealbumin by Costa took place here.

Attempts were made to develop clinical correlations of serum components and disease (is SAA a tumor marker? are there several types of renal amyloid?). The basic science area flourished, - senile cardiac amyloid protein had been isolated; an amyloid degrading serum substance was found; SAA was observed to be an apolipoprotein; possible heterogeneity of AA and SAA were reported; and more definitive studies of AP appeared. Pathogenetic studies continued and the amyloid enhancing factor redefined.

Treatment again was discussed, and the highlight was the fact that colchicine prevented attacks of familial Mediterranean fever (FMF) and seemed to prevent further development of amyloid in FMF. Finally, the nomenclature was extended to include the preliminary term and chemical designation (i.e. AL and $A_{\lambda 1}$ respectively) and reestablish the use of AL, AA, AF, AE, AS and AD (see p. XI-XII, Guidelines for nomenclature).

A social highlight of the meeting, was that in honor of Dr. Andrade and the Symposium, we were visited by the President of Portugal, Ramalho Eanes, who awarded Dr. Andrade his country's highest civilian honor.

Five years after the Portugal meeting, in 1984, the 4th International Amyloid Symposium was held in the United States, at Arden House in Harriman, New York, at a site organized by Dr. Osserman and a committee consisting of himself, Drs. Benditt, Calkins, Cohen, Glenner and Zucker-Franklin. One of the original members of this committee Dr. Franklin died in 1982, a sad personal loss and loss of an outstanding investigator.

Again, the publication exceeded expectation in size. There were 130 listed contributors, 103 papers and the book was 857 pages long (109). Let me merely cite some highlights.

The chemical characterization of amyloid molecules leaped ahead. We now entered the era of molecular biology and genetic cloning. Complementary DNA clones for apoSAA were reported by several groups. Degradation of SAA was extensively reviewed. Experimental models now were used to study regulatory mechanisms, to isolate AEF and to analyze the deposition of AA. Studies on AP have been broadened to include the whole class of pentraxins. Structural studies on AL in several laboratories stressed attempts to determine the reason for their "amyloidogenicity".

The largest burst of information, however, had to do with hereditary amyloidosis, - the identification of the specific amino acid defect (methionine 30 variant) in Portuguese, Japanese and Swedish patients, the existence of other amino acid variants, the prealbumin nature of Danish amyloid cardiomyopathy and of senile systemic amyloid, and finally the role of serum prealbumin levels. Another new hereditary protein, gamma trace (Cystatin C) was reported in Icelandic Hereditary Cerebral Angiopathy.

Many interesting clinical studies were reported, but the other major new emphasis had to do with amyloid and aging, and amyloid and Alzheimer's disease. The early studies of the nature of isolated senile plaques and paired helical filaments were discussed and the possible role of local formation, prion formation, new protein isolates, neuronal origin were discussed in this rapidly developing field. This huge meeting covered an extraordinary number of scientific disciplines and opened new avenues of investigation for many. Its major organizer (Osserman) and major editor (Glenner) are to be congratulated for the scope of this undertaking.

It was decided to defer further discussion of nomenclature until the next, i.e. 5th International Symposium, provisionally to be held in Japan in 1987 to be hosted by Drs. Araki and Kito and their colleagues.

Thus, this extraordinary field has expanded from what would be called a "cottage" industry to modern science and potential genetic engineering within a 25 year period. Our predecessor in the 19th century, Rudolph Virchow, who may not have discovered amyloid, who may not have even named it, was truly the one who opened the door. Virchow publicized amyloid, debated it, and broke down the nomenclature barriers (waxy, lardaceous) that seemed to slow progress. He, however, was a breaker of barriers, for in his lifetime (1821-1902) he was a pioneer advocate for better public health, for social concern in disease as well as a profound scientist. He not only demonstrated that cells derive only from cells, described leukemia, codified oncology, but studied epidemics, designed sewage systems and agitated politically until they were built. Most of his biographies hardly mention amyloid, which work paled beside his many other contributions. In retrospect, he did lead us into a most fascinating field and for this we thank him (110,111).

Acknowledgements

These investigations have been supported by grants from the United States Public Health Service, National Institute of Arthritis, Metabolic and Digestive and Kidney Diseases (AM-04599 and AM-07014), Multipurpose Arthritis Center, National Institutes of Health (AM-20613), the General Clinical Research Centers Branch of the Division of Research Resources, National Institutes of Health (RR-553) and from the Arthritis Foundation.

References

1. Schwartz, P. In Amyloidosis. Cause and manifestation of senile deterioration. Charles C. Thomas, Springfield IL, 1970.
2. Puchtler, H. & Sweat, F. J. Histochem. Cytochem. 14, 123-134, 1966.
3. Letterer, E. In Amyloidosis. Mandema, E., Ruinen, L., Scholten, J.H., Cohen, A.S., Eds. Excerpta Medica, Amsterdam, 3-9, 1968.
4. Aterman, K. Histochemistry 49, 131-143, 1976.
5. Aterman, K. J. Hist. Med. Allied Sci. 31, 431-447, 1976.
6. Cohen, A.S. Int. Rev. Exp. Pathol. 4, 159-243, 1965.
7. Cohen, A.S. N. Engl. J. Med. 277, 522-530, 574-583, 628-638, 1967.
8. Sorenson, G.D., Heefner, W.A. & Kirkpatrick, J.B. In Methods and Achievements in Experimental Pathology, vol. 1. Bajusz, E., Jasmin, G., Eds. Year Book Medical Publishers, Chicago, 514-543, 1966.
9. Virchow, R. Virchows Arch. Pathol. Anat. Physiol. 6, 268-271, 1854.
10. Virchow, R. Virchows Arch. Pathol. Anat. Physiol. 6, 135-137, 1854.
11. Virchow, R. Virchows Arch. Pathol. Anat. Physiol. 8, 364-368, 1855.
12. Virchow, R. In Cellular Pathology (lecture XVII delivered in the Pathological Institute of Berlin on April 17, 1858). John Churchill, London, 1860.
13. Rokitansky, C. In Handbuch der Pathologischen Anatomie, 3. Band. Braumuller and Siedel, Wien, 311, 1842.
14. Budd, G. On Diseases of the Liver. John Churchill, London, 243-244, 1845.
15. Gairdner, W.T. Mon. J. Med. (London) 18, 393-397a, 186-186b, 1854.
16. Meckel, H. Ann. Charite-Krankenhauses, Berlin, 264-320, 1853,
17. Schleiden, M.J. Ann. Physik 43, 391-397, 1838.
18. Harting, P. Bot. Ztg. 5, 337-348, 1847.
19. Busk, G. Virchows Arch. 6, 135, 1853; Quart. J. Microsc. Sci. 2, 101-108, 1854.
20. Cornil, A.V. C.R. Acad. Sci. (Paris) 80, 1288-1291, 1875.
21. Heschl, R. Wien. Med. Wschr. 25, 715-716, 1875.
22. Jurgens, R. Virchows Arch. Pathol. Anat. Physiol. 65, 189-196, 1875.
23. Friedreich N. & Kekule, A. Virchows Arch. Pathol. Anat. Physiol. 16, 50-65, 1859.
24. Oddi, R. Arch. Exp. Path. Pharmakol. 33, 376-388, 1894.
25. Krawkow, N.P. Arch. Exp. Pathol. Pharmakol. 40, 195-220, 1898.
26. Bennhold, H. Munch. Med. Wschr. 69, 1537, 1922.
27. Cohen, A.S. & Skinner, M. In Laboratory Diagnostic Procedures in the Rheumatic Diseases, 3rd Edition. Cohen, A.S., Ed. Grune & Stratton, Orlando FL, 377-399, 1985.
28. Divry, P. & Florkin, M. C.R. Soc. Biol. (Paris) 97, 1808-1810, 1927.
29. Romhanyi, G. Schweiz. Z. Pathol. Bakt. 12, 253-262, 1949.
30. Ladewig, P. Nature (London) 156, 81-82, 1945.
31. Pfeiffer, H.H. Exp. Cell Res. 5, 443-448, 1953.
32. Missmahl, H.P. & Hartwig, M. Virchows Arch. Pathol. Anat. 324, 489-508, 1953.
33. Cohen, A.S., Calkins, E. & Levene, C.I. Am. J. Pathol. 35, 971-989, 1959.
34. Cohen, A.S. & Calkins, E. Nature 183, 1202-1203, 1959.

35.Cohen, A.S., Weiss, L. & Calkins, E. Clin. Res. 6, 237, 1958.
36.Cohen, A.S. & Calkins, E. Arthritis Rheum. 2, 70-71, 1959.
37.Cathcart, E.S., Comerford, F.R. & Cohen, A.S. N. Engl. J. Med. 273, 143-146, 1965.
38.Bladen, H.A., Nylen, M.U. & Glenner, G.G. J. Ultrastruct. Res. 14, 449-459, 1966.
39.Skinner, M. & Cohen, A.S. Biochem. Biophys. Res. Commun. 54, 732-736, 1973.
40.Skinner, M., Cohen, A.S., Shirahama, T. & Cathcart, E.S. J. Lab. Clin. Med. 84, 604-614, 1974.
41.Oliveira, E.B., Gotschlich, E.C. & Liu, T.Y. J. Biol. Chem. 254, 489-502, 1979.
42.Soyka, J. Prag. Med. Wschr. 1, 165-171, 1876.
43.Wild, C. Beitr. Pathol. Anat. 1, 177-199, 1886.
44.Wilks, S. Guys Hosp. Rep. (Series 3) 2, 103-132, 1856.
45.Adams, W. & Dowse, T.S. Trans. Pathol. Soc. (London) 23, 186-187, 1872.
46.Askanazy-Koenigsberg, M. Verhandl. der Deutsch. Path. Gesellsch. 7, 32-34, 1904.
47.Magnus-Levy, A. Z. Klin. Med. 116, 510-531, 1931.
48.Apitz, K. Virchows Arch. Pathol. Anat. 306, 631-699, 1940.
49.Ostertag, B. Zbl. Allg. Pathol. 56, 253-254, 1932.
50.Andrade, C. Brain 75, 408-427, 1952.
51.Siegal, S. Ann. Intern. Med. 23, 1-21, 1945.
52.Heller, H., Sohar, E. & Sherf, L. Arch. Int. Med. 102, 50-71, 1958.
53.Krawkow, N.P. Zbl. Allg. Pathol. 6, 337-342, 1895.
54.Bennhold, H. Verh. Dtsch. Ges. Inn. Med. 34, 313-315, 1922.
55.Kuczynski, M.H. Virchows Arch. Pathol. Anat. 239, 185-302, 1922.
56.Letterer, E. Verh. Dtsch. Ges. Pathol. 20, 301-304, 1925.
57.Teilum, G. Ann. Rheum. Dis. 11, 119-136, 1952.
58.Giles, Jr, R.B. & Calkins, E. J. Clin. Invest. 34, 1476-1482, 1955.
59.Calkins, E. & Cohen, A.S. Bull. Rheum. Dis. 10, 215-218, 1960.
60.Schwartz, P., Kurucz, J. & Kurucz, J. Presse Med. 72, 3341-3344, 1964.
61.Eanes, E.D. & Glenner, G.G. J. Histochem. Cytochem. 16, 673-677, 1968.
62.Bonar, L., Cohen, A.S. & Skinner, M. Proc. Soc. Exp. Biol. Med. 131, 1373-1375, 1969.
63.Glenner, G.G., Terry, W., Harada, M. et al. Science 172, 1150-1151, 1971.
64.Glenner, G.G., Ein, D., Eanes, E.D. et al. Science 174, 712-714, 1971.
65.Natvig, J.B., Westermark, P., Sletten, K. et al. Scand. J. Immunol. 14, 89-94, 1981.
66.Skinner, M., Benson, M.D. & Cohen, A.S. J. Immunol. 114, 1433-1435, 1975.
67.Hermodson, M.A., Kuhn, R.W., Walsh, K.A. et al. Biochemistry 11, 2934-2938, 1972.
68.Levin, M., Franklin, E.C., Frangione, B. & Pras, M. J. Clin. Invest. 51, 2773-2776, 1972.
69.Husby, G., Natvig, J.B., Sletten, K. et al. Scand. J. Immunol. 4, 811-816, 1975.
70.Skinner, M., Cathcart, E.S., Cohen, A.S. & Benson, M.D. J. Exp. Med. 140, 871-876, 1974.
71.Levin, M., Pras, M. & Franklin, E.C. J. Exp. Med. 138, 373-380, 1973.
72.Benson, M.D., Skinner, M., Lian, J.B. & Cohen, A.S. Arthritis Rheum. 18, 315-322, 1975.
73.Sipe, J.D., Vogel, S.N., Ryan, J.L. et al. J. Exp. Med. 150, 597-606, 1979.
74.Benson, M.D. & Kleiner, E. J. Immunol. 124, 495-499, 1980.
75.Sipe, J.D., Vogel, S.N., Sztein, M.B. et al. Ann. N.Y. Acad. Sci. 389, 137-150, 1982.
76.Benditt, E.P. & Eriksen, N. Proc. Natl. Acad. Sci. USA 74, 4025-4028, 1977.
77.Ranløv, P. Acta Pathol. Microbiol. Scand. 70, 321-329, 1967.
78.Janigan, D.T. & Druet, R.L. Am. J. Pathol. 48, 1013-1025, 1966.
79.Axelrad, M.A., Kisilevsky, R. & Beswetherick, S. Am. J. Pathol. 78, 277-284, 1975.
80.Costa, P.P., Figueira, A.S. & Bravo, F.R. Proc. Natl. Acad. Sci. USA 75, 4499-4503, 1978.
81.Skinner, M. & Cohen, A.S. Biochem. Biophys. Res. Commun. 99, 1326-1332, 1981.
82.Benson, M.D. J. Clin. Invest. 67, 1035-1041, 1981.
83.Tawara, S., Nakazato, M., Kangawa, K. et al. Biochem. Biophys. Res. Commun. 116, 880-888, 1984.
84.Saraiva, M.T.M., Birken, S., Costa, P.P. & Goodman, D.S. J. Clin. Invest. 74, 104-119, 1984.
85.Dwulet, F.E. & Benson, M.D. Proc. Natl. Acad. Sci. USA 81, 694-698, 1984.
86.Whitehead, A.S., Skinner, M., Bruns, G.A. et al. Mol. Biol. Med. 2, 411-423, 1984.
87.Cohen, D., Feiner, H., Jensson, O. & Frangione, B. J. Exp. Med. 158, 623-628, 1983.
88.Gejyo, F., Yamada, T., Odani, S. et al. Biochem. Biophys. Res. Commun. 129, 701-706, 1985.
89.Shirahama, T., Skinner, M., Cohen, A.S. et al. Lab. Invest. 53, 705-709, 1985.
90.Westermark, P., Natvig, J.B. & Johansson, B. J. Exp. Med. 146, 631-637, 1977.
91.Terry, R.D. J. Neuropathol. Exp. Neurol. 22, 629-642, 1963.
92.Westermark, P. Ups. J. Med. Sci. 80, 88-92, 1975.
93.Goldfinger, S.E. N. Eng. J. Med. 287, 1302, 1972.
94.Ravid, M., Robson, M. & Kedar, I. Ann. Intern. Med. 87, 568-570, 1977.
95.Shirahama, T. & Cohen, A.S. J. Exp. Med. 140, 1102-1107, 1974.
96.Kedar, I., Ravid, M., Sohar, E. & Gafni, J. Isr. J. Med. Sci. 10, 787-789, 1974.
97.Symposium on Paramyloidosis. Krucke, W., Seitelberger, F., Eds. Acta Neuropathol. (Berl.), Suppl. II, 1-126, 1963.

98. Leukemia Amyloidosis. Proc. 8th Conference International Society of Geographical Pathology. Roulet, F.C., Ed. Pathol. Microbiol. 27, 782-889, 1964.
99. Fortschritte der Amyloidforschung. Bruns, G., Zschiesche, W., Fritsch, S., Eds. Nova Acta Leopoldina 31, 1-141, 1966.
100. Andrade, C., Araki, S., Block, W.D. et al. Arthritis Rheum. 13, 902-915, 1970.
101. Extension Meeting of the IXth International Congress of the International Academy of Pathology. Isr. J. Med. Sci. 9, 849-887, 1973.
102. XXth Colloquium Protides of the Biological Fluids. Peeters, H., Ed. Pergamon Press, Oxford, 55-161, 1973.
103. Amyloidosis E.A.R.S. Tribe, C.R., Bacon, P.A., Eds. John Wright & Sons Ltd., Bristol, 1983.
104. Kushner, I., Volanakis, J.E., Gewurz, H. Ann. N.Y. Acad. Sci. 389, 1-482, 1982.
105. First Symposium on Hereditary Central Nervous System Amyloid Angiopathy, 1985.
106. Amyloidosis. Mandema, E., Scholten, J.H., Ruinen, L., Cohen, A.S., Eds. Excerpta Medica, Amsterdam, 1968.
107. Amyloidosis. Wegelius, O., Pasternack, A., Eds. Academic Press, London, 1976.
108. Amyloid and Amyloidosis. Glenner, G.G., Costa, P.P., Freitas, A.F., Eds. Excerpta Medica, Amsterdam, 1980.
109. Amyloidosis. Glenner, G.G., Osserman, E.F., Benditt, E.P., Calkins, E., Cohen, A.S., Zucker-Franklin, D., Eds. Plenum Press, New York, 1986.
110. Bloch, H. N.Y. State J. Med. 74, 1471-1473, 1974.
111. Hosp. Pract. Feb. 123-140, 1978.

SECTION II

CHEMICAL AND ULTRASTRUCTURAL ASPECTS

sub-editor: Gunnar Husby

II.1 AMYLOID PROTEINS

Gunnar Husby[1] and Knut Sletten[2]

Department of Rheumatology
University Hospital of Tromsø, Tromsø, Norway[1].

Institute of Biochemistry,
University of Oslo, Oslo, Norway[2].

1. Introduction

In 1968 Pras and coworkers (1) published the water extraction method for purification of amyloid fibrils. This method opened up a new area for the understanding of the structural properties of amyloid. It was confirmed, as suggested more than a century ago that amyloid was principally a proteinaceous material. Gel filtration of solubilized amyloid fibrils obtained from different clinical and experimental types of amyloidosis has in many instances revealed an elution pattern consisting of two main protein peaks. One of these represents a material with very high molecular weight, the so-called void volume (Vo) material (2-4). This material is also present in corresponding preparations of normal tissues and appears to contain a variety of macromolecules, among them fibronectin and a protein related to reticulin (4). Its role in amyloid formation is not established. The second peak represents a protein sub-unit with much smaller molecular weight ranging from 4,200 to 31,000 dalton in different amyloid preparations (5).

It is the recognition and characterization of this low molecular weight amyloid protein subunit that has enabled a chemical and immunologic classification of amyloid fibrils. It has been shown that different, apparently completely unrelated proteins can constitute this subunit in different cases of amyloidosis. However, the nature of the protein subunit seems in most cases to be related to specific clinical types of amyloidosis.

It has been postulated that one prerequisite for the genesis of amyloid fibrils is that the proteins making up such fibrils consist of polypeptide chains arranged in a β-pleated sheet conformation (6). The β-pleated sheet pattern as shown by X-ray crystallographic and infra-red analyses seems to be responsible for the unique ultrastructural as well as tinctorial and optical properties of amyloid. The basis for the formation of amyloid may be the presence of excess amounts of fibril protein precursors capable of assuming the β-pleated sheet structure. Certain serum proteins appear to be the fibril precursors in the systemic forms of amyloidosis. The increase in such proteins may be due to either an overproduction and/or a decreased clearance. A very recent report (7), however, questioned whether the β-pleated sheet structure is obligatory for amyloid fibrils.

Table I shows the human amyloid fibril proteins which have been characterized by complete or partial amino acid sequencing, together with their respective clinical correlates and related serum protein. A slight modification of the preliminary nomenclature from the 3rd. International Symposium on Amyloidosis in Portugal in 1979 (8) is used.

Table I: HUMAN AMYLOID FIBRIL PROTEINS[*] VERIFIED BY AMINO ACID SEQUENCING

CLINICAL TYPE	CHEMICAL TYPE	AMYLOID PROTEIN	RELATED PROTEIN
Idiopathic (primary) amyloidosis			
Systemic	AL	A_κ, A_λ	$IgL, (V_\kappa, V_\lambda)$
Localized	AL	A_κ, A_λ	$IgL, (V_\kappa, V_\lambda)$
Myeloma-associated amyloidosis	AL	A_κ, A_λ	$IgL, (V_\kappa, V_\lambda)$
Reactive (secondary) amyloidosis	AA	AA	SAA
Heredofamilial amyloidosis			
Recessive autosomal:			
- Familial Mediterranean fever (FMF)	AA	AA	SAA
Dominant autosomal:			
- Familial amyloid polyneuropathy (FAP)	AFp[**]	Prealbumin variant	Prealbumin
- Familial amyloid cardiomyopathy (FAC)	AFc	Prealbumin like	Prealbumin
- Hereditary cerebral hemorrhage with amyloidosis (HCHWA)	AFb	gamma-trace like	gamma-trace microprotein
Senile cardiac amyloidosis	ASc	Prealbumin like	Prealbumin
Alzheimer's disease		β-protein	?
Down's syndrome		β-protein	?
Endocrine-related amyloidosis	AE		
- Medullary carcinoma of the thyroid	AEt	(pro-?) calcitonin	calcitonin
Amyloidosis with peripheral nerve entrapment in patients on chronic haemodialysis	AH	β_2-microglobulin	β_2-microglobulin

[*] The nomenclature and abbreviations are according to those proposed in ref.8 with small modifications.
[**] p:peripheral nerves/polyneuropathy, c:cardiac, b:brain, t:thyroid.

2. Immunoglobulin light chain (AL) proteins

AL proteins are derived form homogenous immunoglobulin light chains or N-terminal fragments of such chains and are seen in idiopathic (primary) amyloidosis and amyloidosis associated with monoclonal gammopathies (myelomatosis and Waldenstrøm's macroglobulinaemia). The immunoglobulin nature of these forms of amyloid was finally proven by Glenner et al in 1971 (9).

Chemical identity between tissue AL protein and the urinary Bence-Jones proteins from the same patient has been verified by amino acid sequence analysis (10). Free light chains in serum and amyloid fibril protein from the same patient have been shown to carry the same idiotypic determinant (6). Intact light chains as well as different-sized aminoterminal fragments of the same light chains are often present in the same amyloid preparation, indicating that the fragments are the result of an enzymatic cleavage of intact chains rather than being aberrant cellular products (6,11). Such proteolytic degradation appears to make the light chains more prone to fibril formation (6,12). The fragments usually consist of the entire variable (V) region together with a smaller or larger part of the constant region of the light chain (6,11), suggesting that the V region plays a significant role in the formation of AL amyloid fibrils. However, a recent study (13) has demonstrated a V_λII protein lacking the 7 N-terminal residues which made up AL fibrils together with a fragment derived from the constant part of the same lambda protein. Fibrils similar to those of amyloid have also been formed in vitro by enzymatic treatment of some, but not all Bence-Jones proteins (6,14).

Increased numbers of plasma cells in the bone marrow, M-components in serum and Bence-Jones proteinuria are often observed in patients with idiopathic amyloidosis (15,16), suggesting that this disorder belongs to the plasma cell dyscrasias and is the result of the same basic pathogenetic mechanism as in myelomatosis (17). This is also illustrated by the fact that it is, in many cases difficult to distinguish clinically between them, and, indeed a significant number of patients with myeloma will subsequently develop AL amyloidosis (17). The major differences between these disorders are the osteolytic lesions of myelomatosis which are not present in idiopathic amyloidosis. Another difference is that the κ to λ ratio which is approximately 2:1 in myelomatosis is reversed (1:2) in AL type amyloidosis, showing that λ chains are more prone to fibril formation than κ chains, i.e. more readily assume the β-pleated sheet structure of amyloid fibrils (6). This is also the case with the Bence-Jones proteins that form amyloid-like fibrils in vitro; most of them are λ (6,14).

No light chain protein unique for AL amyloid has been found, although one particular variable subgroup of λ chains, namely V_λVI has a striking association with amyloidosis. We have described the amyloid fibril protein AR which is a prototype of λVI proteins (18). Four out of the 5 first λVI proteins described were derived from AL type amyloid fibrils, while the 5th was a Bence-Jones protein from a patient with myelomatosis (5,18,19). This strong association between λVI proteins and AL amyloidosis (20) has later been confirmed and even strengthened by others (21). The λVI AL proteins or λVI Bence-Jones proteins contain a 2-residue V-region insertion between positions 68 and 69 which appear to be unique for λVI proteins (22). Whether this or other structural characteristics make the λVI proteins more "amyloidogenic" than others is not known at the present.

It has also been suggested that certain κIII (23) and also λI, λII and III proteins (for references, see ref. 24) may contain "amyloidogenic" sequences, and in a recent study (23) of 14 AL proteins, 9 of them were found to contain hexosamine which is more than 4 times higher than that reported for Bence-Jones proteins.

25

Evidence for amyloid fibrils consisting of immunoglobulin heavy chains or fragments of such chains have not, to our knowledge, been provided by amino acid sequence studies up to the present.

The mechanisms for the processing of the light chain precursors to amyloid fibrils are not well understood. Indeed, factors other than possible amyloidogenic light chains may well be required. This was clearly indicated by the finding that AL fibrils could be formed in vitro by proteolysis of Bence-Jones proteins from patients not affected by amyloidosis (6,14).

Clearly, proteolysis appears to be important for this process, in which cells belonging to the reticulo-endothelial system may play an important role (6,11,20,21).

Localized, so called "tumour-forming" idiopathic AL type amyloid has been reported to be present in various organs, of which the respiratory and genito-urinary tracts and the skin are most frequent. In such cases, the AL amyloid may be synthesized locally by monoclonal immunoglobulin light chain-producing cells, and again, the majority of these "amyloidomas" are made up of λ light chains (6,11,25). The masses of amyloid often contain numerous phagocytic cells, and it is possible that both the production of the precursor protein and its processing to amyloid fibrils take place locally (11).

3. Amyloid protein AA

The unique amyloid A (AA) protein (6,26-29) which is connected with reactive (secondary) amyloidosis, amyloid associated with the recessively inherited familial Mediterranean fever (FMF), and with reactive and experimental amyloidosis in animals (for references see 5,6) was first described by Benditt and co-workers in 1971 (26). AA is a heterogeneous protein, particularly in the C-terminal end (20,27,28,30) suggesting that it is a fragment of a larger precursor protein. The precursor is serum amyloid A (SAA) (31,32) although direct evidence for this has been lacking up to the present. However, very recent experiments performed in our laboratory (33) provided rather solid evidence that SAA is indeed the precursor of tissue AA. We introduced human SAA to mice during the induction of amyloidosis with endotoxin. Control animals received endotoxin only. Human AA detected with monospecific antisera (not cross-reacting with mouse AA) using immunodiffusion, immunoblot and radioimmunoassay techniques was present in amyloid fibrils isolated from the animals who had received human SAA, while only mouse AA was found in the fibrils obtained from the control animals. The mouse thus converted human SAA to AA and incorporated it in its own amyloid fibrils, and the precursor-product relationship between SAA and AA was thereby established.

SAA consists of 104 amino acid residues corresponding to a molecular weight of about 11,500 dalton and is larger, but otherwise essentially identical to protein AA in its primary structure (34,35). AA is most probably formed by proteolytic cleavage of protein SAA. Interestingly, like the situation for AL proteins, AA is also an N-terminal fragment of its precursor, and AA proteins of varying size have been found among different amyloid preparations as well as in amyloid extracted from a single organ (5,36), with molecular weights reportedly varying from 4,500 to 9,200 dalton (27,5), corresponding to 45-83 amino acid residues. Most human AA proteins consist of 76 amino acid residues (18) thus lacking a 28 amino acid C-terminal segment which has been split off from the precursor SAA molecule.

The functional significance of SAA is largely unknown. It has been suggested to possess immunoregulatory properties (37), but these experiments need to be confirmed using more refined SAA preparations (12).

Being a protein capable of forming amphipathic helices (38) SAA is complexed mainly to high density lipoprotein (HDL) (38-40) and to a less extent to low density lipoprotein and very low density lipoprotein (39) in serum, and may therefore be termed apo SAA (34). The contents of other lipoproteins in the lipoprotein particles appear to be rather unaltered by the binding of different amounts of SAA (39,41). However, a decrease in the phospholipid content has been observed in SAA-rich HDL in the mouse as compared to control HDL low in SAA (41). Also, a recent study (42) suggests that experimentally induced SAA in non-human primates displaces apo A-I and apo A-II or apo C proteins without altering the overall lipid or protein composition of the HDL particle. It appears that the presence of SAA increases the clearance of HDL from serum, and that SAA may help to increase the removal of unwanted materials like toxic microbial products transported by HDL (43).

Recent X-ray crystallographic studies by Turnell et al (44) suggest two binding sites on SAA for HDL. One corresponds to the hydrophobic 12 first N-terminal residues of SAA which bind electrostatically to phospholipid on HDL. The second one is a calcium-dependent binding between a portion of SAA corresponding to residues 48-51, and phospholipid on the HDL particle. This suggests that the C-terminal part of SAA which is not shared by AA is not essential for the binding to HDL. This is highly compatible with our studies (45) showing that small amounts of an AA-like fragment are present on serum HDL in vivo, and that the binding capacity of HDL for AA in vitro is similar to that for SAA. It could further suggest that the 28 C-terminal portion of SAA which is not present in AA is accessible for enzymatic cleavage when SAA circulates as a part of the HDL particle. However, whether this is important for amyloid formation and for the systemic nature of AA type amyloidosis, is not known at present.

It is now well established that SAA behaves like an acute phase protein in man and in various animals (5,6,25,28,39,41,43,46,48-52,54) but the biological significance of this is not clear.

Although the functional role of SAA is rather obscure, its structure is phylogenetically very conservative as revealed by comparative studies of SAA and AA from man and several animal species (20,30,53), which points to an important biological role for the protein.

Increased concentration of SAA appears to be a prerequisite for the formation of AA both in reactive, human amyloidosis (5,51,54) and in different animal models for AA amyloid (46,48). Longstanding inflammation (54) and certain malignancies (47) are known underlying disorders for reactive amyloidosis, and such diseases are associated with increased serum concentration of acute phase proteins including SAA (5,34). It is now clear that the liver (i.e. hepatocytes) is the chief producer of SAA (50) as is the case with most acute phase proteins (51). Normally, the production and the serum concentration of SAA are very low, but increase several hundredfold within 24 hours after certain inflammatory stimuli and during inflammatory diseases known to induce an acute phase response (50). SAA has been shown to constitute up to 48% of the total HDL protein content in acute phase situations in humans (55) and to rise from less than 1% to 25% of HDL proteins following endotoxin administration in the mouse (41). Studies of SAA mRNA in vitro (52) have confirmed that the liver is the chief producer of SAA, and that SAA synthesis can increase to as much as 2,5% of total hepatic protein synthesis during the acute phase response.

The signal for SAA induction is mediated by a monokine, interleukin-I, released by activated mononuclear phagocytes (50). Although the mechanism by which interleukin-I stimulates the liver to SAA production is not known (51), activation of mononuclear phagocytes appears a key phenomenon in the induction, production and hence for the serum concentration of SAA.

However, only a minority of the patients with "amyloid-prone" diseases develop reactive amyloidosis in spite of chronically raised SAA concentrations (5,20,50,51,54). Additional factors must therefore be necessary for the formation of amyloid. SAA is heterogenous (25,39,50, 51,55) i.e. more than one gene codes for the protein, and it has been speculated that only certain molecular species of SAA are precursors of AA, in other words that patients with reactive amyloidosis are those who produce "amyloid-prone" SAA molecules. This assumption is, however, yet to be proven, although AA was recently found to be identical to only one out of two SAA isotypes in the mouse (25,56), and the amyloid-specific isotype was selectively removed from serum during amyloidogenesis (57).

A possible alternative mechanism for AA amyloid fibril formation is a defective enzymatic break-down of SAA. Protein AA appears to be an intermediate protein fragment in the catabolism of SAA (29,58). Insufficient further break-down and removal of protein AA (58) may, therefore, be an additional mechanism for amyloid formation.

Finally, in vitro studies have indicated individual differences in the resolution of already formed AA fibrils, the so-called amyloid degrading activity (59,60), could be another mechanism for reactive amyloidosis. But again, this is also a hypothesis yet to be proven, and thus all the explanations so far offered for the AA amyloid deposition are rather speculative. The availability of complementary DNA probes for murine and human SAA has enabled more detailed studies of the induction, regulation and structure of SAA protein products (61-65). These studies have shown that three (or more) genes code for SAA in both species. This explains the heterogeneity of the protein mentioned before. The covalent structure of SAA as previously elucidated by amino acid sequencing (34,35, 56) has also been largely confirmed (63-65). Also evidence has been provided that the mouse SAA gene is expressed in extra-hepatic sites (62), and that many cell types including macrophages may express the gene. This may indicate that SAA can be induced, synthesized and deposited locally as AA fibrils in organs other than the liver. Studies of the genetic material coding for SAA proteins are now in progress in many centers and the results will no doubt shed new light on the formation of AA type amyloid.

4.Amyloid proteins related to prealbumin

Heredofamilial amyloidosis with polyneuropathy (FAP) has been detected in a considerable number of families. The amyloid fibril protein (AF_p) derived from the Portuguese FAP was first isolated (66) and shown to be a variant of prealbumin, the only difference in the primary structure of these proteins being a single substitution of valine in position 30 of normal plasma prealbumin by a methionin in the variant amyloid protein AF_p (67,68). The same prealbumin variant has also been isolated from FAP patients of Japanese (69) and Swedish (70) origin.

An amyloid fibril protein of prealbumin nature has also been demonstrated in a Jewish form of FAP (67). However, in this case two genetic mutations appear to be present (B. Frangione, personal communication), namely an amino acid substitution of an isoleucine for a phenylalanine at position 33 (71) and glycine for threonine at position 49 (67). Amyloid fibrils made up by prealbumin variants thus seem to have a high affinity for peripheral nerves.

We (72) have recently characterized the structure of amyloid fibrils derived from a patient with familial amyloid cardiomyopathy (FAC) of Danish origin, also most probably inherited autosomal, dominant (73). Fragments, monomers and polymers of a prealbumin-like protein were found in the myocardial amyloid fibril preparation. Preliminary data indicate a substitution of a methionin for a leucine in position 110, the replacement thus being present at another position, than in FAP. One can only speculate whether the different amino acid replacements may determine the different tissue distributions and thereby the clinical picture of the amyloidoses observed among these families. Furthermore, an increased resistance of the prealbumin variants to proteolysis in vivo, may provide a basis for amyloid formation and deposition in these families.

The acquired, senile cardiac amyloidosis is also related to prealbumin as the amyloid protein derived from a patient with this common age-related disorder showed partial sequence homology with normal pre-albumin (74).

5.Endocrine-related amyloid (AE) protein

The presence of fibrils typical of amyloid has been demonstrated locally in a variety of endocrine tumours, and almost invariably so in the calcitonin-producing medullary carcinoma of the thyroid, MCT (36). Sletten and co-workers (22) have demonstrated the presence of a protein (AE_t) with molecular weight 5,700 dalton in the amyloid fibril extracted from MCT. The amino acid sequence of a peptide obtained by cyanogen bromide cleavage of the protein corresponded to residues 9-19 in normal human precalcitonin. There were some differences in the amino acid composition between the AE_t protein and precalcitonin. Also, the molecular weight of AE_t was higher than that of precalcitonin (3,300 dalton). AE_t was therefore thought to represent a proform of calcitonin.

6.Amyloid related gamma-trace alkaline microprotein

Amyloid fibrils isolated from the leptomeninges and meningeal blood vessels from patients with hereditary cerebral hemorrhage with amyloidosis (HCHWA) of Icelandic origin (75) has recently been shown to be made up by polypeptides homologous in their amino acid sequence with fragments of gamma-trace protein (76,77). The alkaline microprotein gamma-trace has a molecular weight of 13,260 dalton and is present in a number of neuro-endocrine cells (75).

7.Amyloid "β-protein"

Recently, Glenner and Wong (78) provided amino acid sequence data on a 4,200 dalton protein purified from an amyloid fibril extract of affected meningeal vessels of patients with Alzheimer's disease (AD). The protein, called "β-protein", appears to be unique, since a computer search could reveal no homology with any protein sequenced.

The amyloid deposits found in Down's syndrome patients over 40 years of age appear very similar to those of AD (78) and Glenner and Wong (79) have established the N-terminal sequence of a protein similarly extracted from meningeal vessels from such patients to be homologous to that of the AD "β-protein" up to position 24.

8.$β_2$-microglobulin

Some patients undergoing chronic haemodialysis develop peripheral nerve entrapment of the median or the ulnar nerve (80) or pathologic fractures (81) caused by the deposition of amyloid in the flexor retinaculum and bone.

Recently (80) amyloid fibrils extracted from tissue obtained at surgery for carpal tunnel syndrome from a patient on haemodialysis, were fractionated by high pressure liquid chromatography. N-terminal amino acid sequence studies of a major protein fraction with molecular weight 11,000 dalton showed that the 16 first residues were identical to those of β_2-microglobulin; also the amino acid compositions were similar, although not identical. A protein homologous to β_2-microglobulin has also been demonstrated in tumoral bone amyloid from a patient on haemodialysis (81). It is believed that amyloid made up by β_2-microglobulin is a result of an excess of this protein, because haemodialysis is not able to remove it from plasma, and biopsy studies indicate that this form of amyloid is systemic in nature (81).

9. Organ-limited/localized forms of amyloidosis

As already stated (Table I), some forms of localized amyloid have been characterized by amino acid sequence studies of extracted amyloid fibrils. These are local forms of idiopathic AL amyloid (6,11), the calcitonin-related amyloid in MCT (71), and amyloids localized to the central nervous system, namely that related to gamma-trace protein in HCHWA (77) and the unique amyloid β-protein in AD and Down's syndrome (78,79).

Other forms on non-systemic amyloidosis like lichen amyloidosis of the skin (82), and microdeposits of amyloid in the aorta and sclerocalcific heart valves (83), joints (84), and the cornea (57,85), appear to be unrelated to known, sequenced amyloid proteins. In such cases, amyloid fibrils may be made up by local tissue protein, perhaps as a result of cell degeneration. In lichen amyloidosis, for example, the amyloid is antigenically related to epidermal keratin (82). But none of the localized amyloids have been characterized by amino acid sequencing of isolated fibril proteins.

Amyloid is present locally also in some non-endocrine tumours. The amyloid in basal cell carcinoma has been suggested to arise from the tumour cells (86). A 15,000 dalton amyloid protein associated with the calcifying odontogenic tumour may be a novel type of amyloid fibril protein (87). But amino acid sequence data are needed to verify and establish the precise nature of these proteins.

10. The amyloid P-component; protein AP

Protein AP is an α-glycoprotein which is present in almost all forms of amyloid deposits, regardless of chemical nature of amyloid fibrils and clinical type of amyloidosis (11,51,88), the only possible exceptions being the amyloid plaques and neurofibrillary tangles in the brain of AD patients (89). AP is not a part of the amyloid fibrils, but is closely bound to them in a calcium-dependent fashion (51,88). It is not known whether AP plays a role for amyloid formation. A normal plasma protein, SAP, is identical to protein AP in structure and binding properties (51), and immunohistochemical studies have revealed that material cross--reacting with AP/SAP is present in normal glomerular basement membranes and in the proximity of elastic fibers in blood vessels (51). AP and SAP monomers (molecular weight 23,500 dalton) aggregate to form pentameric structures and thus belong to a group of proteins called pentaxins (51). However, such structures have not been observed directly in amyloid deposits, but only in extracts of amyloid tissues.

The biological significance of AP/SAP is largely unknown, although purified human AP has been shown to modulate immune responses in vitro (90).

References:

1. Pras, M., Schubert, M., Zucker-Franklin, D., et al. J. Clin. Invest. 47, 924-933, 1968.
2. Husby, G. & Sletten, K. Acta Pathol. Microbiol. Scand. (C) 85, 153-160, 1977.
3. Husby, G., Sletten, K., Michaelsen, T.E. & Natvig, J.B. Scand. J. Immunol. 1, 393-400, 1972.
4. Scott, D.L., Marhaug, G., & Husby, G. Clin. Exp. Immunol. 52, 693-701, 1983.
5. Husby, G. Scand. J. Immunol. 23, 253-265, 1986.
6. Glenner, G.G. N. Eng. J. Med. 302, 1283-1292, 1333-1343, 1980.
7. Turnell, W.G., Sarra, R., Glover, et al. In Amyloidosis. Glenner, G.G., Osserman, E.F., Benditt, E.P., Calkins, E., Cohen, A.S., Zucker-Franklin, D., Eds. Plenum Press, New York, 49-55, 1986.
8. Benditt, E.P., Cohen, A.S., Costa, P.P., et al. In Amyloid and Amyloidosis. Glenner, G.G., Costa, P.P., Freitas, A.F., Eds. Excerpta Medica, Amsterdam, XI-XII, 1980.
9. Glenner, G.G., Terry, W., Harada, M., et al. Science 172, 1150-1151, 1971.
10. Terry, W.D., Page, D.L., Kimura, S. et al. J. Clin. Invest. 52, 1276-1281, 1973.
11. Husby, G., Sletten,K., Blumenkrantz, N. & Danielsen, L. Clin. Exp. Immunol. 45, 90-96, 1981.
12. Pick, A.I., Frölichman, R. & Schreibman, S. In Amyloidosis. Wegelius O., Pasternack, A., Eds. Academic Press, London, New York, Amsterdam, 279-290, 1976.
13. Eulitz, M. & Linke, R. Biol. Chem. Hoppe-Seyler 366, 907-915, 1985.
14. Glenner, G.G., Ein, D., Eanes, E.D., et al. Science 174, 712-714, 1971.
15. Isobe, T. & Osserman, E.F. N. Engl. J. Med. 290, 473-477, 1984.
16. Osserman, E.F., Takatsuki, K. & Talal, N. Semin. Hematol. 1, 3-85, 1964.
17. Kyle, R.A. Clin. Hematol. 60, 429-448, 1982.
18. Sletten, K., Natvig, J.B., Husby, G. & Juul, J. Biochem J. 195, 561-572, 1981.
19. Natvig, J.B., Westermark, P., Sletten, K., et al. Scand. J. Immunol. 14, 89-94, 1981.
20. Husby, G. & Sletten, K. In Amyloid and Amyloidosis. Glenner, G.G., Costa, P.P., Freitas, A.F., Eds. Excerpta Medica, Amsterdam, 266-273, 1980.
21. Solomon, A., Frangione, B. & Franklin, E.C. J. Clin. Invest. 70, 453-460, 1982.
22. Sletten, K., Westermark, P. & Natvig, J.B. J. Exp. Med. 143, 993-997, 1976.
23. Sletten, K., Westermark, P. & Husby, G. In Amyloidosis. Glenner, G.G., Osserman, E.F., Benditt, E.P., Calkins, E., Cohen, A.S., Zucker-Franklin, D., Eds. Plenum Press, New York, 463-475, 1986.
24. Toinoke, H., Kametani, F., Hoshi, A., et al. FEBS Lett. 185, 139-141, 1985.
25. Anders, R.F., Natvig, J.B., Sletten, K., et al. J. Immunol. 118, 229-234, 1977.
26. Benditt, E.P., Eriksen, M., Hermodsen, M.A. & Ericsson L.H. FEBS Lett. 19, 169-173, 1971.
27. Ein, D., Kimura, S. & Glenner, G.G. Biochem. Biophys. Res. Commun. 46, 498-500, 1972.
28. Levin, M., Franklin, E.C., Frangione, B. & Pras, M. J. Clin. Invest. 51, 2773-2776, 1972.
29. Skogen, B. & Natvig, J.B. Scand. J. Immunol. 14, 389-396, 1981.
30. Sletten, K. & Husby, G. Eur. J. Biochem. 41, 117-125, 1974.
31. Husby, G. & Natvig, J.B. J. Clin. Invest. 53, 1054-1061, 1974.
32. Levin, M., Pras, M. & Franklin, E.C. J. Exp. Med. 138, 373-380, 1973.
33. Husebekk, A., Skogen, B., Husby, G. & Marhaug, G. Scand. J. Immunol. 21, 283-287, 1985.
34. Parmelee, D.C., Titani, K., Ericsson, L.H., et al. Biochemistry 21, 3298-3303, 1982.

35.Sletten, K., Marhaug, G. & Husby, G. Hoppe-Seyler's Z. Physiol. Chem., 364, 1039-1046, 1983.
36.Westermark, P., Grimelius, L., Polak, J.M., et al. Lab. Invest. 37, 212-215, 1977.
37.Aldo-Benson, M.A. & Benson, M.D. J. Immunol. 128, 2390-2392, 1982.
38.Benditt, E.P. & Eriksen, N. Proc. Natl. Acad. Sci. USA 74, 4025-4028, 1977.
39.Marhaug, G., Sletten, K. & Husby, G. Clin. Exp. Immunol. 50, 382-389, 1982.
40.Skogen, B., Børresen, A.L., Natvig, J.B., et al. Scand. J. Immunol. 10, 39-45, 1979.
41.Hoffman, J.S. & Benditt, E.P. J. Biol. Chem. 257, 10510-10517, 1982.
42.Parks, J.S., & Rudel, L.L. J. Lipid Res. 26, 82-91, 1985.
43.Benditt, E.P., Hoffman, J.S., Eriksen, N., et al. Ann. N.Y. Acad. Sci. 389, 183-189, 1982.
44.Turnell, W.G., Sarra, R., Baum, J.O. & Pepys, M.B. In XXXIVth Colloquium Protides of the Biological Fluids. Peeters, H., Ed. (In press).
45.Husebekk, A., Skogen, B. & Husby, G. In XXXIVth Colloquium Protides of the Biological Fluids. Peeters, H., Ed. (In press).
46.Anders, R.F., Nordstoga, K., Natvig, J.B. & Husby, G. J. Exp. Med. 143, 678-683, 1976.
47.Husby, G., Marhaug, G. & Sletten, K. Cancer Res. 42, 1600-1603, 1982.
48.Kisilevsky, R., Boudreau, L. & Foster, B. Lab. Invest. 48, 60-67, 1983.
49.Marhaug, G., Permin, H. & Husby, G. Acta Paediatr. Scand. 72, 861-866, 1983.
50.McAdam, K.P.W.J., Li, J., Knowles, J., et al. Ann. N.Y. Acad. Sci. 389, 126-136, 1982.
51.Pepys, M.B. & Baltz, M.L. Adv. Immunol. 34, 141-212, 1983.
52.Stearman, R.S., Lowell, C.A., Pearson, W.R. & Morrow, J.F. Ann. N.Y. Acad. Sci. 389, 106-115, 1982.
53.Waalen, K., Sletten, K., Husby, G. & Nordstoga, K. Eur. J. Biochem. 104, 407-412, 1980.
54.Husby, G. Clin. Exp. Rheumatol. 3, 173-180, 1985.
55.Marhaug, G., Gaudernack, G., Bogen, B. & Husby, G. Clin. Exp. Immunol. 50, 390-396, 1982.
56.Hoffman, J.S., Ericsson, L.H., Eriksen, et al. J. Exp. Med. 159, 641-646, 1984.
57.Meek, R.L., Hoffman, J.S. & Benditt, E.P. J. Exp. Med. 163, 499-510, 1986.
58.Lavie, G., Zucker-Franklin, D., & Franklin, E.C. J. Exp. Med. 148, 1020-1031, 1978.
59.Kedar, I. & Sohar, E. J. Lab. Clin. Med. 99, 693-700, 1982.
60.Wegelius, O., Teppo, A.M. & Maury, C.P.J. Br. Med. J. 284, 617-619, 1982.
61.Ramadori, G., Sipe, J.D., Dinarello, C.A., et al. J. Exp. Med. 162, 930-942, 1985.
62.Ramadori, G., Sipe, J.D. & Colten, H.R. J. Immunol. 135, 3645-3647, 1985.
63.Sack, G.H., Jr., Lease, J.J. & DeBerry, C.S. In XXXIVth Colloquium Protides of the Biological Fluids. Peeters, H., Ed. (In press).
64.Sipe, J.D., Colten, H.R., Goldberger, G., et al. Biochemistry, 24, 2931-2936, 1985.
65.Yamamoto, K., Shiroo, M. & Migita, S. In XXXIVth Colloquium of the Biological Fluids. Peeters, H., Ed. (In press).
66.Costa, P.P., Figueira, A.S. & Bravo F.R. Proc. Natl. Acad. Sci. USA. 75, 4499-4503, 1978.
67.Pras, M., Franklin, E.C., Prelli, F., & Frangione, B. J. Exp. Med. 154, 989-993, 1981.
68.Saraiva, M.J.M., Birken, S., Costa, P.P. & Goodman, D.S. Ann. N.Y. Acad. Sci. 435, 86-100, 1984.
69.Tawara, S., Nakazato, M., Kangawa, et al. Biochem. Biophys. Res. Commun. 116, 880-888, 1983.
70.Dwulet, F.E., & Benson, M.D. Proc. Natl. Acad. Sci. USA 81, 694-698, 1984.
71.Nakazato, M., Kangawa, K., Minamino, N., et al. Biochem. Biophys. Res. Commun. 123, 921-928, 1984.
72.Husby, G., Ranløv, P.J., Sletten, K. & Marhaug, G. Clin. Exp. Immunol. 60, 207-216, 1985.
73.Frederiksen, T.H., Gøtzsche, H., Harboe, et al. Am. J. Med. 33, 328-348, 1962.
74.Sletten, K., Westermark, P. & Natvig, J.B. Scand. J. Immunol. 12, 503-506, 1980.
75.Gudmundsson, G.J., Hallgrimsson, T.A., Jonasson, T.A. & Bjørnason, O. Brain. 95, 387-404, 1972.
76.Grubb, A., Jensson, O., Gudmundsson, G. et al. J. N. Engl. J. Med. 311, 1547-1549, 1984.
77.Cohen, D.H., Feiner, H., Jensson, O. & Frangione, B. J. Exp. Med. 158, 623-628, 1983.
78.Glenner, G.G. & Wong, C.W. Biochem. Biophys. Res. Commun. 120, 885-890, 1984.
79.Glenner, G.G. & Wong, C.W. Biochem. Biophys. Res. Commun. 122, 1131-1135, 1984.
80.Gejyo, F., Yamada, T., Odani, et al. Biochem. Biophys. Res. Commun. 129, 701-706, 1985.
81.Gorevic, P.D., Casey, T.T., Stone, et al. J. Clin. Invest. 76, 2425-2429, 1985.
82.Kobayashi, H. & Hashimoto, K. J. Invest. Dermatol. 80, 66-72, 1983.
83.Goffin, Y.A., Murdoch, W., Cornwell III, G.G. & Sorenson, G.D. J. Clin. Pathol. 36, 1342-1349, 1983.
84.Lagefoged, C. Ann. Rheum. Dis. 42, 659-664, 1983.
85.Gorevic, P.D., Rodrigues, M.M., Krachmer, et al. Am. J. Ophthalmol. 98, 216-224, 1984.
86.Looi, L.M. Cancer 52, 1833-1836, 1983.
87.Isobe, T., Miki, T., Kametani F. & Shinoda, T. In Amyloidosis. Glenner, G.G., Osserman, E.F., Benditt, E.P., Calkins, E., Cohen, A.S., Zucker-Franklin, D., Eds. Plenum Press, New York, 805-812, 1986.

88.Holck, M., Husby, G., Sletten, K. & Natvig, J.B. Scand. J. Immunol. 10, 55-60, 1979.
89.Westermark, P., Shirahama, T., Skinner, M., et al. Lab. Invest. 46, 457-460, 1982.
90.Li, J.J., Pereira, M.E.A., DeLellis, A. & McAdam, K.P.W.J. Scand. J. Immunol. 19, 227-236, 1984.

II.2 CARBOHYDRATE-CONTAINING AL PROTEINS

Knut Sletten

Institute of Biochemistry
University of Oslo, Oslo, Norway.

In a previous chapter the chemical and ultrastructural aspects of amyloid have been discussed. Thus in primary and myeloma-associated amyloidosis, the fibrils consist mainly of immunoglobulin light chains or fragments thereof called AL proteins. Structurally, these amyloid fibril proteins are a very heterogeneous group. The AL proteins are derived from different subgroups of both κ and λ chains and have a molecular mass from about 5 to 22 Kdalton (1,2). A common feature with these proteins is the ability to form fibrils. The structural studies here described were performed on the main fraction of AL proteins. Acid hydrolyzed protein samples were analyzed by an automatic amino acid analyzer. The content of hexosamine was used as an indicator of carbohydrate. Hexosamine is the most commonly found monosaccharide residue directly linked to the polypeptide chain in mammalian proteins and is also the least likely to be removed by glycosidases present in the different amyloid tissues. AL proteins isolated from amyloid fibrils prepared from different organs of 17 patients were characterized by Edman degradation, molecular weight determinations, amino acid composition and by a complete carbohydrate composition. A summary of the results is shown in Table I.

TABLE I: CLASSIFICATION OF AMYLOID FIBRIL PROTEINS OF IMMUNOGLOBULIN LIGHT CHAIN ORIGIN

Patient	Clinical classification	Organ studied	Molecular mass(Kdalton)	Subgroup	Carbohydrate
Es305	Primary amyloidosis	Tongue	12	$V_\kappa I$	?
547/74	Myelomatosis	Spleen	22	$V_\kappa I$	+
594/79	Primary amyloidosis	Heart	15	$V_\kappa I$	?
Wr	Localized amyloidosis	Larynx	13	$V_\kappa I$, or $V_\kappa III$	+
KSA	Localized amyloidosis	Skin	14	$V_\kappa III$	+
So124	Primary amyloidosis	Spleen	17	$V_\kappa III$	+
700	Primary amyloidosis	Spleen	15	$V_\kappa III$	trace
EPS	Macroglobulinaemia	Liver	20	$V_\lambda I$	+
Es492	Primary amyloidosis	Spleen	18	$V_\lambda II$	+
612/80	Primary amyloidosis	Spleen	?	$V_\lambda II$,or $V_\lambda I$	trace
MOL	Primary amyloidosis	Spleen	22	$V_\lambda III$	+
808	Primary amyloidosis	Spleen	18	$V_\lambda III$	+
758	Myelomatosis	Tongue	17	$V_\lambda III$	not tested
GIL	Multiple myeloma	Spleen	16	$V_\lambda IV$	trace
AR	Primary amyloidosis	Spleen	16	$V_\lambda VI$	-
RS	Primary amyloidosis	Spleen	16	$V_\lambda VI$	not tested
145/85	Primary amyloidosis	Spleen	14	$V_\lambda VI$	+

Seven of the AL proteins were derived from κ light chains. They were subgrouped in $V_\kappa I$ and $V_\kappa III$ and found to have a molecular mass between 12 and 22 Kdalton. Four of these 7 AL proteins contained carbohydrate, while the other 3 gave a very low yield of hexosamine. Two of the carbohydrate-containing proteins were isolated from patients with localized amyloidosis, while the other 2 were obtained from patients with primary and myeloma-associated amyloidosis. The other 10 AL proteins were derived from λ light chains and were subgrouped in $V_\lambda I$, $V_\lambda II$, $V_\lambda III$, $V_\lambda IV$ and $V_\lambda VI$. The molecular mass varied between 14 and 22 Kdalton. Samples of the 2 proteins 758 $V_\lambda III$ and RS $V_\lambda VI$ were lost during carbohydrate analysis. Five of the other 8 proteins were found to contain carbohydrate, while 2 others revealed a very low yield of hexosamine. Four of the carbohydrate-containing proteins were isolated from patients with primary amyloidosis. In order to verify the carbohydrate content and to elucidate the location in the polypeptide chain, further structural studies were undertaken.

The primary structure of AL proteins EPS $_\lambda$ I, Es492 $_\lambda$ II, MOL $_\lambda$ III, GIL $_\lambda$ IV, AR $_\lambda$ VI and So124 $_\kappa$ III have been determined. Glycopeptides were isolated and characterized from 4 of these AL proteins as shown in Table II.

TABLE II: THE LOCATION AND THE SEQUENCE AROUND GLYCOSYLATION SITES IN HUMAN AL PROTEINS

AL EPS $_\lambda$ I
```
        99                    104                        110
-Phe-Gly-Gly-Gly-Thr-Asn-Val-Thr-Val-Val-Gly-Gln-
                     |
                    CHO
```

AL Es492 $_\lambda$ II
```
                   30                    35
-His-Ser-Asp-Val-Asn-Phe-Thr-Asx-Ala(Glx,Ser)Trp-
                   |
                  CHO
```
```
    90                    95                   100
-Cys-Ser-Ser-Phe-Thr-Asx-Thr-Thr-Gln-Leu-Val-Val-
                     |
                    CHO
```

AL MOL $_\lambda$ III
```
    86                90
-Cys-Gln-Ala-Trp-Asn-Ser-Ser-Ser-Val-Leu-Phe-Gly-
                 |
                CHO
```

AL So124 $_\kappa$ III
```
    65                         72
-Ser-Gly-Ser-Gly-Thr-Glu-Phe-Asn-Phe-Thr-Ile-Ser-
                           |
                          CHO
```

The numbering system corresponds to that used in ref.3

AL protein EPS $_\lambda$ I revealed an N-glycosylation site in position 104 which is in the J segment. This is the first report on a glycosylation site at this position in a λ chain (4), and an asparagine residue in position 104 has not been reported. In Es492 $_\lambda$ II evidences for 2 glycosylation sites were obtained, namely in positions 30 and 95, which are part of the first and the third hypervariable regions. In MOL λ III, the glycosylation site was in position 90 which again is in the third hypervariable region. In So124 $_\kappa$ III, the glycosylation site was in position 72 which is in the framework region (FR 3) (3). In AL protein GIL, where only traces of hexosamine were observed (Table I), no glycopeptide could be isolated. However, an acceptor sequence for N-glycosylation was observed in positions 90 to 93 and an amino acid sequence identical to that in AL MOL λ III (positions 90, 91 and 92) was found (Table II).

In general, the glycosylation sites here observed, are with the one exception already mentioned, located in areas of the light chains where carbohydrates have occurred from patients supposedly without amyloidosis (4). However, the frequency of carbohydrate in light chains obtained from homogeneous immunoglobulins from patients with multiple myeloma (5), and supposedly without amyloidosis, is much lower than that observed for the AL proteins in this study.

A comparison of the amino acid sequence in the variable region of the AL protein with that of a Bence-Jones protein of the same type and subgroup, showed that the AL proteins have a number of unique amino acid substitutions (6,7). Furthermore, the comparison indicated also that there is a greater homology between an AL protein and a Bence-Jones protein than between AL proteins of the same subgroup (8). The significance of the amino acid substitutions, with or without the attached carbohydrate, for the formation of amyloid fibrils is still obscure.

References

1.Glenner, G.G.. N. Engl. J. Med. 302, 1283-1292, 1333-1343, 1980.
2.Eulitz, M. & Linke, R. Biol. Chem. Hoppe-Seyler 366, 907-915, 1985.
3.Kabat, E.A., Wu, T.T., Bilofsky, H., et al. Sequences of Proteins of Immunological Interest, U.S. Department of Health and Human Services, Washington, 1983.
4.Savvidou, G., Klein, M., Horne, C., et al. Molec. Immunol. 18, 793-805, 1981.
5.Sox, H.C. Jr. & Hood, L. Proc. Natl. Acad. Sci. USA 66, 975-982, 1970.
6.Toft, K.G., Sletten, K. & Husby, G. Biol. Chem. Hoppe-Seyler 366, 617-625, 1985.
7.Tveteraas, T., Sletten, K. & Westermark, P. Biochem. J. 232, 183-190, 1985.
8.Sletten, K., Westermark, P. & Husby, G. In Amyloidosis. Glenner, G.G., Osserman, E.F., Benditt, E.P., Calkins, E., Cohen, A.S., Zucker-Franklin, D., Eds. Plenum Press, New York, 463-475, 1986.

II.3 ENDOCRINE AMYLOID FIBRIL PROTEINS

Per Westermark

Department of Pathology,
University Hospital, S-751 85 Uppsala, Sweden.

1. Introduction

Since long deposition of amyloid has been known to occur more or less frequently in polypeptide hormone producing tissues and tumours originating from such tissues. Well known examples are the islets of Langerhans and medullary carcinoma of the thyroid gland. Peptide hormone expressing tissues that often contain amyloid deposits are listed in Table I.

TABLE I: AMYLOID DEPOSITS KNOWN TO OCCUR FREQUENTLY IN
CERTAIN PEPTIDE HORMONE EXPRESSING TISSUES

Tissue	Benign states correlated to amyloid	Corresponding tumours with amyloid	Amyloid protein identified by sequence	Ref.
Adenohypophysis	Old age	Adenomas producing GH and prolactin	-	19,20
Parathyroid glands	Old age	Adenomas	-	21,22
Thyroid gland	C-cell hyperplasia?	Medullary carcinoma	(pro)calcitonin	10
Islets of Langerhans	Old age and type II diabetes	Tumours producing insulin	"Insulinoma amyloid peptide"	17

In most of the non-neoplastic tissues, amyloid deposits occur frequently in old age. It can be noted that the gastrointestinal tract, which can be regarded as the largest peptide hormone-producing organ, is not a frequent localization for endocrine amyloid. Studies of peptide hormone synthesizing tumours have given valuable knowledge about the connection of certain hormones with amyloid depositions. It has been shown, that tumours producing growth hormone, prolactin, calcitonin and insulin contain amyloid far more often than neoplasms expressing ACTH, vasoactive intestinal peptide or gastrin (1,2). Since peptide hormones can create amyloid-like fibrils, these findings can suggest that growth hormone, prolactin, calcitonin and insulin give rise to amyloid more easily than other peptide hormones.

Peptide hormones were among the first proteins shown to form synthetic fibrils with properties of amyloid (3,4). Insulin can here serve as a prototype. It has been demonstrated already in the 1940's that an acidic insulin solution formed fibrils if it was heated and frozen repeatedly (5). This property of insulin has even been used as a method for its purification (6). When the β-pleated sheet nature of amyloid fibrils was invented, it was also shown that fibrillar insulin had properties fulfilling the criteria of amyloid (3). The exact molecular background of the fibril formation of insulin has not been elucidated but a radical change in secondary structure is probably involved since insulin in its normal conformation contains little β-strand structure (7). Other peptide hormones that can form fibrils resembling amyloid fibrils are glucagon, calcitonin and parathormone (3,8).

2. The nature of the amyloid in medullary carcinoma of the thyroid gland

It was natural to believe that amyloid occurring in endocrine tissues has hormonal origin (9). This possibility has been discussed since long in the calcitonin producing medullary carcinoma of the thyroid gland, which is a C-cell tumour, and in the islets of Langerhans in maturity onset (type II) diabetes mellitus. In both these tissues, localized amyloid deposits are very common. The hormonal nature of the amyloid in medullary carcinoma of the thyroid gland was definitely demonstrated in 1976 (10). A fibril-forming protein (11) was purified from the amyloid of a metastasis of such a tumour (Fig.1).

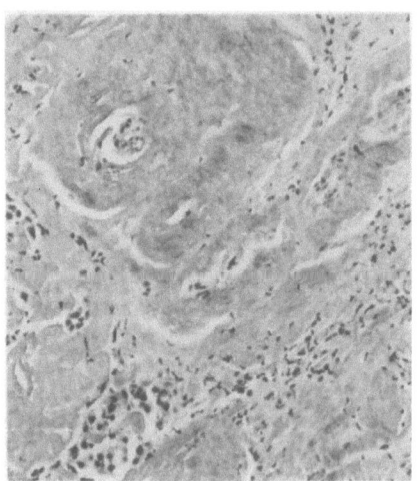 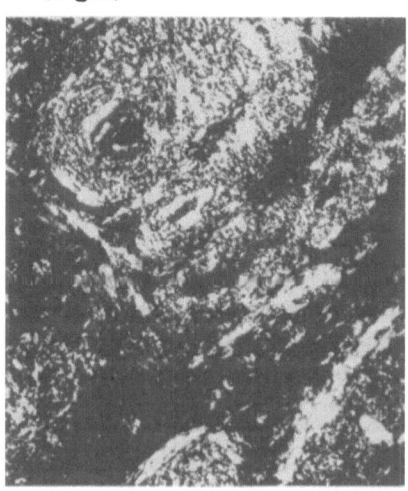

a   b

Figure 1: Lymph node metastasis of medullary carcinoma of the thyroid gland. Amyloid predominates the picture. The main amyloid fibril protein in this tumour showed amino acid sequence homology with calcitonin. Congo red, a. in ordinary light, b. between crossed polars; x 200.

40

The amyloid protein had a blocked N-terminus, but cyanogenbromide cleavage followed by Edman degradation revealed the sequence:

Leu-Gly-Thr-Tyr-Thr-Glx-Asx-Phe-Asx-Lys-Phe-

which corresponds to calcitonin, position 9-19. A peculiar finding, which could not be definitely explained at that time, was the size of the reduced amyloid fibril protein (6,000 dalton compared to 3,400 dalton for calcitonin) (10), and that the blocked N-terminal fragment after cyanogen bromide cleavage had a molecular weight of about 3,000 dalton. Furthermore, the amyloid protein contained significantly more basic amino acid residues than calcitonin. It was therefore suggested that the amyloid protein represents procalcitonin. This theory has been supported by the finding that the mRNA for calcitonin codes for a 141 amino acid residues protein, in which calcitonin is included and flanked by basic amino acids, acting as cleavage points in the generation of calcitonin (12). It is possible that in the genesis of amyloid fibrils in medullary carcinoma of the thyroid gland, a defect processing of the calcitonin precursor is one prerequisite. A part of the N-terminal extension is therefore included in the amyloid fibril protein.

3. The nature of the amyloid in the islets of Langerhans

The nature of the fibril protein in amyloid of the islets of Langerhans is of special interest due to the connection of islet amyloid with maturity onset (type II) diabetes. The close spatial relationship of islet amyloid with the insulin producing β-cells and the common occurrence of amyloid deposits in insulin-producing tumours suggests that insulin is a precursor of this amyloid (13). The ease by which amyloid-like fibrils are formed from insulin gives further support to this hypothesis. The small amounts of extractable insulin in islet amyloid and the mainly negative immunohistochemical results with antisera to insulin (4,14) have therefore been frustrating. Only with an antiserum to a modified insulin, a certain but weak reaction has been obtained with islet amyloid (14,15). A difficulty in the study of islet amyloid is the spotted distribution of the amyloid infiltrated tissue throughout the pancreas. Another great difficulty has been the insolubility of the amyloid in solvents usually used in amyloid protein purification (16). These deviations from most other amyloid deposits have greatly hindered a direct analysis of the islet amyloid. Although amino acid sequence analysis long was impossible, already at an early date the amino acid composition of crude islet amyloid was found not to speak in favour of its origin from insulin or its precursors (11,16).

We have recently had the opportunity to purify amyloid fibrils from an insulin-producing pancreatic tumour (17). The amino acid composition of the amyloid fibrils were similar to that of islet amyloid and had also the same insolubility in the usual solvents. By using other solvent systems in connection with HPLC gel permeation, a major fibril protein was purified. Gas phase amino acid sequence analysis revealed some amino acid positions in the N-terminal part of the molecule. These were:

Lys-?-Asn-?-Ala-?-Ser-Ala-?-Gln-

This embryo of an amino acid sequence does not fit into the pre-pro-insulin molecule (18). The results therefore suggest that the amyloid in insulin producing tumours and probably in the islets of Langerhans in diabetes mellitus is not mainly formed from insulin or its precursors although insulin β-chain seems to constitute a minor part of the deposits (14). Instead, a previously unknown protein is the major constituent of insulinoma amyloid. The nature of this protein is not known at present, but there is reason to believe that it is related to a hormone (17).

From studies performed so far, it can be concluded that the suggestion that the amyloid fibrils in peptide hormone-producing tissues are of hormonal nature, has been verified but as is seen in the islets of Langerhans, the most obvious explanation is not always the right one. It is probable that further elucidation of the composition of endocrine amyloids will give important information not only about the nature of the localized amyloids but also about the physiology of the tissues in which the amyloid appears.

References

1. Westermark, P., Grimelius, L., Polak, J.M., et al. Lab. Invest. 37, 212-215, 1977.
2. Holland, A. In Amyloidosis E.A.R.S. Tribe, C.R. & Bacon, P.A., Eds. John Wright and Sons Ltd., London, 201-204, 1983.
3. Glenner, G.G., Eanes, E.D., Bladen, H.A., et al. J. Histochem. Cytochem. 22, 1141-1158, 1974.
4. Westermark P. Histochemistry 38, 27-33, 1974.
5. Waugh, D.F. J. Am. Chem. Soc. 68, 247-250, 1946.
6. Pettinga, C.W. In Biochemical Preparations. Vestling, C.S., Ed. Wiley, New York, Vol.6, 28-31, 1958.
7. Hodgkin, D.C. & Mercola, D. In Handbook of Physiology, Section 7, Endocrinology, Vol.1, Endocrine Pancreas. Steiner, D.F., Freinkel, N., Eds. Am. Phys. Soc., Washington, D.C. 139-157, 1972.
8. Kedar, I., Ravid, M. & Sohar, E. Isr. J. Med. Sci. 12, 1137-1140, 1976.
9. Pearse, A.G.E., Ewen, S.W.B. & Polak, J.M. Virchows Arch. [Cell Pathol.] 10, 93-107, 1972.
10. Sletten, K., Westermark, P. & Natvig, J.B. J. Exp. Med. 143, 993-998, 1976.
11. Westermark, P. Ups. J. Med. Sci. 80, 88-92, 1975.
12. Amara, S.G., Jonas, V., Rosenfeld, M.G., et al. Nature 298, 240-244, 1982.
13. Westermark, P. Virchows Arch. [A] 359, 1-18, 1973.
14. Westermark, P. & Wilander, E. Diabetologia 24, 342-346, 1983.
15. O'Brien, T., Johnson, K.H. & Hayden, D.W. Am. J. Pathol. 119, 430-435, 1985.
16. Westermark, P. Acta Pathol. Microbiol. Scand. (C) 83, 439-446, 1975.
17. Westermark, P., Wernstedt, C., Wilander, E., et al. manuscript submitted.
18. Bell, G.I., Swain, W.F., Pictet, R., et al. Nature 282, 525-527, 1979.
19. Ravid, M., Gafni, J., Sohar, E., et al. J. Clin. Path. 20, 15-20, 1967.
20. Saeger, W., Warner, R. & Missmahl, H.P. Pathologie 4, 177-182, 1983.
21. Leedham, P.W., Pollock & D.J. J. Clin. Path. 23, 811-817, 1970.
22. Iwata, T., Imada, N., Nakamura, H. et al. Acta Pathol. Jpn. 31, 513-519, 1981.

Mark B. Pepys

MRC Acute Phase Protein Research Group,
Immunological Medicine Unit, Department of Medicine,
Royal Postgraduate Medical School,
Hammersmith Hospital,
Ducane Road, London, W12 OHS, U.K.

1. Introduction

AP is composed of ten identical glycosylated polypeptide subunits which are non-covalently associated in two pentameric disc-like rings interacting face-to-face (1-3). It is identical to the normal serum protein, serum amyloid P component SAP (4-7). Furthermore there is a direct precursor-product relationship between SAP and AP, the latter being derived by deposition of the former from the circulation (8,9). SAP is distinct in its structure and amino acid sequence from all other human proteins with the exception of C-reactive protein (CRP), the classical acute phase protein. CRP and SAP share 51% strict residue for residue identity and when conservative substitutions are taken into account the overall homology is 66% (6,10). No polymorphism of SAP or AP has yet been firmly established.

SAP and CRP are clearly members of the same, unique protein "superfamily", now known as pentraxins (2,5). The genes for both proteins are located on chromosome 1 (6,11) and have presumably been derived by a process of gene duplication. This duplication must have occurred at a very early stage in vertebrate evolution, if not before, since proteins homologous with human SAP and/or CRP are present in all vertebrates in which they have been sought (12-14). A protein homologous with CRP is even present in an invertebrate, Limulus polyphemus, the horseshoe crab (15,16). Such stable conservation during evolution suggests that these proteins have important physiological functions but these have not yet been identified. Reports of immunomodulatory effects of SAP and of its capacity to inhibit proteolysis by elastase have appeared (17,18) but so far have not proved to be reproducible (M.B. Pepys, unpublished observations).

2. Ligand binding by SAP/AP

SAP and AP bind calcium ions and also display specific calcium-dependent ligand binding properties. This was first described in the case of human SAP with respect to agarose (3) and SAP of other species has been isolated and identified on the basis of this same binding specificity. Subsequently SAP was shown to undergo calcium-

-dependent binding to AA and AL-type amyloid fibrils in vitro (19) and the occurrence of this interaction in vivo (8,9) accounts for the presence of AP in amyloid deposits. However SAP has presumably not been conserved in evolution in order to bind either to agarose, a linear galactan hydrocolloid from marine algae, or to amyloid fibrils. Aggregated human SAP expresses new reactivities which are not expressed by native, non-aggregated SAP (20). These reactivities are directed towards two normal plasma proteins, fibronectin and C4-binding protein. When suitably immobilized SAP is exposed to whole normal human serum it selectively binds these two proteins in a strictly calcium-dependent reaction. A pair of SAP molecules, for example bound by an immobilized IgG anti-SAP molecule, binds a single molecule of fibronectin. SAP within the plasma or in serum is not bound to either fibronectin or C4-binding protein and apparently exists freely as single, uncomplexed molecules (21).

The chemical nature of the autologous physiological or even pathophysiological ligand(s) for SAP is not known. SAP does not just bind to any deposit in vivo containing calcium or to any polyanion capable of binding calcium, but displays considerable specificity. In the case of agarose the pyruvate moiety, a variable trace constituent, is essential for SAP binding, and even specific methylation of its carboxyl hydroxyl group is sufficient to abolish uptake of SAP (22). The free 4,6 cyclic pyruvate acetal of methyl β-D-galactose (MOβDG), the form in which pyruvate exists in agarose, has recently been synthesized (22). It inhibits or reverses all the known binding reactions of SAP (22-24), including the binding of AP deposited with amyloid fibrils in vivo. Such activity is strictly dependent on the structure and conformation of MOβDG, presumably reflecting the specific nature of the binding site in the SAP molecule. SAP in normal human serum also binds selectively to bacteria which contain the 4,6 cyclic pyruvate ketal of galactose in their coat but does not bind to those containing the 2,3 cyclic form, non-cyclic ketals or cyclic ketals of glucose (23). SAP is thus a circulating lectin and it also binds to zymosan (yeast cell wall preparation) and various other poorly characterized mannans and galactans (19). However MOβDG itself is not found in mammalian tissues and most amyloid fibrils are formed from non-glycosylated proteins so that the binding specificity of SAP may also be directed to protein structures which stereochemically resemble MOβDG. It is possible that the protein structure in question may be a subclass of those sequences which form β-turns, where polypeptide chains fold back on themselves to allow hydrogen bonded β strands to form a β-pleated sheet. In some of the sequences which form β-turns the end peptide moiety has its peptide acyl oxygen directed nearly perpendicular to the plane of the other atoms and in this exposed position it is able to bind cations, especially calcium with some selectivity over Na^+, K^+ or Mg^{++} (25). Perhaps this conformation is mimicked by that of the pyruvate carboxyl oxygen in MOβDG and related sugars.

Elastin was one of the first proteins in which such β-turns were described and it has a known affinity for binding calcium (25). Amyloid deposits are rich in calcium (26) and, even if not exclusively composed of β-pleated sheets, this structure is evidently present to some extent in all amyloid fibril precursor proteins and fibrils studied so far. Normal elastic fibres throughout the body bear SAP on their surface (27) (see below) and it is therefore possible that SAP is specifically equipped to recognise peptide sequences which include calcium-binding carbonyl groups in appropriate spatial orientation. The presence of these groups may be the feature in common between such apparently diverse protein ligands of SAP as amyloid fibres, elastic fibres, fibronectin and C4-binding protein, and the 4,6 cyclic pyruvate acetal of galactose.

3.Serum levels of SAP

SAP is synthesized by hepatocytes (28,29) and its serum concentration is relatively stable in man, females (mean $\pm$ sd, 33 $\pm$ 10 mg/l) having slightly but significantly lower values than males (43 $\pm$ 14 mg/l) (30). The levels in cord sera are much lower (4 $\pm$ 2 mg/l) (30) but rise rapidly during the first weeks of life to reach the lower part of the adult range, around 10-20 mg/l. In chronic inflammatory or neoplastic diseases in which CRP and SAA levels tend to be raised, the SAP concentration also rises but generally remains within the normal range and does not exceed 100 mg/l (30). Patients with macroglobulinaemia may be exceptional in having higher SAP values than this even with modest rises in acute phase proteins (31,32). In our experience acute stimuli such as major surgery are not followed by any significant or consistent change in SAP levels, however, Hashimoto and Migita (33) have reported a doubling of SAP levels by the third postoperative day in Japanese subjects undergoing surgery.

Amongst the other species in which SAP levels have been measured, mice are exceptional in two respects: firstly, there are marked genetically determined differences in normal levels between different inbred strains and secondly, SAP is a major acute phase reactant in all strains (34). Acute phase levels of mouse SAP are derived largely by de novo synthesis of the protein, in the liver, rather than from release of preformed stocks (35). The T$\frac{1}{2}$ of ^{125}I-SAP measured both by whole body counting and by plasma sampling is about 7.5-9.5 hours in all strains studied (C57BI, CBA, BALB/c, DBA/2), regardless of whether the animals are normal and healthy or are mounting acute phase responses to acute or chronic stimuli, or have established amyloidosis (26). Changes in the plasma level are therefore apparently due to alteration in the rate of synthesis of SAP or of its secretion into the circulation. The turnover and synthesis rates of SAP in man have not been measured directly but observations in individuals undergoing plasma exchange suggest that they are very rapid. It is therefore possible that alterations in overall production and availability of SAP in man could take place in the absence of rises in the plasma level.

4. SAP and amyloidosis

AP has been detected immunochemically using antisera to AP or SAP in deposits or extracts of all forms of amyloid in which it has been sought (37-42), regardless of the chemical nature of the fibril protein, with the exception of intracerebral amyloid plaques (43). Immuno-histochemical staining with anti-SAP therefore provides a valuable aid in the tissue diagnosis of all except the latter form of amyloid. Deposits of experimentally induced amyloid in mice (28) and guinea pigs (44) also contain AP, as do naturally occurring amyloid deposits in cattle (45). In hamsters the counterpart of SAP is known as hamster female protein since its plasma levels are under sex hormonal control, and it too is deposited with amyloid fibrils in experimental (46) and naturally occurring amyloidosis (M.L. Baltz, G. Osborn, M.B. Pepys, unpublished observations).

The mechanism underlying this universal association is that regardless of the chemistry of the subunit proteins, the formed amyloid fibrils all share a common structural feature which happens to be a ligand for SAP. The possible nature of this ligand has been discussed above. SAP of isologous or even heterologous, xenogeneic, origin introduced into the circulation rapidly appears as AP in amyloid deposits (8,9,46). However there may be a more intimate association between AP and the pathogenesis of amyloidosis. For example in man AP is a normal tissue protein located at sites where early amyloid deposition often occurs (see below), whilst in the mouse SAP is an acute phase reactant, levels of which are raised during experimental induction of amyloidosis and correlate more closely with amyloidogenesis than do those of SAA (47).

When isolated pure human SAP is exposed to free ionized calcium it aggregates rapidly and, if the protein concentration is sufficient, it precipitates out (21). The mechanism of this phenomenon is not known although the fact that it is inhibited or reversed by the presence of the cyclic pyruvate acetal of galactose (MOβDG) (24), a specific low molecular weight ligand for SAP (22), suggests that it involves an interaction between the ligand binding site of SAP and a ligand expressed by the SAP itself. It has been suggested that the calcium-dependent aggregation manifested by isolated human SAP may in some way contribute to amyloid fibril deposition (48,49), but it cannot be an essential feature of the pathogenesis since mouse SAP, which is also found in amyloid deposits, does not aggregate in the same way (21). Discovery of the ligand specificity of SAP and availability of MOβDG, and hopefully more active analogues, which are able to dissociate AP from amyloid deposits may in future help to elucidate the role of SAP/AP in amyloidogenesis (22,50).

5.SAP-related material in normal human tissues

Normal human renal glomerular basement membrane (GBM) and the peripheral microfibrillar mantle of elastic fibres in blood vessels and tissues throughout the body contain a protein which binds anti-SAP antibodies immunospecifically (27,39,51-53). It is also present in some other, but not all, vascular basement membranes but is not detectable in renal tubular, dermo-epidermal or other basement membranes (53). The normal tissue AP (TAP) is not present in foetuses nor in children up to the age of 2 years but it then appears and is universally found from 4 years of age onwards (54).

TAP is not eluted from tissue sections except by denaturing solvents which completely destroy tissue architecture, but it can be released in soluble form from isolated GBM by digestion with collagenase. Solubilized TAP from GBM gives reactions of complete identity in gel double immunodiffusion analysis with SAP and anti-SAP. However it is heterogeneous in pI, in molecular size and in polypeptide chain composition. Some of the native material and of the subunits are the same size as SAP but the majority are heavier, suggesting that the TAP is covalently linked to collagen and/or other matrix proteins in the GBM (52). SAP itself has no biochemical similarity or immunochemical cross-reactivity with either collagen or the elastic fibre microfibrillar proteins which have been characterized hitherto (55). The biological significance of TAP in normal tissues is not known but it is possible that the interaction between aggregated AP and fibronectin (see above) may be relevant. It is also of considerable interest that amyloid fibrils are very often located in close relationship to elastic fibres in the skin and elsewhere (56,57).

Immunohistochemical studies with anti-SAP of renal biopsies in various forms of renal disease show distinctive abnormal staining patterns in the GBM and such staining is a simple and sensitive marker for glomerular pathology (58,59). When used routinely for examination of renal biopsies it also has the advantage of detecting small amounts of amyloid which may otherwise be missed unless Congo red staining is included. Anti-SAP is also a useful reagent for the demonstration of abnormalities in the structure and distribution of elastic fibres in skin biopsies (60).

6.Crystallographic studies of SAP

SAP has been crystallized in the presence of calcium ions by precipitation with high molecular weight glycol (61). The crystals took about 15 days to grow and some achieved dimensions of 1.0 x 0.5 x 0.5 mm. SDS-polyacrylamide gel electrophoresis of the crystalline material confirmed the presence of the intact protomer in the crystals. X-ray precession photographs showed that the contents of the crystal were well ordered to at least 2Å resolution. The crystal system was monoclinic, space group $P2_1$ and the cell constants were a = 69.0, b = 99.3, c =

96.8Å, β = 96.1°. X-ray data for the native protein was collected on a four circle diffractometer, to a resolution of 5.6Å.

From this preliminary work the prospects for attaining a molecular model of SAP seem rather good. This model should show the Ca^{++} co-ordination geometry clearly. It may subsequently be possible to co-crystallize SAP with putative calcium-binding peptides and thereby shed some light on the interaction of SAP with amyloid fibril components.

7. Conclusions

There has been much progress in knowledge of the structure and properties of SAP although its in vivo biological role(s) remains elusive. The almost universal nature of its association, as AP, with amyloid fibrils remains most intriguing for the "amyloidologist". AP is not there just as a non-specific accumulation of plasma protein but is specifically and selectively deposited from the circulation as fibrils are formed and appear in detectable quantities. The only amyloid deposits which do not seem to contain AP are plaque cores and the paired helical filaments within the brain. This may reflect a failure of SAP to pass the blood-brain barrier and it certainly suggests that amyloid or amyloid-like fibrils can be formed in the absence of AP; though it should be noted that paired helical filaments have a very different ultrastructure from all other amyloid fibrils and are also intracellular. On the other hand cellular and catabolic processes within the brain are significantly different from those elsewhere and the persistence of intracerebral amyloid in the absence of AP does not vitiate the hypothesis that AP may contribute to the persistence of amyloid deposits laid down in other sites, including the cerebral vasculature itself. Just how AP could effect such a function remains a matter for speculation but possibilities include actions as an enzyme inhibitor, a simple structural effect creating or reinforcing a resistant matrix of fibrils, or the provision of a "native" "autologous" mask shielding the "abnormal" configuration of amyloid fibrils from the cellular or molecular recognition mechanisms necessary for catabolism. Fortunately the experimental tools for investigation of these ideas are now at hand.

References

1. Pinteric, L., Assimeh, S.N., Kells, D.I.C. & Painter, R.H. J. Immunol. 117, 79-83, 1976.
2. Osmand, A.P., Friedenson, B., Gewurz, H. et al. Proc. Natl. Acad. Sci. USA 74, 739-743, 1977.
3. Pepys, M.B., Dash, A.C., Munn, E.A. et al. Lancet i, 1029-1031, 1977.
4. Skinner, M., Pepys, M.B., Cohen, A.S. et al. In Amyloid and Amyloidosis. Glenner, G.G., Costa, P.P., Freitas, A.F., Eds. Excerpta Medica, Amsterdam, 384-391, 1980.
5. Pepys, M.B. & Baltz, M.L. Adv. Immunol. 34, 141-212, 1983.
6. Mantzouranis, E.C., Dowton, S.B., Whitehead, A.S. et al. J. Biol. Chem. 260, 7752-7756, 1985.
7. Prelli, F., Pras, M. & Frangione, B. J. Biol. Chem. 260, 12895-12898, 1985.

8.Baltz, M.L., Caspi, D., Rowe, I.F. et al. In Amyloidosis. Glenner, G.G., Osserman, E.F., Benditt, E.P., Calkins, E., Cohen, A.S., Zucker-Franklin, D., Eds. Plenum Press, New York, 101-108, 1986.
9.Baltz, M.L., Caspi, D., Evans, D.J. et al. Clin. Exp. Immunol. (In press).
10.Woo, P., Korenberg, J.R. & Whitehead, A.S. J. Biol. Chem. 260, 13383-13388, 1985.
11.Whitehead, A.S., Bruns, G.A.P., Markham, A.F. et al. Science 221, 69-71, 1983.
12.Pepys, M.B., Dash, A.C., Fletcher T.C. et al. Nature 273, 168-170, 1978.
13.Baltz, M.L., de Beer, F.C., Feinstein, A., et al. Ann. N.Y. Acad. 389, 49-75, 1982.
14.Robey, F.A., Tanaka, T. & Liu, T.Y. J. Biol. Chem. 258, 3889-3894, 1983.
15.Pepys, M.B., Dyck, R.F., de Beer, F.C. et al. Lancet i, 1029-1031, 1977.
16.Liu, T.Y., Robey, F.A. & Wang, C.M. Ann. N.Y. Acad. 389, 151-161, 1982.
17.Li, J.J. & McAdam, K.P.W.J. Scand. J. Immunol. 20, 219-226, 1984.
18.Li, J.J., Perreira, M.E.A., DeLellis, R.A. & McAdam, K.P.W.J. Scand. J. Immunol. 19, 227-236, 1984.
19.Pepys, M.B., Dyck, R.F., de Beer, F.C. et al. Clin. Exp. Immunol. 38, 284-293, 1979.
20.De Beer, F.C., Baltz, M., Holford, S. et al. J. Exp. Med. 154, 1134-1149, 1981.
21.Baltz, M.L., de Beer, F.C. Feinstein, A. & Pepys, M.B. Biochim. Biophys. Acta 701, 229-236, 1982.
22.Hind, C.R.K., Collins, P.M. & Pepys, M.B. J. Exp. Med. 59, 1058-1069, 1984.
23.Hind, C.R.K., Collins, P.M., Baltz, M.L. & Pepys, M.B. Biochem. J. 225, 107-111, 1985.
24.Hind, C.R.K., Collins, P.M. & Pepys, M.B. Biochim. Biophys. Acta 802, 148-150, 1984.
25.Urry, D.W. In Arterial Mesenchyme and Arteriosclerosis. Wagner, W.D., Clarkson, T.B., Eds. Adv. Exp. Med. Biol. 43, Plenum Press, New York, 211-243, 1974.
26.Kula, R.W., Engel, W.K. & Line, B.R. Lancet i, 92-93, 1977.
27.Breathnach, S.M., Melrose, S.M., Bhogal, B. et al. Nature 293, 652-654, 1981.
28.Baltz, M.L. de Beer, F.C., Feinstein, A. & Pepys, M.B. Biochim. Biophys. Acta 701, 229-236, 1982.
29.Tatsuta, E., Sipe,J.D., Shirahama, T. et al. J. Biol. Chem. 258, 5414-5418, 1983.
30.Pepys, M.B., Dash, A.C., Fletcher, T.C. et al. Nature 273, 168-170, 1978.
31.Jensson, O., Bjornsson, O.G., Arnason, A. et al. Acta Med. Scand. 211, 341-345, 1982.
32.Strachan, A.F. & Johnson, P.M. J. Clin. Lab. Immunol. 8, 153-156, 1982.
33.Hashimoto, S. & Migita, S. Nippon Ket. Gak. Zas. 42, 667-677, 1979.
34.Pepys, M.B. Baltz, M., Gomer, K. et al. Nature 273, 168-170, 1979.
35.Baltz, M.L., Rogers, S.L., Gomer, K. et al. In Amyloid and Amyloidosis. Glenner, G.G., Costa, P.P., Freitas, A.F., Eds. Excerpta Medica, Amsterdam, 534-542, 1980.
36.Baltz, M.L., Dyck, R.F. & Pepys, M.B. Clin. Exp. Immunol. 59, 235-242, 1985.
37.Pepys, M.B., Baltz, M.L., de Beer, F.C. et al. Ann. N.Y. Acad. Sci. 389, 286-297, 1982.
38.Pitkänen, P., Westermark, P., Cornwell III, G.G. & Murdoch, W. Am. J. Pathol. 110, 64-69, 1983.
39.Breathnach, S.M., Bhogal, B., Dyck, R.F. et al. Br. J. Dermatol. 107, 443-452, 1981.
40.Breathnach, S.M., Melrose, S.M., Bhogal, B. et al. Clin. Exp. Dermatol. 8, 355-362, 1983.
41.Wheeler, G.E. & Eiferman, R.A. Exp. Eye Res. 36, 181-186, 1983.
42.Rowe, I.F., Jensson, O., Lewis, P.D. et al. Neuropathol. Appl. Neurol. 10, 53-61, 1984.
43.Shirahama, T., Skinner, M., Westermark, P. et al. Am. J. Pathol. 107, 41-50, 1982.
44.Skinner, M. & Cohen, A.S. In Amyloidosis. Wegelius, O., Pasternack, A., Eds. Academic Press, London, 220-252, 1976.
45.Maudsley, S., Rowe, I.F., de Beer, F.C. et al. Clin. Exp. Immunol. (In press).
46.Coe, J.E. & Ross, M.J. J. Clin. Invest. 76, 66-74, 1985.
47.Baltz, M.L., Gomer, K., Davies, A.J.S. et al. Clin. Exp. Immunol. 39, 355-360, 1980.
48.Pinteric, L. & Painter, R.H. Canad. J. Biochem. 57, 727-736, 1979.
49.Painter, R.H., de Escallon, I., Massey, A. et al. Ann. N.Y. Acad. Sci. 389, 199-213, 1982.
50.Hind, C.R.K., Collins, P.M., Caspi, D. et al. Lancet ii, 376-378, 1984.
51.Houser, M.T., Scheinman, J.I., Basgen, J. et al. J. Clin. Invest. 69, 1169-1175, 1982.
52.Dyck, R.F., Evans, D.J., Lockwood, C.M. et al. J. Exp. Med. 152, 1162-1174, 1980.
53.Breathnach, S.M., Melrose, S.M., Bhogal, B. et al. J. Invest. Dermatol. 80, 86-90, 1983.
54.Khan, A.M. & Walker, F. J. Path. 143, 183-186, 1984.
55.Sear, H.J., Grant, M.E. & Jackson, D.S. Biochem. J. 194, 587-598, 1981.
56.Shirahama, T., Cohen, A.S., Rubinow, A. & Rodgers, O.G. In Amyloid and Amyloidosis. Glenner, G.G., Costa, P.P., Freitas, A.F. Eds. Excerpta Medica, Amsterdam, 132-138, 1980.
57.Yamamoto, K.I. & Migita, S. Proc. Natl. Acad. Sci. USA 82, 2915-2919, 1985.
58.Dyck, R.F., Evans, D.J., Lockwood, C.M. et al. Lancet ii, 606-609, 1980.
59.Orfila, C., Rakotoarivony, J., Segonds, A. & Suc, J.M. Histochemistry 74, 347-354, 1982.
60.Breathnach, S.M., Melrose, S.M., Bhogal, B. et al. Br. J. Dermatol. 107, 443-452, 1982.
61.Oliva, G., O'Hara, B.P., Wood, S. et al. In Protides of the Biological Fluids XXXIV. Peeters, H., Ed. (In press).
62.Rossman, M.G. & Blow, D.M. Acta Cryst. 15, 24-31, 1961.

II.5 A BRIEF REVIEW OF THE ULTRASTRUCTURE OF AMYLOID

Tsuranobu Shirahama and Alan S. Cohen

The Arthritis Center, Boston University School of Medicine,
and the Thorndike Memorial Laboratory
and the Division of Medicine,
Boston City Hospital,
Boston, MA 02118, U.S.A.

1. Introduction

Amyloid consists of a group of chemically diverse proteinaceous substances whose definition depends upon the physico-morphologic characteristics shared commonly amongst them; i.e. characteristic tinctorial properties, unique fibrillar ultrastructure, and cross-β crystallographic configuration.

Since it was first reported by Cohen and Calkins in 1959 (1), the ultrastructural definition of amyloid has been widely used for identification of amyloid. Due to this clear identification, ultrastructural studies have contributed in a great deal towards the clarification of the nature of amyloid and its pathogenesis.

In this article, we shall briefly review those studies.

2. Fine structure of amyloid fibrils

Through electron microscopic examination of amyloid deposits in tissue ultrathin sections from several different patients, it was originally reported in 1959 that amyloid deposits consisted of fine fibrils about 5-14 nm wide, rigid, nonbranching and of indeterminate length (1). Subsequently, the fine structure of amyloid fibrils has been analyzed by many investigators in many different human and animal tissues using a number of different electron microscopic techniques. The ultrastructural analyses were initially carried out on the amyloid fibrils in ultra-thin tissue sections (1-43), and later, when isolation techniques for amyloid fibrils became available, using high resolution electron microscopy on shadow-casted and negatively stained amyloid fibrils (44-57). These studies amply confirmed the fibrillar nature of amyloid and the fibrillar ultrastructure has become one of the most reproducible criteria for the definition of amyloid (58-66).

While some disagreement exists among the reports as to the exact ultrastructural configuration and dimensions of the amyloid fibril and its subunits, it would not be unreasonable to summarize the findings as follows (Figs. 1 and 2).

51

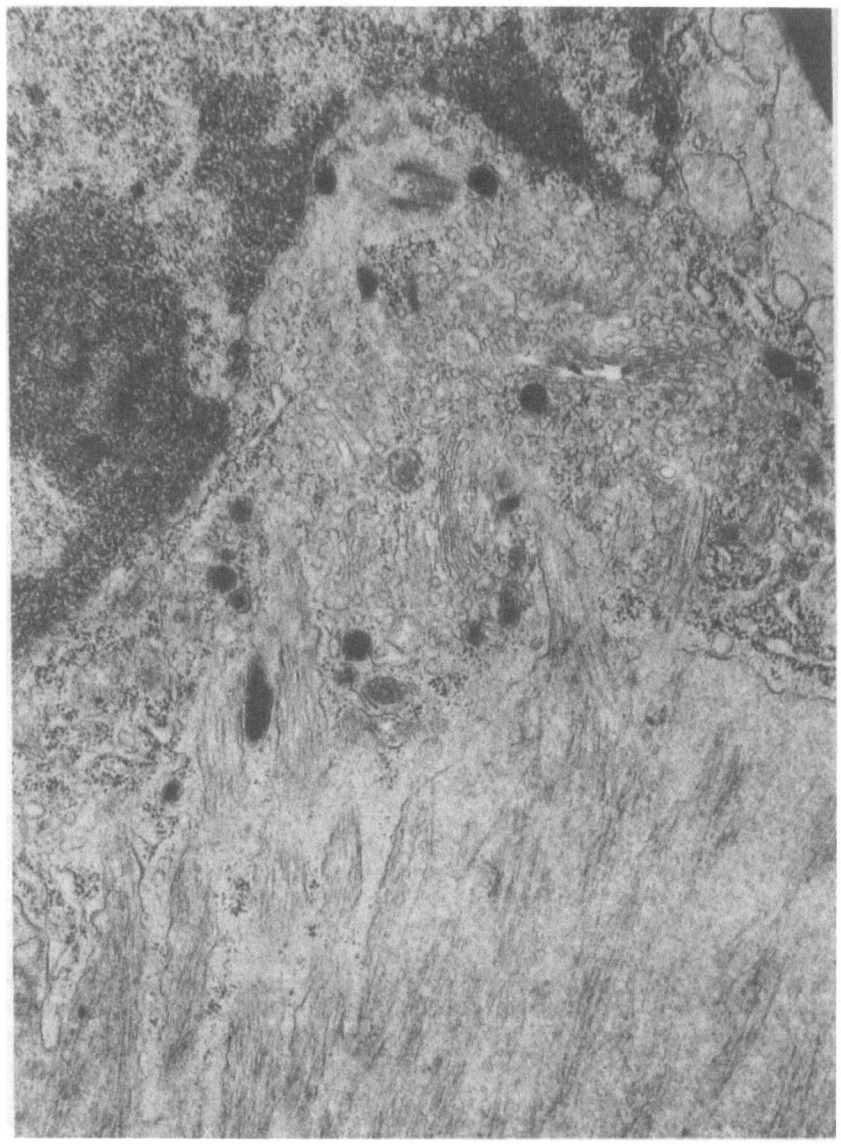

Figure 1: Electron micrograph of a mouse liver in an early stage of casein-induced amyloidosis, showing a portion of a Kupffer cell and an amyloid deposit. At the interphase, the Kupffer cell forms numerous deep invaginations which contain bundles of well-oriented amyloid fibrils. The Kupffer cell displays a well-developed Golgi complex, rough and smooth endoplasmic reticulum, and many dense bodies. Magnification x 30,000.

1. A unit fibrillar structure of amyloid, which has been called "the amyloid fibril" (or "the amyloid filament"), indeed exists.
2. The amyloid fibril is 7.5-10 nm in width and of indeterminate length.
3. The amyloid fibril is composed of two or more filamentous sub-units which run in parallel to and which loosely twist about each other along the long axis of the fibril.
4. The subunit measures 2.5-3.5 nm in diameter.

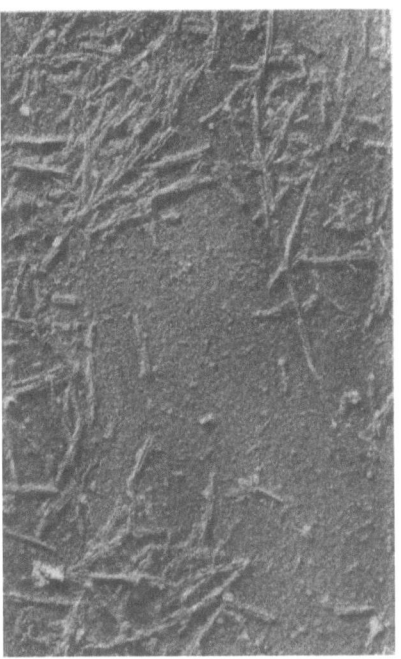

Figure 2: Human AA amyloid fibrils isolated through a sucrose-density gradient centrifugation method, and shadow-casted with platinum-palladium (55). The fibrils are about 10 nm in width. Some fibrils show twisting appearance. Linear subunits of 2.5-3.5 nm width are resolved in portions of the fibrils. Magnification x 60,000.

3. Ultrastructural aspects of amyloidogenesis

a. Sites of amyloid formation

In an attempt to uncover the cells responsible for amyloid production and the subcellular mechanism involved in the amyloid fibril formation, a variety of amyloidotic human and animal tissues have been studied. Proximity of cells and amyloid deposits, ultrastructural changes in the cells neighbouring amyloid deposits, unusual and regular line-up of amyloid fibrils etc. have been used as circumstantial evidence for certain types of amyloid fibril formation (Fig. 1).

Various cell types have been reported to be responsible for amyloid fibril formation, including reticuloendothelial cells (1, 5-7, 10-17, 20, 22, 33-41, 43, 67-71), fibroblasts (21,32), plasma cells (71,72), smooth muscle cells (73) and so on (71,74,75). Clearly as knowledge of the chemical and biological nature of amyloid has advanced, these concepts have been altered to separate sites of amyloid synthesis from the mechanisms of fibrillogenesis.

While amyloid fibrils are usually arranged in a random array, they occasionally line up parallel to one another in well oriented bundles. These bundles of amyloid fibrils are often positioned very close and perpendicular to an invaginating plasma membrane. This type of ultrastructural complex was considered to be the site of amyloid formation by Gueft and Ghidoni (20), and the idea has been widely accepted (58-66)

(Fig. 1). Early on, spleen explants derived from animals on an amyloid inducing regimen were studied by electron microscopic autoradiography, and the results were interpreted as demonstrating production of amyloid fibrils by the reticuloendothelial cells in the culture (4,17).

Intracytoplasmic fibrils that were observed in plasma cells and other cell types from amyloidotic humans and animals were on occasion interpreted as amyloid fibrils and thus the evidence of intracellular formation of amyloid fibrils (71,72,76,77).

Unusual intracellular inclusions being round- to long-fusiform in shape, measuring 0.3-0.8 μm in width 0.5 μm to several micrometers in length, and having varying electron density were observed in the reticuloendothelial cells that showed an intimate relationship to newly formed amyloid deposits in an experimental murine model. In the inclusions, well-organized fibrils comparable with the extracellular amyloid fibrils were often revealed. The inclusions demonstrated lysosomal enzyme activity by histochemistry, and by an immunocytochemical method the fibrils that were observed in the inclusions reacted with anti-mouse AA antisera. These findings have been regarded as evidence for intralysosomal formation of amyloid fibrils, probably the process of intralysosomal proteolytic cleavage of SAA to form AA and finally the AA fibril (69,70,78).

b. Resorption of amyloid

Although amyloid deposits appear to remain static for a long period of time, there are clinical and experimental findings that support the idea that absorption of amyloid deposits can indeed occur (58-66). Through electron microscopy of amyloid laden tissues, phagosomes that contained amyloid fibrils in a random arrangement were observed in phagocytes that were located within or adjacent to amyloid deposits, suggesting phagocytosis of the amyloid (34). Using in vitro systems where amyloid fibrils were incubated with macrophages and polymorphonuclear leukocytes, such phagocytosis of amyloid was demonstrated (79-81). Shirahama and Cohen further observed the process of intraphagosomal digestion of amyloid fibrils (80).

c. In vitro synthesis of amyloid fibrils

Strong evidence to support the concept that serum proteins such as immunoglobulin light chain and SAA are the precursors for amyloid proteins such as AL and AA has been produced by successful creation of amyloid fibrils from the putative precursor proteins in in vitro system. Glenner et al (82) successfully constituted amyloid-like fibrils in vitro from Bence-Jones proteins through peptic cleavage of the proteins and precipitation of the variable segments. This phenomenon was confirmed by several subsequent studies (83-85). Electron micrscopic studies of these synthesized fibrils found that they closely resembled the native amyloid fibrils in ultrastructure. Shirahama et al (85) also observed that in the process of formation of fibrils from variable segments of the immunoglobulin light chains, thinner filamentous structures of an order comparable to the amyloid protofibrils seemed to be formed first and then take on a laterally aggregated appearance to form the fibrils. More recently, a substance that bore tinctorial and ultrastructural characteristics of amyloid was created in vitro from native β_2-microglobulin (86).

d. Electron microscopic immunocytochemistry

Recent advances in immunocytochemical technology and the development of antisera to various amyloid proteins have made it possible to localize amyloid proteins by electron microscopy. Using anti-AA, Shirahama et al (87) demonstrated that some non-fibrillar deposits in secondary amyloidotic tissues reacted positively with anti-AA, thus suggesting the possibility of deposition of amyloid proteins in a non--fibrillar form in the tissues, possibly representing deposition of the precursors or unpolymerized AA-proteins.

In recent years, SAA has been defined as an acute phase reactant and the liver as the major site of SAA biosynthesis. Light microscopic immunohistochemical studies localized a positive reaction to anti-AA in liver tissue sections from stimulated mice (88,89). The positive reaction of anti-AA in the mouse liver was further defined by electron microscopic immunocytochemistry to subcellular components of the hepatocytes, i.e. rough endoplasmic reticulum, Golgi complex and cytoplasmic vesicles, confirming that SAA is indeed synthesized in hepatocytes and that it follows the usual way of synthesis and intracellular pathways as observed with many other proteins (90-92).

4. Final remarks

Electron microscopic studies have established as one of the essential criteria for the definition of amyloid the nonbranching fibrils of 7.5-10 nm width and indeterminate length. This identity has been used for further ultrastructural studies, and has contributed to the elucidation of the pathogenesis of amyloid. Advances in amyloid research in other disciplines and in histochemical and immunohistochemical methodologies have made it possible to identify the localization of amyloid proteins in tissues at light and electron microscopic levels. These recent developments have broadened the applicability of electron microscopy in amyloid research, making it possible to study more dynamic aspects of amyloidogenesis.

Acknowledgements

Supported by grants from the United States Public Health Service, National Institute of Arthritis, Diabetes, Digestive and Kidney Disease (AM-04599 and AM-07014), National Institutes of Health Multipurpose Arthritis Center (AM-20613), the General Clinical Research Centers Branch of the Division of Research Resources, National Institutes of Health (RR-533) and the Arthritis Foundation.

References

1.Cohen, A.S. & Calkins, E. Nature 183, 1202-1203, 1959.
2.Abrahams, C., Pirani,.C.L. & Pollak, V.E. J. Pathol. Bacteriol. 92, 220-225, 1966.
3.Albores-Saavedra, J., Ròse, G.G., Ibanez, M.L. et al. Lab. Invest. 13, 77-93, 1964.
4.Bari, W.A., Pettengill, O.S. & Sorenson, G.D. Lab. Invest. 20, 234-242, 1969.
5.Battaglia, S. Klin. Wochenschr. 39, 795-798, 1961.
6.Battaglia, S. Beitr. Pathol. Anat. 126, 300-320, 1962.
7.Ben-Ishay, Z. & Zlotnik, A. Isr. J. Med. Sci. 4, 987-994, 1968.
8.Bergstrand, A. & Bucht, H. J. Pathol. Bacteriol. 81, 495-503, 1961.
9.Bradburg, S. & Micklem, H.S. Am. J. Pathol. 46, 263-277, 1965.
10.Caesar, R. Z. Zellforsch. 52, 653-673, 1960.
11.Caesar, R. Pathol. Microbiol. (Basel) 24, 387-396, 1961.
12.Caesar, R. Frankfurt Z. Pathol. 72, 506-516, 1963.
13.Caesar, R. In Fortschritte der Amyloidforschung. Bruns, G., Zschiesche, W., Fritsch, S., Eds. Nova Acta Leopoldina 31 (175), 87-97, 1966.
14.Cohen, A.S. & Calkins, E. J.Exp. Med. 112, 479-490, 1960.
15.Cohen, A.S., Weiss, L. & Calkins, E. Am. J. Pathol. 37, 413-431, 1960.
16.Cohen, A.S., Frensdorff, A., Lamprecht, S. & Calkins, E. Am. J. Pathol. 41, 567-578, 1962.
17.Cohen, A.S., Gross, E. & Shirahama, T. Am. J. Pathol. 47, 1079-1111, 1965.
18.Fruehling, L., Kempf, J. & Porte, A. C.R. Acad. Sci. (Paris) 250, 1385-1386, 1960.
19.Gafni, J., Merker, H.J., Shibolet, S. et al. Ann. Intern. Med. 65, 1031-1044, 1966.
20.Gueft, B. & Ghidoni, J.J. Am. J. Pathol. 43, 837-854, 1963.
21.Hashimoto, K., Gross, B.G. & Lever, W.F. J. Invest. Dermatol. 45, 204-219, 1965.
22.Heefner, W.A. & Sorenson, G.D. Lab. Invest. 11, 585-593, 1962.
23.Hinglais, N. & DeMontera, H. Pathol. Biol. (Paris) 12, 176-191, 1964.
24.Hinglais, N., Zweibaum, A. & Richet, G. Nephron 1, 16-30, 1964.
25.Hjort, G.H. & Christensen, H.E. Acta Rheum. Scand. 7, 65-68, 1961.
26.Kidd, M. Nature, 197, 192-193, 1963.
27.Letterer, E., Caesar, R. & Vogt, A. Deutsch. Med. Wschr. 85, 1909-1910, 1960.
28.Marx, A.J., Gueft, B. & Maskal, J.F. Arch. Pathol. 80, 487-494, 1965.
29.Merker, H.J., Shibolet, S., Sohar, E. et al. Nature 211, 1401-1402, 1966.
30.Movat, H.Z. Arch. Pathol. 69, 323-332, 1960.
31.Schrodt, G.R. & Murray, M. Arch. Pathol. 82, 518-525, 1966.
32.Shibolet, S., Merker, H.J., Sohar, E. et al. Br. J. Exp. Pathol. 48, 244-249, 1967.
33.Shimamura, T. & Sorenson, G.D. Am. J. Pathol. 46, 645-656, 1965.
34.Shirahama, T. & Cohen, A.S. Am. J. Pathol. 51, 869-911, 1967.
35.Shirahama, T. & Cohen, A.S. Lab. Invest. 19, 122-131, 1968.
36.Shirahama, T. & Cohen, A.S. Exp. Mol. Pathol. 11, 300-322, 1969.
37.Sorenson, G.D. & Bari, W.A. In Amyloidosis. Mandema, E., Ruinen, L., Scholten, J.H., Cohen, A.S., Eds. Excerpta Medica, Amsterdam, 58-70, 1968.
38.Sorenson, G.D. & Shimamura, T. Lab. Invest. 13, 1409-1417, 1964.
39.Suzuki, Y., Churg, M., Grisham, E. et al. Am. J. Pathol. 43, 555-578, 1963.
40.Terry, R.D., Gonatas, N.K. & Weiss, M. Am. J. Pathol. 44, 269-297, 1964.
41.Thiery, J.P. & Caroli, J. Rev. Int. Hepat. 12, 207-251, 1962.
42.Trump, B.F. & Benditt, E.P. Lab. Invest. 11, 753-781, 1962.
43.Uchino, F. Acta Pathol. Jap. 17, 48-82, 1967.
44.Benditt, E.P. & Eriksen, N. Lab. Invest. 26, 615-625, 1972.
45.Benditt, E.P., Eriksen, N. & Berglund, C. In Amyloidosis. Mandema, E., Ruinen, L., Scholten, J.H., Cohen, A.S., Eds. Excerpta Medica, Amsterdam, 206-214, 1968.
46.Boere, H. Ruinen, L. & Scholten, J.H. J. Lab. Clin. Med. 66, 943-951, 1965.
47.Cohen, A.S. Lab. Invest. 15, 66-80, 1966.
48.Cohen, A.S. In Amyloidosis. Mandema, E., Ruinen, L., Scholten, J.H., Cohen, A.S., Eds. Excerpta Medica, Amsterdam, 149-167, 1968.
49.Cohen, A.S. Shirahama, T., Skinner, M. et al. in Protides of Biological Fluids, Vol. 20, ed. Peeters, H., Pergamon Press,Oxford, 73-80, 1973.
50.Emeson, E.E., Kikkawa, Y. & Gueft, B. J. Cell Biol. 28, 570-576, 1966.
51.Glenner, G.G. & Bladen, H.A. In Amyloidosis. Mandema, E., Ruinen, L., Scholten, J.H., Cohen, A.S., Eds. Excerpta Medica, Amsterdam, 216-226, 1968.
52.Pras, M., Schubert, M., Zucker-Franklin, D. et al. J. Clin. Invest. 47, 924-933, 1968.
53.Ruinen, L., Van Bruggen, E.F.J., Scholten, J.H. et al. In Amyloidosis. Mandema, E., Ruinen, L., Scholten, J.H., Cohen, A.S., Eds. Excerpta Medica, Amsterdam, 194-204, 1968.
54.Shirahama, T. & Cohen, A.S. Nature 206, 737-738, 1965.
55.Shirahama, T. & Cohen, A.S. J. Cell Biol. 33, 679-708. 1967.
56.Sorenson, G.D. & Finke, E. In Amyloidosis. Mandema, E., Ruinen, L., Scholten, J.H., Cohen, A.S., Eds. Excerpta Medica, Amsterdam, 184-190, 1968.
57.Westermark, P. Virchows Arch. Pathol. Anat. 373, 161-166, 1977.
58.Cohen, A.S. Int. Rev. Exp. Pathol. 4, 159-243, 1965.
59.Cohen, A.S. New Engl. J. Med. 277, 522-530, 574-583, 628-638, 1967.

60. Cohen, A.S., Shirahama, T. & Skinner, M. In Electron Microscopy of Proteins, Vol. 3. Harris J.R., Ed. Academic Press, London, 165-206, 1982.
61. Franklin, E.C. & Zucker-Franklin, D. Adv. Immunol. 15, 249-304, 1972.
62. Glenner, G.G. New Engl. J. Med. 302, 1283-1292, 1333-1343, 1980.
63. Amyloid and Amyloidosis. Glenner, G.G., Costa, P.P., Freitas, A.F., Eds. Excerpta Medica, Amsterdam, 1980.
64. Amyloidosis. Mandema, E., Ruinen, L., Scholten, J.H., Cohen, A.S., Eds. Excerpta Medica, Amsterdam, 1968.
65. Shirahama, T., Cohen, A.S. & Skinner, M. In Advances in Immunohistochemistry. DeLellis, R.A., Ed. Masson Publishing, New York, 277-302, 1984.
66. Amyloidosis. Wegelius, O., Pasternack, A., Eds. Academic Press, London, 1976.
67. Seixas Duarte, M.I., Sesso, A. & de Brito, T. Am. J. Pathol. 92, 85-98, 1978.
68. Shirahama, T. & Cohen, A.S. Am. J. Pathol. 73, 97-114, 1973.
69. Shirahama, T. & Cohen, A.S. Am. J. Pathol. 81, 101-116, 1975.
70. Shirahama, T. & Cohen, A.S. In Amyloidosis. Wegelius, O., Pasternack, A., Eds. Academic Press, London, 361-370, 1976.
71. Zucker-Franklin, D. & Franklin, E.C. Am. J. Pathol. 59, 23-42, 1970.
72. Kjeldsberg, C.R., Eyre, H.J. & Totzke, H. Blood, 50, 493-504, 1977.
73. Shirahama, T., Cohen, A.S., Rubinow, A. & Rodgers, O.G. In Amyloid and Amyloidosis. Glenner, G.G., Costa, P.P., Freitas, A.F., Eds. Excerpta Medica, Amsterdam, 132-138, 1980
74. Cohen, A.S. & Benson, M.D. In Peripheral Neuropathy. Dyck, P.T., Thomas, P.K., Lambert, E.H., Eds. W.B. Saunders, Philadelphia, 1076-1091, 1975.
75. Hashimoto, K. & Kobayashi, H. In Amyloid and Amyloidosis. Glenner, G.G., Costa, P.P., Freitas, A.F., Eds. Excerpta Medica, Amsterdam, 426-447, 1980.
76. Chai, C.K. Am. J. Pathol. 85, 49-72, 1976.
77. Ranløv, P. & Wanstrup, J. In Amyloidosis. Mandema, E., Ruinen, L., Scholten, J.H. Cohen, A.S., Eds. Excerpta Medica, Amsterdam, 74-79, 1968.
78. Shirahama, T., Skinner, M. & Cohen, A.S. In 35th Ann. Proc. Electron Microscopy Soc. Am. Bailey, G.W., Ed. Claitor's Publishing Division, Baton Rouge, 542-543, 1977.
79. Shirahama, T., Cohen, A.S. & Rodgers, O.G. Exp. Mol. Pathol. 14, 110-123, 1971.
80. Shirahama, T. & Cohen, A.S. Am. J. Pathol. 63, 463-485, 1971.
81. Zucker-Franklin, D. J. Ultrastruct. Res. 32, 247-257, 1970.
82. Glenner, G.G., Ein, D., Eanes, E.D. et al. Science, 174, 712-714, 1971.
83. Epstein, W.V., Tan, M. & Wood, I.S. J. Lab. Clin. Med. 84, 107-110, 1974.
84. Linke, R.P., Zucker-Franklin, D. & Franklin, E.C. J. Immunol. 111, 10-23, 1973.
85. Shirahama, T., Benson, M.D., Cohen, A.S. & Tanaka, A. J. Immunol. 110, 21-30, 1973.
86. Connors, L.H., Shirahama, T., Skinner, M. et al. Biochem. Biophys. Res. Commun. 131, 1063-1068, 1985.
87. Shirahama, T., Skinner, M. & Cohen, A.S. In Amyloid and Amyloidosis. Glenner, G.G., Costa, P.P., Freitas, A.F., Eds. Excerpta Medica, Amsterdam, 278-282, 1980.
88. Benson, M.D. & Kleiner, E. J. Immunol. 124, 495-499, 1980.
89. Shirahama, T., Skinner, M. & Cohen, A.S. Cell Biol. Int. Reports 8, 849-856, 1984.
90. Miura, K., Takahashi, Y. & Shirasawa, H. Lab. Invest. 53, 453-463, 1985.
91. Shirahama, T. & Cohen, A.S. Am. J. Pathol. 118, 108-115, 1985.
92. Takahashi, M., Yokota, T., Yamashita, Y. et al. Lab. Invest. 52, 220-223, 1985.

SECTION III

CLINICAL ASPECTS

sub-editor: Alan S. Cohen

III.1   CLINICAL EVALUATION OF AA AND AL AMYLOID DISEASE

Sven Janssen, Martin H. van Rijswijk, Sijtze Meijer,
Lucas Ruinen and Gjalt K. van der Hem

Department of Internal Medicine, University Hospital Groningen,
The Netherlands.

1. Introduction

In recent years major advances have been made in elucidating the nature of the amyloid fibril proteins and the pathogenesis of the different
amyloid syndromes. The most frequently encountered amyloid diseases
are those associated with plasma cell dyscrasia or chronic inflammatory
diseases. In amyloidosis associated with chronic diseases (AA
amyloidosis) the amyloid protein AA is derived from the acute phase
serum protein SAA, whereas in amyloidosis associated with monoclonal
gammopathy the major protein component AL consists of amino terminal
fragments of light polypeptide chains of immunoglobulin origin (1).
Amyloidosis remains a disease of which few clinicians gain a large experience. Because of the multisystemic character of amyloidosis and the
variety of underlying conditions the evaluation and the treatment of
amyloidotic patients challenge the ingenuity of the physician. In this
report we attempt to provide a diagnostic framework for the evaluation
of amyloidotic patients with special emphasis to the reliability of biopsy
procedures, the immunohistochemical classification, and the non-invasive
assessment of the degree of organ function loss.

2. Clinical spectrum in AA and AL disease

The clinical features at the time of diagnosis in 91 patients with AA
and 53 patients with AL amyloidosis seen at the Department of Internal
Medicine are given in Table I. AA and AL amyloidosis were differentiated histochemically using the potassium permanganate ($KMnO_4$) method. From this table it is apparent that, although AA amyloidosis is dominated by kidney involvement, clinically significant impairment of other
organ systems does occur; in AL amyloidosis the clinical picture is more
diverse, comprising among others the kidneys, the heart, the nervous
system and the gastrointestinal tract. AA and AL amyloidosis differ not
only with regard to the clinical pattern of organ involvement, but also
with respect to prognosis (Figure 1) and mode of death (Table II).

TABLE I: CLINICAL FEATURES IN 91 PATIENTS WITH SYSTEMIC AA AND 53 PATIENTS WITH SYSTEMIC
AL AMYLOIDOSIS [n (%)]

	AA	AL
Nephropathy:		
Renal function loss (CrCl <100 ml/min)	77 (85)	43 (81)
Proteinuria (>0.5 g/24 hrs)	77 (85)	39 (74)
Cardiomyopathy:		
Heart failure with LV-ECG	6 (7)	29 (55)
Heart failure without LV-ECG	2 (2)	8 (15)
LV-ECG without heart failure	0 (0)	5 (9)
Enteropathy:		
Macroglossia	0 (0)	17 (32)
Prepyloric obstruction	1 (1)	1 (2)
Pseudo-obstruction	3 (3)	2 (4)
Diarrhea with malabsorption	7 (8)	1 (2)
Diarrhea without malabsorption	7 (8)	4 (8)
Malabsorption without diarrhea	4 (4)	3 (6)
Hepatomegaly	17 (19)	30 (57)
Neuropathy:		
Polyneuropathy	2 (2)	19 (36)
Orthostatic hypotension	2 (2)	14 (26)
Carpal tunnel syndrome	0 (0)	4 (8)
Miscellaneous:		
Sicca syndrome	1 (1)	2 (4)
Goiter with hypothyroidism	1 (1)	0 (0)
Goiter without hypothyroidism	2 (2)	2 (4)
Hypothyroidism without goiter	1 (1)	3 (6)
Arthropathy	0 (0)	2 (4)
Myopathy	1 (1)	1 (2)
Dermopathy	0 (0)	1 (2)

LV-ECG = low voltage electrocardiogram; CrCl = creatinine clearance (ml/min).

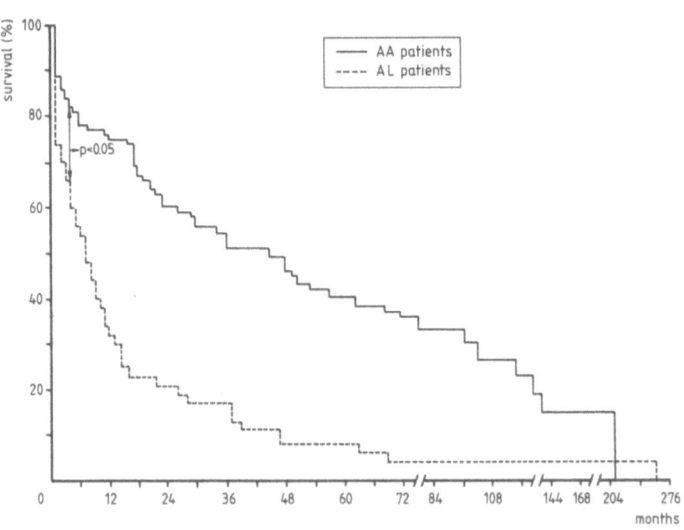

Figure 1: Survival of 91 patients with systemic AA and 53 patients with systemic AL
amyloidosis. From 4 months after diagnosis, the prognosis was worse in AL compared with AA
disease. Reprinted with permission from the Neth. J. Med.

TABLE II: CAUSE OF DEATH IN 63 PATIENTS WITH AA AND 51 PATIENTS WITH AL AMYLOIDOSIS

	AA	AL
Cardiac disorder	5 (8)	33 (65)
Renal disorder	22 (35)	8 (16)
Intestinal disorder	6 (10)	4 (8)
Infection	11 (17)	2 (4)
Bleeding	5 (8)	2 (4)
Miscellaneous	4 (6)	0 (0)
Unknown	10 (16)	2 (4)

3. Evaluation of amyloidosis: a protocol

At the moment patients presenting with amyloidosis are evaluated according to the following guidelines:

1. Immunohistochemistry: Congo red stain, $KMnO_4$ test, immunofluorescence using the following antisera: anti-AA, anti-kappa, anti-lambda (anti-prealbumin and anti-β_2 microglobulin).

2. Quantification of the acute phase response: serum levels of CRP and/or SAA.

3. Search for a monoclonal component: bone marrow examination, immunofluorescence of bone marrow cells, immunofixation of serum and concentrated urine.

4. ^{99m}Tc-methylene diphosphonate scintigraphy.

5. Renal function tests: degree and selectivity of proteinuria, kidney size, glomerular filtration rate, effective renal plasma flow, relative clearance of ^{99m}Tc-dimercaptosuccinate.

6. Cardiac function: electrocardiography, chest X-ray, echocardiography, systolic time intervals.

7. Liver function tests: alkaline phosphatase, transaminases, gamma-glutamyl transferase, cholinesterase.

8. Coagulation tests: bleeding time, activates partial thromboplastin time, prothrombin time, antithrombin III.

9. Thyroid function tests: serum levels of free thyroxin and thyroid stimulating hormone.

10. Absorption tests: D-xylose test, Schilling test.

11. Nerve conduction velocity.

The immunohistochemical classification of the amyloid syndromes, radionuclide imaging of amyloid infiltration, the assessment of renal and cardiac involvement, and therapeutic implications will be discussed in more detail.

4. Diagnosis and immunohistochemical classification

The diagnosis of amyloidosis depends on the demonstration of amyloid deposits by Congo red staining of biopsy specimens. Only the birefringence after staining with Congo red and under examination with polarized light is specific. Staining techniques employing thioflavin S and T and methyl violet lack the required specificity to be conclusive (2). Until the 1950th amyloidosis was seldom diagnosed during life. The development of biopsy techniques has resulted in obtaining histological proof of clinically suspected disease. The ideal routine biopsy technique for the diagnosis of amyloidosis should be based on the following principles: a) a readily available involved organ, b) operative ease assuring adequate specimen, c) absence of complications and d) minimal discomfort to the patient. With these objectives in mind biopsy of rectal mucosa, introduced by Gafni and Sohar (3), appears to be the best diagnostic procedure in cases of suspected amyloidosis. To be adequate, the biopsy specimen must contain submucosa, because this tissue is involved more often than the mucosa.

In our series amyloidosis was diagnosed during life in 94% of cases. Of 137 rectal biopsies performed in 119 patients (80 AA, 39 AL) 110 (80%) gave positive results. 75/93 (81%) rectal biopsies in the AA group showed amyloid deposits, compared with 35/44 (80%) in the AL group. Of importance is the finding that 17/27 (63%) of the negative rectal biopsies were adequate, i.e. contained submucosa. Before the introduction of the rectal biopsy procedure, gingival biopsies were favored for diagnosing of amyloidosis; the results, however, were disappointing, showing amyloid deposition in 19-60% of cases (4-6), which is in concordance with our results (42% positive). If the rectal biopsy is adequate but negative, tissue should be obtained from a suspected involved organ. Both liver and renal biopsies often reveal amyloid, but these procedures are more difficult and liver biopsy is reported to produce bleeding in patients with gross hepatomegaly (7). Sural nerve biopsy is a high-yield diagnostic procedure in patients suspected of amyloid neuropathy (8). Bone-marrow biopsy, small-bowel biopsy, skin biopsy, fine-needle biopsy of subcutaneous abdominal fat, prostatic biopsy, aspiration biopsy of the spleen and endomyocardial biopsy have been used to diagnose amyloidosis (9-14).

It is of importance to make an accurate histochemical classification with regard to the type of amyloid involved, since AA and AL amyloidosis differ considerably with regard to prognosis and therapeutic approach (1). Two histochemical techniques are available for differentiating between AA and AL amyloidosis: the $KMnO_4$ test (15) and immunohistochemical methods using antibodies to protein AA. Whereas an accurate histological diagnosis of AA amyloidosis can be made by the use of specific anti-AA antiserum, the demonstration of AL amyloid by histochemical techniques is more complex, because AL deposits of different patients appear to have individual specificity and usually do not show cross-reactivity (1).

Recently we have shown that the results of the $KMnO_4$ test are in accordance with the immunohistochemical typing of amyloid, i.e. anti-AA antibodies stained $KMnO_4$ sensitive amyloid deposits (see Figure 2), whereas $KMnO_4$ resistant deposits remained unstained (16). This finding is of importance since it confirms the reliability of the $KMnO_4$ test, which is a simple procedure and can be performed in every laboratory in contrast to immunohistochemical methods requiring antisera, which are difficult to raise and need extensive purification by affinity chromatography. With regard to the $KMnO_4$ test two remarks should be made. Firstly, it is a prerequisite for the proper interpretation of the $KMnO_4$ test that the histological structure is unaffected. Secondly, in a recent publication Shirahama et al (17) reported hemodialysis-associated amyloid, which is derived from β_2-microglobulin and is characterized by carpal tunnel syndrome and arthropathy, to be a second form of $KMnO_4$ sensitive amyloid. It is our opinion that greater efforts are required to make anti-AA antiserum widely available, thereby opening the possibility to distinguish the major amyloid syndromes using a panel of antisera (anti-AA, anti-lambda, anti-kappa, anti-β_2-microglobulin, anti-pre-albumin).

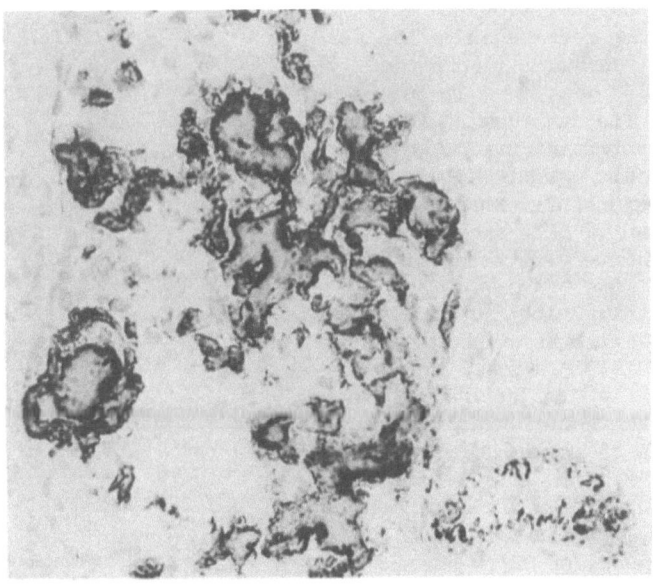

Figure 2: Kidney of a patient with amyloidosis associated with rheumatoid arthritis. PAP-stained tissue with rabbit anti-AA, showing positive reaction of amyloid deposits in glomerulus and blood vessel.

5. Radionuclide imaging of amyloid infiltration

Soft-tissue uptake (especially in the heart and the liver) on scanning with ^{99m}Tc-labeled phosphates has been attributed to the presence of amyloid in a number of cases of AL amyloidosis (18). This prompted us to investigate whether scintigraphy using with [99m]technetium-labelled methylene-diphosphonate (^{99m}Tc-MDP) and pyrophosphate (^{99m}Tc-PYP) might provide a reliable non-invasive test for the extent of organ involvement in amyloid disease. ^{99m}Tc-MDP and ^{99m}Tc-PYP scintigraphy was performed in 19 patients with systemic amyloidosis (9 AA, 9 AL, 1 FAP) and 2 patients with local dermal and local bronchial amyloid (19).

Scanning with ^{99m}Tc-labeled phosphates appeared to be a sensitive non--invasive screening test for the extent and the distribution of organ involvement in both systemic AA and AL amyloid (see Figure 3) as well as in localized amyloid, although echocardiography was more sensitive for demonstrating cardiac involvement than ^{99m}Tc-MDP or ^{99m} Tc-PYP scintigraphy. The scintigraphic pattern of organ involvement in AA amyloid was multisystemic, which is compatible with the histological distribution of amyloid. There was no difference in the extent or the intensity of soft-tissue uptake between the ^{99m}Tc-MDP and ^{99m}Tc--PYP, although the ^{99m}Tc-MDP images generally showed a better contrast than ^{99m}Tc-PYP images, which may be explained by the biologic characteristics of the agents. With regard to the mechanism of amyloid affinity for phosphates we were able to demonstrate that in vitro ^{99m}Tc-MDP was only bound to isolated AA and AL fibrils in the presence of both serum amyloid P-component (SAP) and calcium (20). So, the calcium-dependent binding of SAP to amyloid fibrils seems to be res-

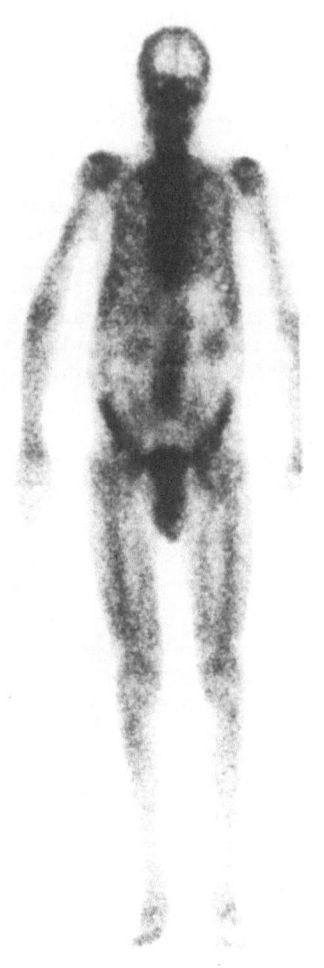

Figure 3: ^{99m}Tc-MDP scintigraphy in a patient with systemic AL amyloidosis, showing uptake of tracer in the thyroid gland, the abdominal area and in the limbs.

ponsible for visualization of amyloid deposits on "bone-scanning". In this context it should be noted that cerebral amyloid, which is reported to lack amyloid P component, displays affinity for ^{99m}Tc-MDP (21).

In conclusion: ^{99m}Tc-MDP scintigraphy is a sensitive non-invasive test in evaluating the extent of organ involvement in amyloid diseases except for cardiomyopathy and may provide a tool to substantiate amyloid infiltration.

6. Renal amyloidosis

Although a growing number of investigations have supplied information on the clinical and pathological characteristics of renal amyloidosis,
there remains contradiction with regard to basic data concerning the
picture of amyloid nephropathy (22). In a retrospective study we have
compiled data concerning the renal status in 57 (46 AA, 11 AL)
amyloidotic patients in whom a renal biopsy was performed (23). Our
aim was to describe the basic clinical characteristics of amyloid nephropathy. The results (neither positive nor negative) of appropriate
(submucosa containing) rectal biopsy were not conclusive with regard to
renal amyloid involvement. So, a renal biopsy should be performed on
suspicion of renal amyloidosis particularly in patients with rheumatoid
arthritis, since in 7% of AA patients nephropathy was caused by vas-
culitis or drugs and not by amyloid deposition despite a positive rectal
biopsy.

Hypertension was not an infrequent finding and occurred in 19% of
the patients. Proteinuria was more massive in the AL than in the AA
patients, whereas 5% of the AA patients presented with renal function
loss in the absence of proteinuria. On the other hand, once the
nephrotic syndrome has developed, it shows no tendency for remittance.
Even in advanced renal failure or in patients on regular hemodialysis
treatment proteinuria may be massive. Initially proteinuria is selective
and becomes non-selective with progression of renal function loss
(creatinine clearance < 30 ml/min). There appeared to be a positive
correlation between kidney size and renal function, with small kidneys
being a regular finding in renal failure and enlarged kidneys occurring
only in renal vein thrombosis. With regard to renal replacement therapy
in amyloid nephropathy, hemodialysis treatment and renal transplantation appeared to alter the course and prognosis favourably, although
survival rates after entry into hemodialysis treatment were relatively
low compared to a general hemodialysis population and recurrence of
amyloid in the renal allograft did occur.

With respect to the mechanism of renal function loss, histological
studies indicate that renal failure might develop not mainly as the result
of glomerular, but as the consequence of vascular amyloid deposition,
resulting in interstitial fibrosis with concomitant tubular atrophy
(24-26). This would imply that tubular function is impaired in renal
amyloidosis and that measurement of the degree of tubular dysfunction
might provide information on the degree of interstitial fibrosis. To test
this hypothesis we studied proximal tubular function in 22 patients with
biopsy proven renal amyloidosis (27). Proximal tubular function was
measured by the relative clearance of ^{99m}Tc-dimercaptosuccinate
(^{99m}Tc-DMSA), which is handled in the kidney by glomerular filtration
and subsequent tubular reabsorption. An accelerated urinary excretion
of ^{99m}Tc-DMSA indicates proximal tubular dysfunction (28, 29).
Proximal tubular dysfunction, measured by enhanced clearance of ^{99m}
Tc-DMSA, appeared to be a frequent (in 86% of cases) finding in

amyloid nephropathy. Furthermore, the degree of interstitial fibrosis as observed in the renal biopsies showed a distinct positive correlation with the degree of proximal tubulopathy. These findings confirm the value of the relative clearance of ^{99m}Tc-DMSA as a non-invasive test for the degree of interstitial fibrosis in amyloid nephropathy and contribute to a better understanding of the mechanism of renal function loss in renal amyloidosis.

7.Cardiac amyloidosis

Cardiac involvement has been known for a long time to be a major manifestation and cause of death in amyloidosis associated with immunocyte dyscrasia (AL amyloidosis) (1, 8, 30). In amyloidosis associated with chronic inflammatory diseases (AA amyloidosis) cardiomyopathy due to amyloid infiltration is regarded to be very uncommon (1). However, in most clinical surveys on cardiac involvement in systemic amyloidosis the amyloid protein involved has not been characterized and hence the clinical classification is not reliable (31, 32). Clinically manifest cardiac disease was found by Brandt and Cohen in 54-60% of patients with amyloidosis secondary to inflammatory conditions; the nature of the cardiac deterioration was not defined (30, 33). Browning reported marked cardiac amyloid deposition to be present at autopsy in 14% of cases with histochemically proven AA amyloidosis (34).

In clinical practice, the diagnosis of cardiac amyloidosis is usually suggested by the combination of congestive heart failure and low QRS voltage at electrocardiography (8, 31-34); other electrocardiographic abnormalities may be a pseudo-infarction pattern or disturbance of rhythm and conduction (31, 32, 35). Clinical and electrocardiographic abnormalities may be indicative for the existence of an infiltrative cardiomyopathy, but are in no way specific for amyloid cardiomyopathy. Echocardiography might provide a valuable aid in the non-invasive diagnosis of cardiac amyloidosis. Echocardiographic findings may include increased thickness of heart walls, decreased wall motion and reduced systolic thickening (36-39). We have analyzed the clinical, electrocardiographic, and echocardiographic features in 30 AA and 24 AL patients firstly to determine the characteristics of AL amyloid cardiomyopathy and secondly to evaluate the cardiac status in AA amyloid (23).

In AL amyloidosis echocardiographic changes appeared to be related to the degree of clinical heart disease. In the asymptomatic phase of cardiac involvement, amyloid may be detected by echocardiography and is manifested by mild or moderate increase in wall thickness; in clinically significant cardiac dysfunction echocardiography discloses more or less severe thickening and hypokinesis of posterior and septal wall. Although the results of electrocardiography were not predictable with regard to cardiac amyloid involvement, the combination of a low voltage electrocardiogram and increased thickness of heart walls appeared to be of distinct differential diagnostic value, since in other conditions an increased cardiac mass is accompanied by increased electrocardiographic voltage (40). In AA amyloid clinically significant amyloid heart disease occurred in a minority (7%) of patients; the characteristics of cardiac AA amyloidosis resemble those of AL cardiomyopathy (see Figure 4). In AA amyloidosis associated with rheumatoid arthritis, cardiac dysfunction must be differentiated from cardiomyopathy related to the inflammatory condition itself.

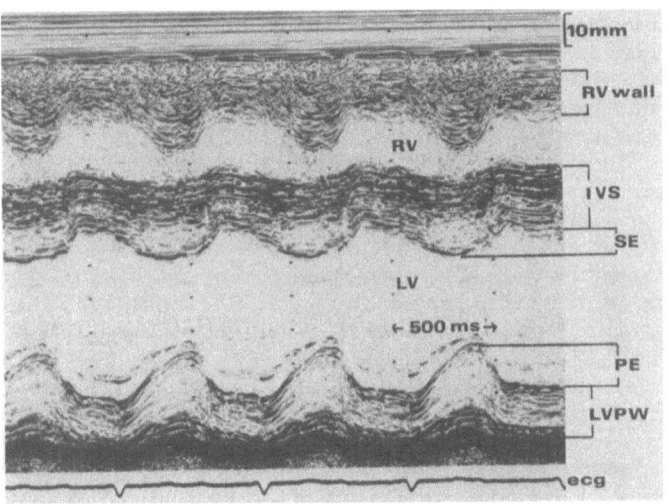

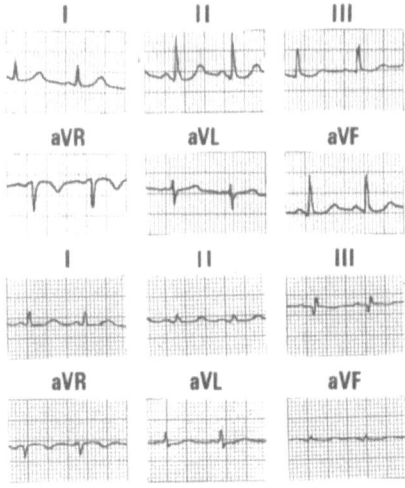

Figure 4: M-mode echocardiographic recording (top) of a patient with AA amyloidosis. The recording was made in anteroposterior direction at the level of the tip of the mitral valve. The heart walls are strongly thickened. The motion pattern was good. In the absence of hypertension and the development of a low voltage electrocardiogram (left: upper ECG September 1980; lower ECG November 1984), the picture fits in a diagnosis of cardiac AA amyloidosis. RV= right ventricle; LV= left ventricle IVS= interventricular septum; LVPW= left ventricular posterior wall; SE= septal excursion; PE= excursion of the left ventricular posterior wall.

8. Therapeutic approach

Treatment for AL amyloidosis is not satisfactory. The results of treatment with melphalan/prednisone or colchicine are inconclusive. Data obtained by Cohen et al. suggest that colchicine may be effective in blocking AL amyloidogenesis, thereby increasing survival in AL amyloidosis (41). Kyle and Greipp reported some benifit to patients with AL nephropathy treated with melphalan/prednisone, although there was no difference in survival in comparison with untreated patients (42). A recent study suggests that melphalan/prednisone potentially is superior to colchicine in the treatment of AL amyloidosis (43), whereas another study (44) indicates the existence of a subset of patients with AL amyloidosis associated with multiple myeloma with prolonged survival due to melphalan/prednisone. At present we think it is justified to treat AL patients with melphalan/prednisone since AL amyloid is derived from light chains produced by plasma cells and this regimen is effective against proliferation of neoplastic plasma cells. Treatment of AA amyloidosis is directed towards the suppression of inflammatory activity i.e. SAA production, since the presence of a significant amount of the precursor protein is a prerequisite for AA formation. The effect of anti-inflammatory therapy should be monitored by measurement of serum acute phase proteins. CRP is to date most widely used in monitoring chronic inflammatory diseases. SAA, however, has even greater sensitivity than CRP in reflecting changes of inflammatory activity since it shows a greater incremental range compared to CRP (see Figure 5) (45). Reduction of the acute phase response by corticosteroids and cytostatics may stop the progression of AA amyloid. At present we treat patients with AA nephropathy, who have still a reasonable renal function (glomerular filtration rate > 20 ml/min) with prednisolone and azathioprine. In case of preterminal renal insufficiency (glomerular filtration rate < 20 ml/min) we consider treatment with dimethylsulfoxide the therapy of choice. Treatment with dimethylsulfoxide may favourably alter the course of AA nephropathy firstly by reducing the interstitial inflammatory reaction, which accompanies renal vascular amyloid deposition (short-term effect), and secondly because of its anti-inflammatory effect (long-term effect) (46). Furthermore, treatment of hypertension and reduction of dietary protein and phosphate load may be of value in the maintenance of reduced renal function (47). The observation by Zemer et al., who demonstrated the prophylactic and therapeutic efficacy of uninterrupted daily administration of colchicine in AA nephropathy associated with familial Mediterranean fever (48), is of great interest not only with regard to the treatment and the prevention of AA amyloidosis associated with familial Mediterranean fever. Further studies are warranted to establish whether colchicine is beneficial in the prevention and the treatment of renal amyloidosis secondary to other inflammatory conditions, e.g. rheumatoid arthritis.

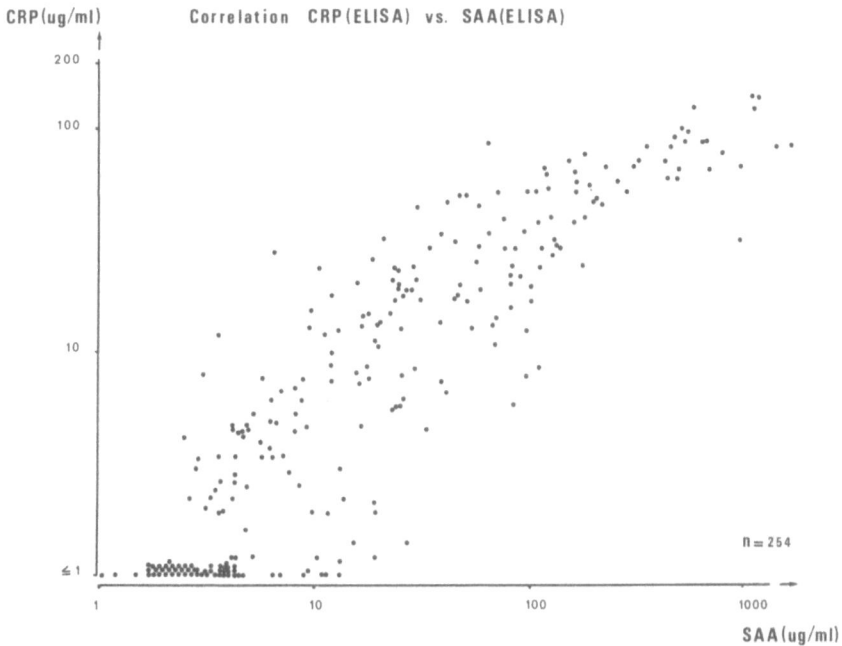

Figure 5: SAA versus CRP levels in 254 patients with chronic inflammatory conditions, showing the greater incremental range of SAA compared to CRP. Reprinted with permission of Pergamon Press Limited.

Acknowledgement

This study was supported by a grant from the Dutch Kidney Foundation.

References

1. Glenner, G.G. N. Engl. J. Med. 302, 1283-1292 and 1333-1343, 1980.
2. Cooper, J.H. In Amyloidosis. Wegelius, O. & Pasternack, A., Eds. Academic Press, London, 61-69, 1976.
3. Gafni, J. & Sohar, E. Am. J. Med. Sci. 240, 332-336, 1960.
4. Trieger, N., Cohen, A.S. & Calkins, E. Arch. Oral. Biol. 1, 187-192, 1959.
5. Calkins, E. & Cohen, A.S. Bull. Rheum. Dis. 10, 215-218, 1960.
6. Lehner, T. Isr. J. Med. Sci. 4, 1000-1004, 1968.
7. Stauffer, M.H., Gross, J.B., Foulk, W.T. & Dahlin, D.C. Gastroenterology. 41, 92-96, 1961.
8. Kyle, R.A. & Greipp, P.R. Mayo Clin. Proc. 58, 665-683, 1983.
9. Conn Jr, R.B. & Sundberg, R.D. Am. J. Pathol. 38, 61-71, 1961.
10. Monteiro, J.G. Gastroenterologia 99, 118-122, 1963.
11. Rubinow, A. & Cohen, A.S. Ann. Intern. Med. 88, 781-785, 1978.
12. Westermark, P. & Stenkvist, B. Arch. Intern. Med. 132, 522-523, 1973.
13. Wilson, S.K., Buchanan, R.D., Stone, W.J. & Rhamy, R.K. J. Urol. 110, 322-323, 1973.

14. Swanton, R.H., Brooksby, I.A.B., Davies, M.J., et al. Am. J. Cardiol. 39, 658-664, 1977.
15. Van Rijswijk, M.H. & Van Heusden, C.W.G.J. Am. J. Pathol. 97, 43-58, 1979.
16. Janssen, S., Elema, J.D., Van Rijswijk, M.H., et al. Appl. Pathol. (In Press).
17. Shirahama, T., Skinner, M., Cohen, A.S., et al. Lab. Invest. 53, 705-709, 1985.
18. Janssen, S., Van Rijswijk, M.H., Piers, D.A. & Jong, G.M.Th. de. Eur. J. Nucl. Med. 9, 538-541, 1984.
19. Janssen, S., Piers, D.A., Van Rijswijk, M.H., et al. (submitted).
20. Janssen, S., Van Rijswijk, M.H. & Piers, D.A. (unpublished results).
21. Moreno, A.J., Brown, J.M., Brown, T.J., et al. Clin. Nucl. Med. 8, 528-530, 1983.
22. Brenner, B.M., Rector, F.C., Eds. The kidney. Vol II. W.B.Saunders Company, Philadelphia, 1528-1533, 1981.
23. Janssen, S. Clinical and diagnostic features of amyloidosis. Thesis. Groningen, 1985. ISBN 90-9001079-3.
24. Mackensen, S., Grund, K.E., Bader, R. & Bohle, A. Virchows Arch. [A]. 375, 159-168, 1977.
25. Törnroth, T., Falck, H.M., Wafin, F. & Wegelius O. In Amyloid and Amyloidosis. Glenner, G.G., Costa, P.P., Freitas, A.F., Eds. Excerpta Medica, Amsterdam, 191-199, 1980.
26. Gise, H. von, Gise, V. von, Stark, B. & Bohle, A. Klin. Wochenschr. 59, 75-82, 1981.
27. Janssen, S., Meijer, S., Piers, D.A., et al. Kidney Int. (In Press).
28. Van Luijk, W.H.J., Ensing, G.J. & Piers, D.A. Eur. J. Nucl. Med. 8, 404-405, 1983.
29. Van Luijk, W.H.J., Meijer, S., Donker A.J.M. et al. Kidney Int. 26, 528, 1984.
30. Cohen, A.S. N. Engl. J. Med. 277, 522-530, 574-583, 628-638, 1967.
31. Buja, L.M., Khoi, N.B. & Roberts, W.C. Am. J. Cardiol. 26, 394-405, 1970.
32. Roberts, W.C. & Waller, B.F. Am. J. Cardiol. 52, 137-146, 1983.
33. Brandt, K., Cathcart, E.S. & Cohen, A.S. Am. J. Med. 44, 955-969, 1968.
34. Browning, M.J., Banks, R.A., Tribe, C.R., et al. Q. J. Med. 54, 215-227, 1985.
35. Bernreiter, M. Am. J. Cardiol. 1, 644-647, 1958.
36. Borer, J.S., Henry, W.L. & Epstein S.E. Am. J. Cardiol. 39, 184-188, 1977.
37. Child, J.S., Krivokapich, J. & Abbasi, A.S. Am. J. Cardiol. 44, 1391-1395, 1979.
38. Siqueira-Filho, A.G., Cunha, C.L.P, Tajik, A.J., et al. Circulation. 64, 188-196, 1981.
39. Cueto-Garcia, L., Tajik, A.J., Kyle, R.A., et al. Mayo Clin. Proc. 59, 589-597, 1984.
40. Carroll, J., Gaasch, W.H. & McAdam K.P.W.J. Am. J. Cardiol. 49, 9-14, 1982.
41. Cohen, A.S., Rubinow, A., Kayne, H. et al. In Amyloidosis. Glenner, G.G., Osserman, E.F., Benditt, E.P., Calkins, E., Cohen, A.S., Zucker-Franklin, D., Eds. Plenum Press, New York, 559-565, 1986.
42. Kyle, R.A. & Greipp, P.R. Blood 52, 818-827, 1978.
43. Kyle, R.A., Greipp, P.R., Garton, J.P. & Gertz M.A. Am. J. Med. 79, 708-716, 1985.
44. Fielder, K. & Durie, B.G.M. Am. J. Med. 80, 413-418, 1986.
45. Janssen, S., Limburg, P.C., Bijzet, J., et al. In XXXIVth Colloquium Protides of the Biological Fluids. Peeters, H., Ed. Pergamon Press Ltd, Oxford (In Press).
46. Van Rijswijk, M.H., Ruinen, L., Donker, A.J.M., et al. Ann. NY. Acad. Sci. 411, 67-83, 1983.
47. Rosman, J.B., Ter Wee, P.M., Meijer, S., et al. Lancet. ii, 1291-1296, 1984.
48. Zemer, D., Pras, M., Sohar, E., et al. J. N. Engl. J. Med. 314, 1001-1005, 1986.

III.2 CARDIAC INVOLVEMENT IN AMYLOIDOSIS

Rodney H. Falk

Department of Clinical Cardiology
Boston City Hospital
Boston University School of Medicine
Boston, MA 02118, U.S.A.

1. Introduction

Amyloid infiltration of the heart is the leading cause of death in patients with systemic amyloidosis. Symptoms of congestive heart failure are frequently the presenting feature of AL amyloidosis, but, because of the rarity of the disease the etiology may go unrecognized unless the clinician is particularly alert. Prior to the widespread use of echocardiography, cardiac amyloidosis was often initially diagnosed as constrictive pericarditis because of several shared clinical features. Attempts to differentiate these two entities by hemodynamic characteristics found at cardiac catheterization were generally unrewarding, due to an overlap in supposedly "specific" abnormalities (1-4).

In the past decade, M-mode and two-dimensional echocardiography have become routine tools for the assessment of cardiac disease. Echocardiography has been able to distinguish cardiac amyloid from constrictive pericarditis, and several features have been described which, when present, are considered to be highly suggestive of cardiac amyloid (5,6). Additional methods for the diagnosis of cardiac amyloid have also been described utilizing radionuclide techniques (technetium - 99m - pyrophosphate) (7), electrocardiographic criteria (8), computerized tomography of the heart (9) or endomyocardial biopsy (10). In this chapter the emphasis will be on the clinical manifestations of cardiac amyloidosis and its diagnosis. However, for a more complete understanding of the spectrum of cardiac amyloidosis a brief review of its prevalence in the various forms of systemic amyloidosis is in order.

2. Cardiac involvement in the various forms of amyloidosis

Microscopic deposits of amyloid in various body tissues is a normal accompaniment of aging. In the cardiovascular system three distinct types of age-related amyloid have been described. These are senile aortic amyloid (11), isolated atrial amyloid and senile cardiac amyloid (12). In an unselected group of 85 hearts, taken consecutively from autopsies on patients aged 80 years and above (13), senile aortic amyloid was present in all patients. Isolated atrial amyloid (IAA) usually involving both atria to a very mild degree was present in 78% of cases. One-quarter of the hearts studied had evidence of senile cardiac amyloid (ASC1) which involving both the atria and ventricles. Cardiac involvement was generally in the form of discrete focal interstitial or vascular deposits and did not appear to have been clinically significant in the patient group studied.

Senile cardiac amyloid may, in rare instances, be associated with heart failure. In such cases myocardial infiltration is extreme. Unless this diagnosis is borne in mind the rarity of involvement of extracardiac tissues may make premortem diagnosis difficult.

Primary and myeloma-associated (AL) amyloidosis is the form of amyloidosis most frequently associated with cardiac involvement. Up to 90% of patients with AL amyloid have evidence of cardiac infiltration, and approximately half of all cases will die of cardiac disease (14,15). The presence of congestive heart failure in AL amyloid is the least favorable of all clinical features (including nephrotic syndrome and orthostatic hypotension). Cardiac symptoms correlate with echocardiographic abnormalities which generally indicate extensive myocardial amyloid infiltration (16-18). In patients with AL amyloid dying of congestive heart failure the heart is typically firm and rubbery, with thickened walls and a normal ventricular chamber size. The atrial septum may show considerable thickening due to infiltration (Fig. 1) and microscopic examination of myocardium may show massive replacement of cardiac tissue by sheets of amyloid. Unlike senile cardiac amyloid, cardiac AL amyloid is usually associated with extracardiac amyloid deposition although this may, on occasion be subclinical.

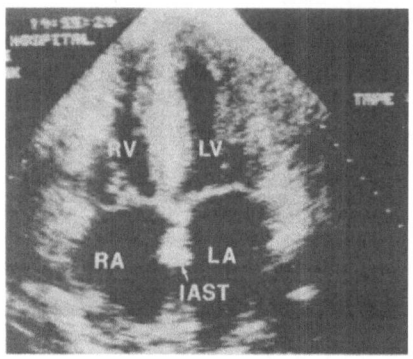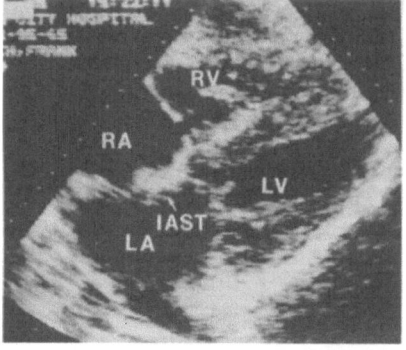

Figure 1: Typical echocardiogram in AL cardiac amyloidosis. Left panel shows the heart viewed from the cardiac apex, and right panel from the subcostal view.
The right and left ventricular cavities (RV and LV) are normal in size with an increased wall thichness. The right and left atria (RA and LA) are somewhat dilated with a marked interatrial septal thickening (IAST) of 12-15 mm (normal < 5 mm). The left ventricular walls show the granular, increased echogenicity typical of cardiac amyloid (echocardiogram courtesy of Dr. Jonathan Plehn).

Familial amyloid polyneuropathy (FAP) very frequently involves the heart although clinical heart failure is much less common than in AL amyloidosis. In autopsy studies cardiac involvement is almost always present, and echocardiographic and scintigraphic abnormalities have been found in the majority of patients, despite lack of cardiac symptoms (19). The poor prognosis associated with evidence of cardiac involvement in AL amyloidosis (even in asymptomatic patients) does not seem to apply to patients with FAP. In contrast to the predominance of heart failure in AL amyloidosis, disorders of cardiac conduction account for the major morbidity in FAP. This is discussed in greater detail below.

Secondary (AA) amyloid is uncommonly associated with significant cardiac involvement, either clinically or histologically. When symptomatic cardiac involvement does occur, it tends to present features similar to those seen in AL amyloidosis (14).

3. Clinical features of cardiac amyloidosis

The predominant symptoms of cardiac amyloidosis are those related to congestive heart failure. Dyspnea on exertion, fatigue and peripheral edema are common complaints, whereas acute pulmonary edema is rare. Physical examination reveals signs of predominant right-sided failure with markedly elevated jugular venous pressure, hepatomegaly and leg edema. Pleural effusions may also be present but only the minority of cases have pulmonary rales. The pulse is of normal or low volume. If atrial fibrillation is present the ventricular response may be surprisingly well controlled (less than 100 beats per minute) even in the absence of digoxin, due to impaired atrioventricular nodal conduction. Examination of the wave form of the jugular venous pulse may reveal a variety of patterns e.g. steep X and Y descent typically seen with constrictive pericarditis, or the V waves typical of tricuspid regurgitation. The latter may occur even when tricuspid regurgitation is absent (21).

The apex beat is undisplaced or displaced slightly laterally, but is rarely markedly displaced as ventricular dilation is not a feature of cardiac amyloid. Palpation of the apical impulse may be difficult owing to its reduced force. The heart sounds are usually of normal intensity but may be soft. Contrary to some textbook descriptions of cardiac amyloid, we have found a fourth heart sound to be very uncommon in cardiac amyloid, presumably due to impaired contraction of the disease atrium. Recent noninvasive data using Doppler echocardiography have supported our clinical impression of impaired atrial function in amyloidosis (22). A third heart sound is uncommon and if present, is usually soft. A cardiac murmur suggestive of mild mitral regurgitation is quite common and, less frequently, tricuspid regurgitation may exist. Peripheral edema can be extensive and ascites may occur. In assessing peripheral edema in amyloidosis is important to distinguish between that due to cardiac involvement and that due to nephrotic syndrome. Heavy proteinuria and hypoalbuminemia in the absence of jugular venous distension suggest a primary renal cause for edema, whereas elevated jugular pressure and minimal or no proteinuria implicates the heart. When renal and cardiac involvement coexist the edema may be particularly troublesome as the high venous pressures accelerate the extravasation of the hypoalbuminemic fluid into the tissues.

Patients with cardiac amyloid may on occasion have cardiac symptoms other than those of heart failure. These may occur in isolation or in conjunction with congestive heart failure. Angina pectoris, while relatively uncommon, may be due to concomitant atherosclerotic heart disease or amyloid involvement of the coronary arteries or arterioles (23). In the latter case coronary angiography may be normal, even though exercise testing reveals changes typical of ischemia (24). Pericardial effusions are detected in about one-third of patients with cardiac amyloid. They are usually of mild to moderate size and cause no clinical problem (5). Very rarely pericardial tamponade may occur requiring periocardiocentesis (25). Atrial and ventricular arrhythmias occur in about 70% of patients with echocardiographic evidence of cardiac amyloid undergoing 24 hour Holter monitoring (18). Symptomatic tachyarrhythmias are rare, but the presence of ventricular couplets or ventricular tachycardia on Holter monitoring may correlate with subsequent sudden death (18). Bradyarrhythmias, due to sinus node dysfunction or atrioventricular block, are more common in familial than AL amyloid (20). Recurrent syncope, particularly if non-postural, should alert the physician to the possibility of intermittent bradycardia (Fig. 2).

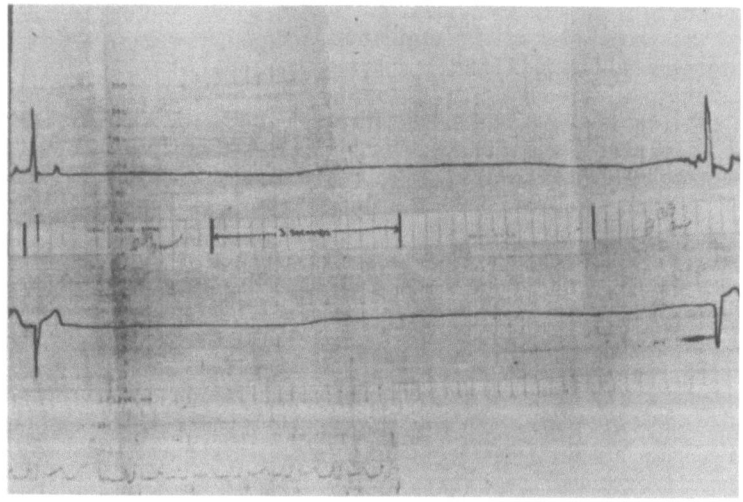

Figure 2: Recording from a Holter monitor in a patient of Portuguese descent with familial amyloid polyneuropathy and occasional non-postural dizzy spells. There is a pause of twelve seconds due to sinus node arrest without an escape rhythm. The patient was supine and asymptomatic at the time of this recording. Her 12-lead ECG showed left bundle branch block with a normal P-R interval. An A-V sequential pacemaker was inserted, leading to abolition of dizzy spells.

4.Diagnostic tests

The chest X-ray in cardiac amyloid shows non-specific abnormalities with mild to moderate cardiomegaly often with evidence of congestive heart failure. The electrocardiogram in AL amyloidosis frequently shows low voltage in the limb leads (Fig. 3). Low voltage in familial amyloid is less common, even in the presence of significant cardiac involvement. Intraventricular conduction block occurs in approximately one-third of cases and a pseudo-infarction pattern (Q waves on the precordial leads) is often seen (18,26). Apart from first-degree atrioventricular block, the commonest conduction abnormality is left anterior hemiblock. Surprisingly we have found left bundle branch block to be a very unusual manifestation of AL amyloid, a fact which appears to be borne out by other studies (26). In familial amyloid, however, left bundle branch block may occur.

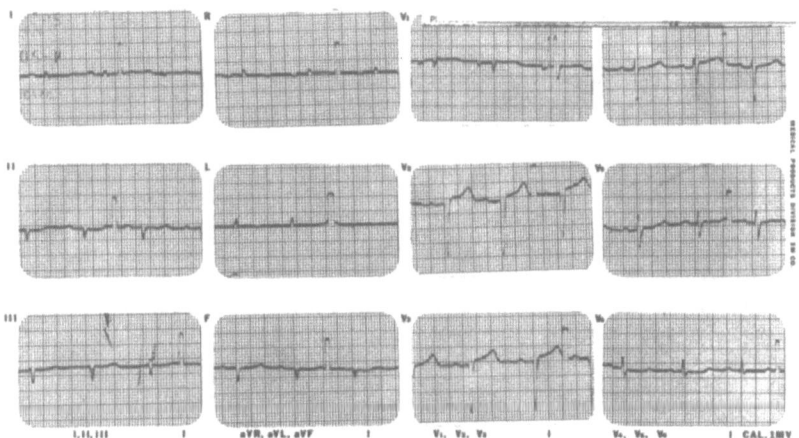

Figure 3: Typical electrocardiogram in primary cardiac amyloidosis. There is extremely low voltage in the limb leads, left anterior hemiblock, first-degree atrioventricular block and an anteroseptal pseudo-infarction pattern (calibration: 1 mV).

Although the electrocardiogram in severe cardiac amyloid may be suggestive of the disease, the diagnosis cannot be made by electrocardiography alone. Echocardiography has proven to be a sensitive tool for diagnosing amyloidosis. The most consistent finding on echocardiography is a thick-walled ventricle with a normal or reduced ventricular cavity size. The calculated ejection fraction may be within normal limits despite clinically significant heart failure, since the predominant functional disturbance in amyloid is severely impaired cardiac relaxation (1,3,6). A thick walled ventricle with a small cavity may be seen in hypertensive heart disease or hypertrophic cardiomyopathy, and is thus not diagnostic for amyloidosis.

Other echocardiographic features occur which are more specific for amyloid. Segueira-Filho et al described an unusual highly refractile appearance of the myocardium in patients with severe cardiac amyloid (5). This appearance, which they termed "granular sparkling", is assumed to be due to the abnormal echogenicity of the amyloid-laden myocardium and was initially thought to be a highly specific finding. Subsequent studies have described this appearance in patients with chronic renal failure and hypertrophic cardiomyopathy (when it is usually localized to the septum rather than uniformly spread throughout the myocardium (27)). Increased myocardial echogenicity does not occur in the absence of left ventricular thickening (17). Most cases of left ventricular thickening are due to left ventricular hypertrophy, whereas the thickening in amyloid is due to infiltration. This results in a decrease in electrocardiographic voltage in amyloid compared to an increase in true left ventricular hypertrophy. Based on this concept, Carroll et al (18) suggested that a distinctive ratio of electrocardiographic voltage and left ventricular mass (calculated from the echocardiogram) distinguishes patients with cardiac amyloidosis from those with true causes of left ventricular hypertrophy. Other authors, including our group, have confirmed this finding (28).

We have found the presence of increased myocardial echogenicity to be 87% sensitive and 81% specific for diagnosing cardiac amyloid (28). When echocardiograms of patients with documented cardiac amyloid were compared, blindly, to those with left ventricular hypertrophy, the corresponding figures for a voltage/mass ratio greater than 1.5:1 was 82% specific and 83% sensitive for diagnosing AL amyloid (voltage = sum of S in V1+R in V5 or V6; "mass" = $(R+Th)^2 - R^2$ divided by body surface area, where R = ventricular radius and Th is ventricular thickness). We also found atrial septal thickness to be a highly sensitive, though less (60%) specific marker of cardiac amyloid. In a patient with thickened left ventricular walls, increased myocardial echogenicity and an increased atrial septal thickness we believe the diagnosis of cardiac amyloid is virtually certain (Fig. 1).

Doppler echocardiography is a recently introduced technique capable of measuring the velocity of blood flow across cardiac valves. Little data are available on Doppler abnormalities in cardiac amyloid. However, information from Plehn et al (22) suggest that this technique may reliably distinguish amyloid infiltration from true left ventricular hypertrophy. In a preliminary study of a small group of patients, the atrial contribution of diastole was markedly reduced in cardiac amyloid as opposed to an increased component in ventricular hypertrophy. This presumably represent the impaired atrial contraction in amyloidosis due to atrial involvement with the disease.

5.Isotope studies

Technetium-99m pyrophosphate is a radioisotope which is normally taken up by the bones and kidneys but not by the normal heart. In AL amyloidosis, severe enough to produce echocardiographic evidence of left ventricular thickening, diffuse myocardial pyrophosphate uptake is present and may be intense (7) (Fig. 4). The abnormal isotope uptake may be related to the fact that amyloid is an avid binder of calcium, and technetium pyrophosphate uptake is correlated with abnormal tissue calcium accumulation. Technetium pyrophosphate scans may also be positive in patients with familial amyloid polyneuropathy (29) and abnormal echocardiograms, but are negative in secondary amyloidosis even when cardiac involvement is clinically apparent (30). Since technetium pyrophosphate scintigraphy may occasionally be negative in amyloid, or (rarely) diffusely and strongly positive in other diseases, this study is not recommended as the sole diagnostic test. However, as an adjunct to the diagnosis of amyloid in a patient in whom the disease is suspected but not firmly diagnosed, a positive pyrophosphate scan is strong additional evidence for cardiac amyloidosis.

Other cardiac imaging studies of the heart, such as CT scanning have been investigated in amyloidosis (9). Inadequate data are available at present to comment on their diagnostic value.

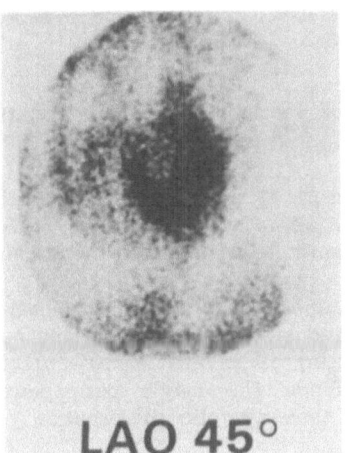 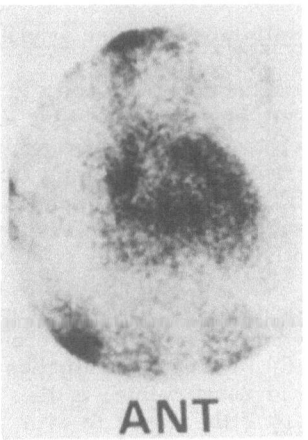

Figure 4: Technetium pyrophosphate cardiac scintigram in severe AL cardiac amyloid. The ventricular walls are outlined by avid isotope uptake, seen as dark black image. The lighter central portion of the image represents the ventricular cavity. LAO = left anterior oblique view; ANT = anterior view.

6. Cardiac arrhythmias

Sudden cardiac death accounts for about one-half of all cardiac-related amyloid deaths. In other forms of cardiac disease sudden death is most frequently caused by ventricular fibrillation. Long-term (24-28 hour) electrocardiographic monitoring (Holter monitoring) in patients with various cardiac diseases has shown an association with the presence of nonsustained ventricular tachycardia and subsequent sudden cardiac death. In a series of 27 patients with AL amyloidosis complex ventricular arrhythmias (ventricular couplets or tachycardia) were virtually limited to the 17 with an abnormal echocardiogram (18). Although the number of sudden cardiac deaths was too small to draw statistical conclusions all sudden deaths occurred in patients with complex ventricular arrhythmias. Of note was the fact that clinically significant bradycardia was rare (1 subject) in this series, despite the frequent presence of conduction defects on the electrocardiogram. This contrasts with the findings in familial amyloidosis, where autonomic nervous system involvement may be severe and symptomatic bradycardia is common (20). Invasive electrophysiologic testing in primary amyloid has been undertaken in isolated cases only and their prognostic value cannot be determined.

Several studies in different groups of familial amyloid polyneuropathy have demonstrated defective autonomic regulation of the heart. However, the conduction system infiltration, rather than defective innervation, is considered to be the predominant cause of bradyarrhythmias in this disease (31).

7. Treatment of cardiac amyloidosis

Unfortunately, no specific treatment of cardiac amyloidosis exists at present, and thus therapy is directed against symptoms of heart failure rather than the underlying disease.

Certain principles apply to the treatment of congestive heart failure due to amyloidosis, which do not usually apply to other forms of heart disease. Patients with amyloidosis have long been noted to be unusually sensitive to the toxic effects of digoxin, but it is only recently that this observation has been explained. Rubinow et al (32) demonstrated that amyloid fibrils avidly bind digoxin and suggest that this may result in toxic levels in the myocardium, resulting in severe impairment of an already diseased conduction system. Since the major component of amyloid heart failure is diastolic rather than systolic dysfunction there is very little reason to ever use digoxin.

Diuretic use is also fraught with hazards in amyloidosis. In patients with nephrotic syndrome vigorous diuresis may result in intravascular depletion and severe hypotension. In patients in whom normal renal function exists, diuretics should be used to reduce cardiac edema but care must be exercised not to produce overdiuresis. Careful attention must be paid to the jugular venous pressure, which should be allowed to remain slightly to moderately elevated. Since the ventricular volume is low in cardiac amyloidosis, patients may be very sensitive to overdiuresis with a resultant fall in cardiac output. It is therefore prudent to leave patients with some peripheral edema, provided this is not too uncomfortable. They should be advised to weigh themselves daily and may increase the diuretics temporarily if excessive (> 1 kg) weight gain occurs.

The role of vasodilators in amyloid heart failure is unclear. In patients with autonomic involvement, peripheral resistance is abnormally low and vasodilators would be expected to have little effect or even adverse effects. Hypotension per se, without a postural blood pressure fall, is not an absolute contraindication to vasodilator use and a marked symptomatic improvement may be seen after the initiation of captopril therapy.

Antiarrhythmic therapy, in an attempt to prevent subsequent sudden death, is of unproven value in cardiac amyloid. Unless sustained symptomatic arrhythmias occur -a rare event- there seems to be no indication for such therapy. Ventricular arrhythmias on Holter monitoring, although often of high-grade (couplets or ventricular tachycardia), are uncommonly associated with frequent premature ventricular contractions. Thus, the assessment of antiarrhythmic therapy by serial Holter monitoring becomes impossible in most cases. In addition, little is known of the binding of various antiarrhythmic drugs to amyloid fibrils nor whether these drugs are more toxic in amyloidosis than in other heart disease.

In other cardiac diseases which affect cardiac relaxation, specifically hypertrophic cardiomyopathy, calcium-channel blocking agents (verapamil, nifedipine, diltiazem) are beneficial in improving ventricular relaxation and hence symptoms of heart failure (33). The functional disorder in cardiac amyloid - namely extensive myocardial infiltration - differs greatly from hypertrophic cardiomyopathy and it would be unwise to extrapolate potential benefits of these drugs from one disease to the other. Indeed the few isolated reports of the use of calcium-channel blocking agents in amyloid indicate an adverse rather than a positive effect of them (34,35). Thus, these drugs appear to have no role on amyloid heart disease.

8.Heart transplantation

Although kidney transplants have been performed in selected patients with renal amyloid (36) there have been no reports, to date, of heart transplants. Since amyloidosis is a generalized disease most patients have multiple organ involvement, thereby excluding them from most transplant criteria. However in the occasional young patient with apparently isolated severe cardiac amyloid, transplantation may offer some hope of survival. The feasibility of such transplants remains to be seen.

References

1.Chew, C., Ziady, G.M., Raphael, M.J. & Oakley, C.M. Am. J. Cardiol. 36, 438-444, 1975.
2.Meaney, E., Shabetai, R., Bhargava, V. et al. Am. J. Cardiol. 38, 547-556, 1976.
3.Swanton, R.H., Brooksby, I.A.B., Davies, M.J. et al. Am. J. Cardiol. 39, 658-664, 1977.
4.Tyberg, T.L., Goodyer, A.V.N., Hurst III, V.W., et al. Am. J. Cardiol. 47, 791-796, 1981.
5.Sigueira-Filho, A.G., Cunha, C.L.P., Tajik, A.J. et al. Circulation 63, 188-196, 1981.
6.St. John Sutton, M.G., Reichek, N., Kastor, J.A. & Giullani, E.R. Circulation 66, 790-799, 1982.

7.Falk, R.H., Lee, V.W., Rubinow, A. et al. Am. J. Cardiol. 51, 826-830, 1983.
8.Carroll, J.D., Gaasch, W.H. & McAdam, K.P.W.J. Am. J. Cardiol. 49, 9-13, 1982.
9.Sekiya, T., Foster, C.J., Isherwood, L. et al. Br. Heart J. 51, 519-522, 1984.
10.Schroeder, J.S., Billingham, M.E. & Rider, A.K. Am. J. Med. 59, 269-273, 1975.
11.Cornwell III, G.G., Westermark, P., Murdoch, W. & Pitkanen, P. Am. J. Pathol. 108, 135-139, 1982.
12.Westermark, P., Johansson, B. & Natvig, J.B. Scand. J. Immunol. 10, 303-308, 1979.
13.Cornwell III, G.G., Murdoch, W.L., Kyle, R.A. et al. Am. J. Med. 75, 618-623, 1983.
14.Brandt, K., Cathcart, E.S. & Cohen, A.S. Am. J. Med. 44, 955-969, 1968.
15.Kyle, R.A. & Griepp, P.R. Mayo Clin. Proc. 58, 665-683, 1983.
16.Smith, T.J., Kyle, R.A. & Lie, J.T. Mayo Clin. Proc. 59, 547-555, 1984.
17.Cueto-Garcia, L., Tajik, A.J., Kyle, R.A. et al. Mayo Clin. Proc. 59, 589-597, 1984.
18.Falk, R.H., Rubinow, A. & Cohen, A.S. J. Am. Coll. Cardiol. 3, 107-113, 1984.
19.Hongo, M. & Ikeda, S.L. Circulation 73, 249-256, 1986.
20.Olofsson, B.O., Andersson, R. & Furberg, B. Acta Med. Scand. 208, 77-80, 1980.
21.Gowda, S., Salem, B.L. & Haikal, M. Cathet. Cardiovasc. Diagn. 11, 483-491, 1985.
22.Plehn, J.F., Skinner, M., Cohen, A.S. & Apstein, C.S. J. Am. Coll. Cardiol. 7, 97A, 1986.
23.Saffitz, J.E., Sazama, K. & Roberts, W.C. Am. J. Cardiol. 51, 1234-1235, 1983.
24.Cueto-Garcia, L., Tajik, A.J., Kyle, R.A. et al. Am. J. Cardiol. 55, 606-607, 1985.
25.Brodarick, S., Paine, R., Higa, E. & Carmichael, K.A. Am. J. Med. 73, 133-135, 1982.
26.Roberts, W.C. & Waller, B.F. Am. J. Cardiol. 52, 137-146, 1983.
27.Bhandari, A.K. & Nanda, N.C. Am. J. Cardiol. 51, 817-825, 1983.
28.Falk, R.H., Plehn, J.F., Deering, T. et al. Am. J. Cardiol. (In press).
29.Falk, R.H., Lee, V.W., Rubinow, A. et al. Am. J. Cardiol. 54, 1150-1151, 1984.
30.Leinonen, H., Totterman, K.J., Korppi-Tommola, T. & Korhola, O. Am. J. Cardiol. 53, 380-381, 1984.
31.Eriksson, P., Karp, K., Bjerle, P. & Olofsson, B.O. Br. Heart J. 51, 658-662, 1984.
32.Rubinow, A., Skinner, M. & Cohen, A.S. Circulation 63, 1285-1288, 1981.
33.Bonow, R.O., Rosing, D.R., Bacharach, S.L. et al. Circulation 64, 787-796, 1981.
34.Griffiths, B.E., Hughes, P., Dowdle, R. & Stephens, M.R. Thorax 37, 711-712, 1982.
35.Gertz, M.A., Falk, R.H., Skinner, M. et al. Am. J. Cardiol. 55, 1645-1646, 1985.
36.Jones, N.F. Clin. Nephrol. 6, 459-464, 1976.

III.3   HEMODIALYSIS-ASSOCIATED AMYLOID OF β_2-MICROGLOBULIN NATURE

Tsuranobu Shirahama, Alan S. Cohen and Martha Skinner

The Arthritis Center, Boston University School of Medicine,
the Thorndike Memorial Laboratory,
and the Division of Medicine,
Boston City Hospital,
Boston, Massachusetts 02118, U.S.A.

1. Introduction

With the widespread use of long-term hemodialysis to maintain patients with end-stage renal disease, a number of complications have been recognized. Among them, carpal tunnel syndrome (CTS) and osteoarthropathy have received increasing attention recently because of their persistence, severe disabling effects and unclarified etiology. Recently, amyloid has been implicated in a possible cause of these phenomena (1-13). The type (biochemical nature) of the amyloid had not been elucidated. Early in 1984 we instituted studies of hemodialysis-associated amyloid (AH), analyzed the clinical and pathologic picture, successfully identified the chemical nature of the amyloid through histochemical, immunohistochemical and biochemical analyses, and carried out some additional studies in order to elucidate its etiology (14-16). We were fortunate in the development of the chain of events that led to our conclusions and will describe them in a personal chronologic fashion.

2. Clinical and pathological aspects

Although we had been aware of the complication of CTS and osteoarthropathy in maintenance hemodialysis and the implication of amyloid in these conditions through published literature and personal communications (1-13), our intense study on this subject started in 1984 after having a series of discussions with Dr. F. Gejyo of Niigata University, Japan that led to our collaboration. As the person in charge of hemodialysis program at the university's Kidney Center (one of the oldest and largest hemodialysis centers in Japan), he was facing a serious problem in that an increasing number of their patients under chronic hemodialysis developed CTS. Carpal release operations had been performed on 7 patients until then (June, 1984), and amyloid deposits were found in all surgical tissues examined.

Based on the information available at the time, we assessed the circumstances with regard to amyloid as follows:
1. The association of amyloid deposition in this hemodialysis-associated CTS is quite high, and therefore amyloid may have a significant etiologic role.
2. The issue as to whether the amyloidosis associated with chronic hemodialysis be systemic or localized has not been clearly settled.
3. This amyloidosis develops as a complication of chronic hemodialysis which is an aggressive treatment in a sense, and therefore may turn out to be secondary (acquired) amyloidosis. In addition, the cuprophan membrane used in hemodialysis evokes interleukin-1 production and subsequently an acute phase reaction (17) which in turn creates high levels of SAA. These conditions tend to support the hypothesis that this amyloid may be of AA-type. On the other hand, while CTS is known to associate with amyloidosis, there have been no proven cases of CTS associated with secondary AA amyloidosis reported so far (18-23). Therefore, the clinical picture of this amyloidosis does not fit well that of any known type of amyloidosis. We set the goals of our study to answer these questions.

3. Histologic aspects in regard to distribution of amyloid

Using Congo red and hematoxylin staining, we initially examined the tissues collected at carpal release operation from 5 patients who all also underwent diagnostic rectal biopsy. Substantial amyloid deposits were observed in all the carpal tissues, i.e. synovia and perineural connective tissue. Deposition of amyloid was also found in rectal biopsies from three of the five patients. Amyloid deposition was however minute in all three cases, and was restricted in the walls of small rectal blood vessels (16). Besides CTS, destructive osteoarthropathy was recently added to the list of prominent manifestations caused by deposition of amyloid associated with chronic hemodialysis. Many different joints can be affected. Large cystic lesions have been noted in the humerus at the shoulder joint, in the femur adjacent to the hip and in the carpal bones at the wrist joint. Arthralgias in other joints suggest they may also be involved. Clinical symptoms can widely vary from acute and chronic articular and para-articular inflammatory episodes in multiple joints to femoral neck fracture as the results of destructive osteoarthropathy (3,7,8,10).

Our finding of amyloid deposits in the rectal biopsies in three of five cases (16) and the involvement of multiple joints (1-13) indeed support the possible systemic involvement of this type of amyloidosis. While systemic amyloid deposition was indeed observed in a few cases, there are also reports that extensive examination of cases with hemodialysis-associated amyloidosis did not reveal visceral amyloid deposition (1,6,7,9,10, and personal communications). In our own more recent experience, among 5 autopsy cases whose records we had access to

84

through collaboration with Dr. T. Bardin, Paris, France and Dr. A.Z. Fenves, Dallas, Texas, only one had extensive visceral amyloid deposition. Clarification of the issue as to whether involvement of this type amyloidosis is localized, selective to certain tissues, or systemic, should wait until much more comprehensive studies of autopsy cases have accumulated.

4.Identity of AH in relation to the known amyloid types

In 1984, no information was available on the nature of this type of amyloid. Our initial approach was to examine formalin-fixed paraffin sections by histochemical and immunohistochemical means, and to decide whether it has an identity with any of the known types of amyloid. With the permanganate treatment (24,25) the Congophilia of the amyloid deposits was drastically reduced. In the tissues of our initial 5 cases, the degree of the reduction of Congophilia by the permanganate treatment was comparable to that seen with AA-amyloid, and the amyloid was therefore judged as sensitive to the permanganate treatment (16). At this point, we suspected that the AH could be of the AA-type.

However, in the immunohistochemical preparations in a controlled system, the AH failed to react not only with anti-human AA antisera but also with antisera to other known amyloid protein types tested (16).

These histochemical and immunohistochemical findings combined led us to the conclusion that the AH was a new form of amyloid, and eventually to our effort for definitive chemical analysis of the protein.

5.Chemical identity of AH as β_2-microglobulin

At the first opportunity that the tissue became available after the above-mentioned observations had been made, about 0.5 gram wet weight of amyloid laden tissue obtained at carpal release operation was subjected to chemical analysis. Amyloid fibrils were isolated through a "waterextraction" procedure. Solubilized in guanidine HCl, a significant amount of the protein was located in a homogenous low molecular weight fraction. The protein was found to be identical to β_2-microglobulin (β_2-M) with regard to its molecular weight of 11,000 dalton, amino acid composition and 16 amino-terminal amino acids (15):

Ile-Gln-Arg-Thr-Pro-Lys-Ile-Gln-Val-Tyr-Ser-Arg-His-Pro-Ala-Glu-

The results indicate that AH is indeed a new form of amyloid and of β_2-M nature, and that the amyloid protein probably represents an intact or nearly intact β_2-M molecule for their molecular weight is comparable and no variation was indicated in amino acid sequence up to the position 16. This view was confirmed by others in a study where AH was analyzed and the N-terminal amino acids were sequenced up to position

30 (26), and by in vitro studies noted below. Very recently, a smaller (7 Kdalton) protein bearing amino acid sequence homology with β_2-M was reported as the major constituent of amyloid in urinary calculi from uremic patients, suggesting that fragments of β_2-M can also form amyloid fibrils (27).

6.Generality of β_2-M nature of AH in different cases

After the chemical identity of AH as β_2-M was established in one case (15), attempts to carry out further chemical analyses were limited by the minute amounts of tissue available. We therefore examined formalin--fixed paraffin sections from different AH cases using histochemical and immunohistochemical methods.

In addition to the initial 5 cases (16), we have so far examined tissues from 26 cases with AH that were made available to us through collaboration with Dr. T. Bardin and Dr. A.Z. Fenves. The tissues were collected from various areas including carpal tissues from patients with CTS, synovial membranes, cartilages and contents of bone cysts from femoral heads, and tissues obtained from the areas of destructive spondyloarthropathy. All amyloid deposits in these tissues from 31 cases reacted positively with anti-human β_2-M in immunohistochemical preparations, indicating the presence of β_2-M (Fig. 1). Immunohistochemically positive reaction of AH amyloid deposits with anti-β_2-M has also been confirmed by others (26,27).

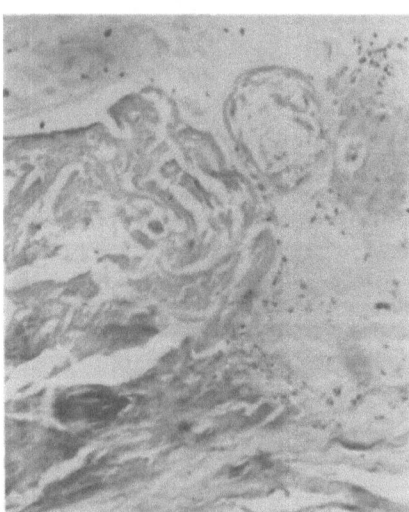 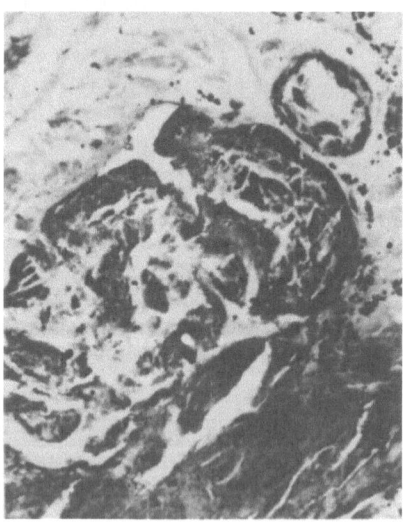

Figure 1: a.(left): Tissue obtained from a cystic lesion in the femoral neck of a patient on chronic hemodialysis. Congo red and hematoxylin staining reveals that about 50% of the tissue area is covered by Congophilic amyloid. b.(right): An adjacent section, immuno-histochemically stained with anti-human β_2-microglobulin using an avidin-biotin peroxidase method. The amyloid shows a positive reaction. Magnification: x 140.

The "permanganate test" on the amyloid deposits of our initial 5 AH cases showed that they were all "sensitive". Through examination of amyloid deposits in our subsequent 26 cases, however, we have found that they not all are sensitive to the permanganate treatment. Although the majority of AH deposits were judged to be sensitive, reduction of Congophilia by permanganate treatment was observed only 20-50% with amyloid deposits in some tissue sections. In addition, the permanganate test is often subtle and preparatory variations often affect the results. Although our permanganate treatment preparations are performed under a strictly controlled system, we can not be sure whether the different reactions observed among different AH deposits to the permanganate treatment is due to the chemical and/or physical variation among them or resulted from minor preparatory variations in our test procedure.

7. Etiologic consideration of AH

β_2-M is a low molecular weight (11,800 dalton)) protein normally present in biological fluids (28-31). Its entire sequence of 99 amino acids is known and shows significant homology to that of the constant domain of IgG, while antigenic cross-reactivity between the two has not been observed (32). β_2-M is known to contain the β-pleated sheet configuration (33,34), which is one of the essential properties of amyloid (21,24,35). Functionally, this protein is the smaller surface protein of the class 1 major histocompatibility complex antigens (36). It is also known that β_2-M readily forms crystals or insoluble compounds given certain conditions, e.g. high protein concentration and low salt solvent (33,34). In addition, renal insufficiency creates high serum levels of this protein and hemodialysis cannot sufficiently lower the levels (37,38). Combined these informations and the biochemical characteristics of the AH amyloid protein, one may postulate that the chronically high levels of β_2-M in hemodialysis patients can be an important factor in etiology of hemodialysis-associated amyloidosis.

This concept gained strong support from our study that created amyloid fibrils from intact β_2-M in vitro (14). However, the high levels of β_2-M concentration may not be the sole etiologic factor for AH. Recent study by Gejyo et al found no significant difference in β_2-M serum levels between the groups of patients under chronic hemodialysis with and without CTS (39).

8. Final remarks

Studies on AH have so far indicated the following:
1. Various rheumatic complications that develop during chronic hemodialysis are often associated with amyloid deposition.
2. The amyloid is "sensitive" to the "permanganate treatment" in the majority of cases, and does not react with antisera to other known

amyloid proteins in immunohistochemical preparations.

3. The AH amyloid protein is chemically and immunologically identical with β_2-M.

4. High levels of β_2-M concentration in the patients undergoing chronic hemodialysis may be an important etiologic factor of the amyloidosis.

5. There is no significant difference in β_2-M serum levels between patients undergoing hemodialysis with and without amyloidosis, and therefore high levels of β_2-M may not be the sole etiologic factor for AH.

With the above knowledge, it would clearly be possible to develop measures to prevent this complication of hemodialysis. Studies of a change in the hemodialysis membrane from cuprophane is already underway in several laboratories.

Acknowledgements

Supported by grants from the United States Public Health Service, National Institute of Arthritis, Diabetes, Digestive and Kidney Disease (AM-04599 and AM-07014), National Institutes of Health Multipurpose Arthritis Center (AM-20613), the General Clinical Research Centers Branch of the Division of Research Resources, National Institutes of Health (RR-533) and the Arthritis Foundation.

References

1. Altmeyer, P., Kachel, H.G. & Runne, U. Hautarzt 34, 277-285, 1983.
2. Bardin, T., Kuntz, D., Zingraff, J. et al. Arthritis Rheum. 28, 1052-1058, 1985.
3. Brown, E.A. & Gower, P.E. Clin. Nephrol. 18, 247-250, 1982.
4. Clanet, M., Mansat, M., Durroux, R. et al. Rev. Neurol. 137, 613-624, 1981.
5. Delmez, J.A., Holtmann, B., Sicard, G.A. et al. Nephron 30, 118-123, 1982.
6. Herve, J.P., Cledes, J., Bourbigot, B. et al. Nephron 40, 494, 1985.
7. Hillion, D., Villeboeuf, J., Hillion, Y. et al. Nephron 41, 127-128, 1985.
8. Huaux, J.P., Noel, H., Bastien, P. et al. Rev. Rheum. Mal. Osteoartic. 52, 179-182, 1985.
9. Kachel, H.G., Altmeyer, P., Baldamus, C.A. & Koch, K.M. Contrib. Nephrol. 36, 127-132, 1983.
10. Kuntz, D., Naveau, B., Bardin, T. et al. Arthritis Rheum. 27, 369-375, 1984.
11. Schwarz, A., Keller, F., Seyfert, S. et al. Clin. Nephrol. 22, 133-137, 1984.
12. Spertini, F., Wauters, J.P. & Poulenas, I. Clin. Nephrol. 21, 98-101, 1984.
13. Warren, D.J. & Otiemo, L.S. Postgrad. Med. J. 51, 450-452, 1975.
14. Connors, L.H., Shirahama, T., Skinner, M. et al. Biochem. Biophys. Res. Commun. 131, 1063-1068, 1985.
15. Gejyo, F., Yamada, T., Odani, S. et al. Biochem. Biophys. Res. Commun. 129, 701-706, 1985.
16. Shirahama, T., Skinner, M., Cohen, A.S. et al. Lab. Invest. 53, 705-709, 1985.
17. Henderson, L.W., Koch, K.M., Dinarello, C.A. & Shaldon, S. Blood Purification 1, 3-8, 1983.
18. Benson, M.D., Cohen, A.S., Brandt, K.D. & Cathcart, E.S. Lancet i, 10-12, 1975.
19. Benson, M.D. & Dwulet, F.E. Arthritis Rheum. 26, 1493-1498, 1983.
20. Cohen, A.S. N. Engl. J. Med. 277, 522-530, 574-583, 628-638, 1967.
21. Glenner, G.G. N. Engl. J. Med. 302, 1283-1292, 1330-1345, 1980.
22. Lambird, P.A. & Hartmann, W.H. Am. J. Clin. Pathol. 52, 714-719, 1969.
23. Rukavina, J.G., Block, W.D., Jackson, C.E. et al. Medicine 35, 239-334, 1956.
24. Shirahama, T., Cohen, A.S. & Skinner, M. In Advances in Immunohistochemistry. DeLellis, R.A. Ed. Masson, New York, 277-302, 1984.
25. Wright, J.R., Calkins, E. & Humphrey, R.L. Lab. Invest. 36, 274-281, 1977.
26. Gorevic, P.D., Casey, T.T., Stone, W.J. et al. J. Clin. Invest. 76, 2425-2429, 1985.
27. Linke, R.P., Bommer, J., Ritz, E. et al. Biochem. Biophys. Res. Commun. 136, 665-671, 1986.
28. Berggård, B., Björck, L., Cigen, R. & Lögdberg, L. Scand. J. Clin. Lab. Invest. 40, (Suppl. 154) 13-25, 1980.

29.Berggård, I. & Bearn, A.G. J. Biol. Chem. 243, 4095-4103, 1968.
30.Bernier, G.M. Vox Sang. 38, 323-327, 1980.
31.Karlsson, F.A., Wibell, L. & Evrin, P.E. Scand. J. Clin. Lab. Invest. 40, (Suppl. 154), 27-37, 1980.
32.Cunningham, B.A., Wang, J.L., Berggård, I. & Peterson, P.A. Biochemistry 12, 4811-4822, 1973.
33.Becker, J.W. & Reeke, G.N.Jr. Proc. Natl. Acad. Sci. USA 82, 4225-4229, 1985.
34.Karlsson, F.A. Immunochemistry 11, 111-114, 1974.
35.Cohen, A.S., Shirahama, T., Sipe, J.D. & Skinner, M. Lab. Invest. 48, 1-4, 1983.
36.Kindt, T.J. & Robinson, M.A. In Fundamental Immunology, Paul, W.E. Ed. Raven Press, New York, 347-377, 1984.
37.Vincent, C., Revillard, J.P., Galland, M. & Traeger, J. Nephron 21, 260-268, 1978.
38.Wibell, L., Evrin, P.E., & Berggård, I. Nephron 10, 320-331, 1973.
39.Gejyo, F., Homma, N., Suzuki, Y. & Arakawa, M. N. Engl. J. Med. 314, 585-586, 1986.

III.4 AMYLOID P-COMPONENT: CLINICAL IMPLICATIONS

Martha Skinner, Tsuranobu Shirahama and Alan S. Cohen

The Thorndike Memorial Laboratory and Division of Medicine,
Boston City Hospital, and
The Arthritis Center,
Boston University School of Medicine,
Boston, MA 02118, U.S.A.

1. Introduction

In the course of studying the isolation of amyloid fibril proteins, the structural protein P-component was identified. In 1965 an antibody was made to a solubilized fraction of amyloid fibrils that were isolated by a technique of sucrose gradient centrifugation (1). The antibody cross reacted with a circulating plasma alpha globulin and was called P (plasma) component. This plasma component was isolated from amyloid rich tissues from patients with primary (AL) and secondary (AA) types of amyloidosis and identified as a pentagonally structured protein separate from the amyloid fibrils (2,3). Subsequent studies have shown that AP can be extracted uniquely from amyloid tissue and is identical with normal α-1-glycoprotein (4,5). Thus, AP has been the term used for the P-component associated with amyloid tissues and SAP for the P-component found in serum (6). The two proteins are believed to be completely identical and the terms AP and SAP simply denote the site from which P-component has been isolated. AP has been found associated with amyloid fibrils in primary AL (immunoglobulin light chain), secondary AA, and heredofamilial AF (prealbumin) forms of systemic amyloid disease. In addition, it has been found on all deposits of the various localized forms of amyloid with the possible exception of the intracerebral amyloid plaques and neurofibrillary tangles associated with Alzheimer's disease (7).

Amyloid P-component has a distinctive ultrastructural appearance consisting of a parallel pair of pentagonally arranged subunits (Fig. 1) each of approximately 23,000 dalton, with a total molecular weight of 230,000 dalton (8,9). By electron microscopy each P-component protein measures approximately 90 Å in outside diameter and 40 Å in inside diameter. Each of the five subunits measures 25-30 Å in diameter. On side view each pentagonally structured protein is 25 Å high and occasionally stacked on each other to form a short rod (10). AP belongs to a unique family of proteins termed pentraxins which include C-reactive protein (CRP) and the recently described hamster female protein (FP) (11). The three proteins have an ultrastructural similarity to AP with non-covalently bound subunits. Human CRP is usually seen as a single pentameric disc with only very occasional pairs and no tendency to stack (12). Its subunit size is comparable to that of SAP. Hamster female protein is a pentamer of five 30,000 dalton subunits, which usually appears as a single pentagonal structure. A considerable amount of sequence homology exists among the three proteins, yet they remain immunologically distinct. A stable evolutionary conservation suggests that SAP may be functionally important, although its physiologic role is as yet unknown. SAP has been found in all vertebrate species where it has been sought, including the mouse, rabbit, pig, goat, sheep, donkey, human, cow, marine toad, plaice, flounder and dogfish (12).

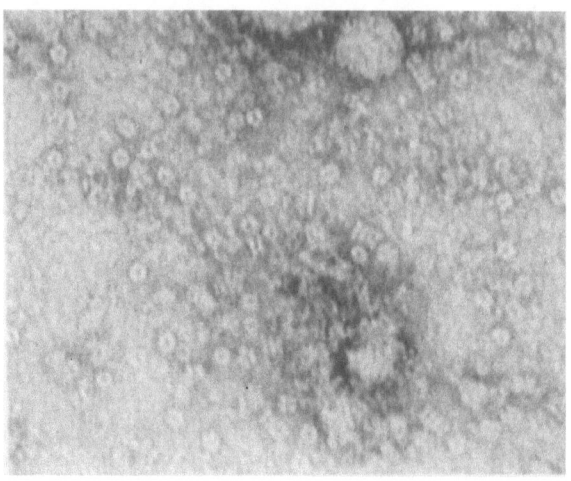

Figure 1: Electron micrograph of human amyloid P-component negatively stained with 1% sodium phosphotungstate. Ring structures measured 90 Å in outside diameter, 40 Å in inside diameter and appeared to be pentagonally shaped. They occasionally appeared stacked, forming short rods (x 320,000).

2. Chemical characterization

A partial amino acid sequence of AP in 1974 identified an amino terminus of histidine and a sequence to 23 residues unlike any known protein sequence (10). In 1980, a partial sequence of SAP showed complete homology to AP and a 50% homology to CRP (13). In 1982, the sequence of SAP was extended (14) and very recently the complete primary structure of SAP was reported by Prelli et al (15) as glycoprotein consisting of 204 amino acids. It is known to have a single disulfide bridge linking Cys 36 and Cys 95 and a carbohydrate attached to Asn 32. The sequence is identical to the complete nucleotide and derived amino acid sequence of SAP determined by Mantzouris et al (16), who have found pre-SAP biosynthesis to be regulated by a 1.1 kilobase mRNA and the human SAP gene to be on chromosome 1 (as is the gene for CRP). The identity of the carbohydrate portion is not clear. A 12% carbohydrate content in the human serum protein (SAP) and a 1.5% sialic acid and 2% hexose content in the rat SAP have been reported (5,17).

Synthesis of SAP takes place in the liver and it can be produced by mouse hepatocytes in tissue culture (18). The half-life of AP is 7.5-8.5 hours suggesting a rapid continuous production to maintain a stable and significant serum level of 40-50 μg/ml (19-21). The level in men is approximately 10 μg/ml higher than that of women. SAP is increased slightly in malignancy, in Waldenström's macroglobulinemia, in rheumatoid arthritis and at the end of pregnancy (22-25). It is decreased in all types of liver disease (26). In umbilical cord sera the SAP level is very low, 4±2 μg/ml, and it rises rapidly to normal values in the infant during the first weeks of life (21).

In the mouse, SAP acts as an acute phase protein (27). There appear to be marked genetically determined differences in the normal SAP levels within inbred mouse strains ranging from 10-100 μg/ml. However, in all strains SAP is a major acute phase protein. The SAP level begins to rise after an inflammatory stimulus and peaks at 24-48 hours. The rise is induced by a monokine which is probably interleukin-1 and varies over a ten fold range (28,29).

AP has been found in amyloid rich tissues of humans as well as in the mouse and guinea pig (30). It is always bound to the amyloid fibrils of the amyloid-rich tissue in a calcium dependent fashion and often in large amounts of up to 20% of the isolated weight of the fibril protein (31). By immunohistochemistry, AP has been identified in normal human renal glomerular basement membranes, in the basement membrane of the parietal wall of the rat yolk sac (Reichert's membrane) and in elastic fiber microfibrils throughout the body (32,33). Using a chelating technique for isolation of calcium bound proteins, large amounts of AP were isolated and identified in the Engelbreth-Holm-Swarm (EHS) mouse basement membrane tumor (34).

In the presence of calcium, SAP has been found to bind to a number of other substances including fibronectin (35) and the C4-binding protein (36). Both AP and SAP will bind to plain unsubstituted agarose and to zymosan in the presence of calcium (37). The very selective and specific binding to certain ligands has aided in the isolation of these proteins and is likely to be important in its as yet unknown physiologic role.

Very recently, Hind et al (38) have shown that pyruvate, a trace contaminant of agarose, is actually the ligand to which SAP binds and this binding can be abolished by methylation of the carboxylic acid of pyruvate. They found that a synthesized pyruvate acetal at the 4,6 positions of galactose will inhibit calcium dependent binding of SAP to agarose, amyloid fibrils, fibronectin and C4-binding protein. Furthermore millimolar amounts of the methyl 4,6-0-(1-carboxyethylidene)- -β-D-galactopyranoside (MOβDG), will dissociate AP from human and mouse amyloid deposits in vitro (39). Similar pyruvate acetals are known to be present in the cell walls of some microorganisms. Hind et al (40) found that SAP binds to bacteria which contain the 4,6-cyclic pyruvate acetal of galactose, i.e. Klebsiella rhinoscleromatis and group A Streptococcus pyogenes and more weakly to others containing the

93

mannose counterpart, i.e. Xanthomonas campestres.

Potempa et al (41) found that the binding of SAP to the polysaccharide ligands of zymosan occurs not only in the presence of calcium but also the divalent cations copper, zinc and cadmium. However no binding occurs with the cations barium, cobalt, manganese, magnesium or nickel. The calcium dependent binding to zymosan decreases as the pH decreases to 5, the copper binding increases at the lower pH values, while the zinc binding remains unchanged.

3.AP binding to amyloid tissues

Amyloid rich tissues provide an excellent source for the isolation of AP protein. AP is found in amounts of 10-20% of the weight of the isolated amyloid fibrils and is known to be bound to all chemical types of amyloid in a calcium dependent fashion. The exact binding site on the amyloid fibrils is unknown, but since fibrils are not glycosylated, it is likely that the autologous ligand is a stereochemically similar structure to the galactoside ligand reported by Hind et al (40). It was orginally thought that AP was present in only minute quantities in association with amyloid fibrils of all three systemic types of amyloidosis. Later, regardless of type the polyanionic nature of all fibrils was recognized as well as their tendency to bind positively charged substances. The P-component protein and blood clotting factors are known to be bound in a calcium dependent fashion and can be dissociated from the fibrils by gentle chelating agents (42). Interestingly, some chemical substances such as digoxin and nifedipine have been found to bind to amyloid fibrils by a non-calcium dependent mechanism (43,44). Very recently, an elastase with the characteristics of human neutrophil elastase was found closely associated with all amyloid fibrils (45). This elastase was not bound by calcium and could be eluted with salt solutions. It is likely that other proteins and positively charged chemical substances may be bound to the fibrils.

The isolation of AP from amyloid-rich tissues is carried out by multiple gentle homogenizations of the tissue containing insoluble amyloid fibrils. The amyloid fibril isolation procedure involving saline washes is used (46) with the addition of citrate washes (31) to free more efficiently the calcium dependent AP protein from the fibril (Table I) (47). AP is isolated from the first 6 saline and citrate supernatants of the amyloid rich tissue after Step 1. Amyloid fibrils are isolated from the sediment.

A number of techniques are available for the further purification of the crude AP obtained from the dialyzed and lyophilized supernatants 1-6. The procedure of choice is outlined in steps 2 and 3 of Table I (47). The same procedure can also be used for the isolation of SAP from serum or plasma. It takes advantage of the binding of AP or SAP to agarose in the presence of calcium. When other soluble proteins have been washed away, P-component can be freed from agarose by EDTA.

TABLE I: ISOLATION OF AMYLOID P-COMPONENT (AP) FROM TISSUE

Step 1

      Amyloid rich tissue (20 gram wet weight)
            homogenize with 200 ml normal saline
            centrifuge at 15,000 rpm (27,000 x g) at $4^{o}C$
            save supernatant (supernatant 1)
            repeat procedure (supernatant 2)

      Tissue sediment
            homogenize (200 ml 0.05 M sodium citrate, TBS, pH 8.0)
            centrifuge and save supernatant (supernatant 3)
            repeat procedure (supernatant 4)

      Tissue sediment
            rehomogenize with 200 ml of normal saline
            centrifuge and save supernatant (supernatant 5)
            repeat until OD_{280} of supernatant < 0.1 (supernatant 6)

      Supernatants 1-6   Tissue sediment
            dialyze vs. H_2O continue with water washing
            lyophilize (crude AP)   for fibril isolation (41)

Step 2

      Crude AP
            dissolve in 0.002 M $CaCl_2$ TBS, centrifuge
            supernatant added to Biogel A (1.5 m column)
            wash with 0.002 M $CaCl_0$ TBS
            elute with 0.01 M EDTA-TBS

Step 3

      Partially purified AP
            Ultragel ACA34 chromatography in 0.02 M EDTA-TBS

      Pure AP

4.Measurement of AP and SAP

The difference between the pentraxins, CRP and SAP, are most notable in their serum levels. CRP is only a trace protein in human adults with levels of 5 µg/ml or lower. It behaves as an acute phase protein which within 24 hr can increase up to several hundredfold in response to inflammation or cell necrosis. In contrast to CRP, SAP circulates at a higher level of 40-50 µg/ml. The SAP level does not vary with age; levels in men, however, are approximately 10 µg/ml higher than those for women. This stable level is attained soon after birth and does not increase in the acute phase situation, except in the mouse species where the increase is approximately tenfold.

Three methods are most widely used for the quantitation of SAP. These are rocket immunoelectrophoresis, radioimmunoassay, and rate nephelometry (21,25,48). The technique of rate nephelometry appears to be the method of choice because it is rapid, reproducible and technically simple. It utilizes the nephelometer, an instrument available in most clinical laboratories where it is used to measure immunoglobulin levels. This instrument measures the intensity of light scattered particles formed by the immunoprecipitation reaction in a polymer-enhancing buffer, that occurs when antibody reacts with specific antigen. An internal microprocessor differentiates the light scatter signal to a rate signal. When the reaction conditions are defined, the peak rate value will be proportional to the antigen concentrations (48). By rocket immunoelectrophoresis, AP is quantitated from the surface area of the precipitate formed when it migrates by electrophoresis in an agarose gel containing antibody to AP. The size of the rocket shaped precipitate is proportional to the amount of AP in the sample (Fig. 2). Excellent descriptions of this method are found in the original paper by Laurell (49) and it has been used by a number of investigators for the measurement of AP and SAP (19,21).

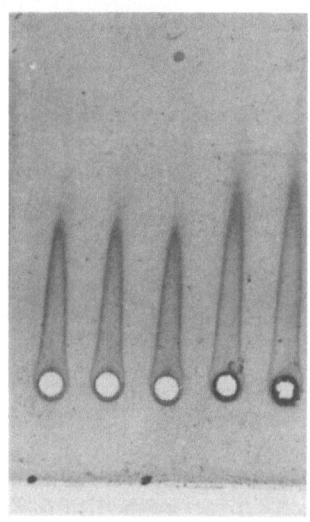

Figure 2: Rocket immunoelectro-phoresis of amyloid P-component in agar containing anti-human AP. The rocket height is proportional to the concentration of AP in the sample.

5. Immunohistochemical reactions

The presence of AP in intimate association with the amyloid fibrils of all types leads to the common belief that fibrils could be identified in tissue deposits by their reaction with antibody to AP. A recent comprehensive immunohistochemical study of multiple tissues from two systemic types of amyloid (secondary and hereditary) suggested that AP may not be an optimal universal marker (50). Although amyloid deposits generally showed moderate reactions with anti AP, these were not always clearly distinguished from the surrounding non-amyloid tissue elements which often stained as well. Basement membrane structures often showed stronger reaction to anti AP than adjacent amyloid deposits. Liver tissue demonstrated a high overall reaction to anti AP, often to such a degree that the reaction of anti AP on amyloid deposits was obscured.

6. Summary

Since its discovery twenty years ago, P-component has undergone thorough ultrastructural and chemical characterization. It has been found to be composed of a parallel pair of pentagonally shaped discs. Each disc has five non-covalently bound subunits of 23,000 dalton. Along with C-reactive protein and hamster female protein which have similar ultrastructures, it has been termed a pentraxin. Biochemically it has been found to be a glycoprotein with 204 amino acids whose sequence has been determined. Its hepatic synthesis is regulated by a SAP gene on chromosome 1. The SAP serum level remains stable at 40-50 μg/ml, with slightly lower levels consistently found in women. The half-life is approximately 8 hours, suggesting a rapid continuous production to maintain a stable and significant serum level. For the mouse species, SAP has an acute phase nature, elevating tenfold with an inflammatory stimulus.

AP binds to amyloid fibrils of all types in a calcium dependent fashion. It also binds to basement membrane structures and elastic fiber microfibrils throughout the body. There are no clinical implications associated with the presence of P-component in the amyloid fibril. The binding of calcium to the amyloid fibril has provided a substrate for a number of substances including P-component, to bind to the fibril. The technetium pyrophosphate bone-seeking radionuclide (^{99m}Tc-PYP), is thought to bind to amyloid fibrils due to their high calcium content (51). It is not known wether or not ^{99m}Tc-PYP displaces P-component when it binds to the fibril. The bone scan test has frequently shown uptake of radionuclide over soft tissue which has correlated well with other tests indicating amyloid deposition. It has thus been useful clinically as a measure of the presence of amyloid within tissues.

In spite of extensive knowledge that has been gained on the structural and biochemical nature of this protein, its site of synthesis, serum concentration and unique association with amyloid fibrils, the functional properties remain obscure. The evolutionary conservation of SAP, however, suggests that it may be functionally important.

Acknowledgements

Supported by grants from the United States Public Health Service, NIAMDD (AM 04500 and AM 07014), from the General Clinical Research Centers Branch of the Division of Research Resources, National Institutes of Health (RR 533), Multipurpose Athritis Center, National Institutes of Health (Am 20613), and the Arthritis Foundation.

References

1. Cathcart, E.S., Comerford, F.R. & Cohen, A.S. New Eng. J. Med. 273, 143-146, 1965.
2. Bladen, H.A., Nylen, M.U. & Glenner, G.G. J. Ultrastruct. Res. 14, 449-459, 1966.
3. Cathcart, E.S., Shirahama, T. & Cohen A.S. Biochim. Biophys. Acta 147, 392-393, 1967.
4. Cathcart, E.S., Wollheim, F.A. & Cohen, A.S. J. Immunol. 99, 376-385, 1967.
5. Haupt, H., Heimburger, N., Kranz, T. & Baudner, S. Hoppe-Seyler's Z. Physiol. Chem. 353, 1841-1849, 1972.
6. Cohen, A.S., Franklin, E.C., Glenner, G.G. et al. In Amyloidosis. Wegelius O., Pasternack, A., Eds. Academic Press, New York, p.ix. 1976.
7. Westermark, P., Shirahama, T., Skinner, M. et al. Lab. Invest. 46, 457-460, 1982.
8. Pinteric, L. & Painter, R.H. Can. J. Biochem. 57, 727-736, 1979.
9. Painter, R.H., DeEscallon, I., Massey, A. et al. Ann. N.Y. Acad. Sci. 389, 199-215, 1982.
10. Skinner, M., Cohen, A.S., Shirahama T. & Cathcart, E.S. J. Lab. Clin. Med. 84, 604-614, 1974.
11. Coe, J.E. Contemporary Topics in Molecular Immunology 9, 211-238, 1983.
12. Pepys, M.B., Dash, A.C., Fletcher, T.C. et al. Nature 273, 168-170, 1978.
13. Skinner, M., Pepys, M.B., Cohen, A.S. et al. In Amyloid and Amyloidosis. Glenner, G.G., Costa, P.P. & Freitas, A.F., Eds. Excerpta Medica, Amsterdam, 384-391, 1980.
14. Anderson, J.K. & Mole, J.E. Anal. Biochem. 123, 413-421, 1982.
15. Prelli, F., Pras, M. & Frangione B. J. Biol. Chem. 260, 12895-12898, 1985.
16. Mantzouranis, E.C., Dowton, S.B., Whitehead, A.S. et al. J. Biol. Chem. 260, 7752-7756, 1985.
17. Pontet, M., D'Asnieres, M., Gache, D. et al. Biochim. Biophys. Acta 671, 201-210, 1981.
18. Tatsuta, E., Sipe, J.D., Shirahama, T. et al. J. Biol. Chem. 258, 5414-5418, 1983.
19. Skinner, M., Sipe, J.D., Yood, R.A. et al. Ann. N.Y. Acad. Sci. 389, 190-198, 1982.
20. Thompson, A.R. & Enfield, D.L. Biochemistry 17, 4304-4311, 1978.
21. Pepys, M.B., Dash, A.C., Markham, R.E. et al. Clin. Exp. Immunol. 32, 119-124, 1978.
22. Strachan, A.F. & Johnson, P.M. J. Clin. Lab. Immunol. 8, 153-156, 1982.
23. Jensson, O., Bjornsson, G., Arnason, A. et al. Acta Med. Scand. 211, 341-345, 1982.
24. Sipe, J.D. & Cohen, A.S. Fed. Proc. 41, 4985, 1982.
25. Skinner, M., Vaitukaitis, J.L., Cohen, A.S. & Benson, M.D. J. Lab. Clin. Med. 94, 633-638, 1979.
26. Levo., Y, Shalit, M. & Tur-Kaspa, R. Am. J. Gastroenterol. 77, 427-430, 1982.
27. Pepys, M.B., Baltz, M.L., Gomer, K. et al. Nature 278, 259-261, 1979.
28. Le P.T., Muller, M.T. & Mortensen, R.F. J. Immunol. 129, 665-672, 1982.
29. Mortensen, R.T., Beisel, K., Zeleznik, N.J. & Le, P.T. J. Immunol. 129, 385-430, 1983.
30. Skinner, M., Cathcart, E.S., Cohen, A.S. & Benson, M.D. J. Exp. Med. 140, 871-876, 1974.
31. Skinner, M., Shirahama, T., Cohen, A.S. & Deal, C.L. Prep. Biochem. 12, 461-476, 1983.
32. Dyck, R.F., Lockwood, C.M., Kershaw, M. et al. J. Exp. Med. 152, 1162-1174, 1980.
33. Inoue, S., Leblond, C.P. & Laurie, G.W. J. Cell. Biol. 97, 1524-1537, 1983.
34. Inoue, S., Skinner, M., Leblond, C.P. et al. Biochem. Biophys. Res. Commun. 134, 995-999, 1986.
35. DeBeer, F.C., Baltz, M., Holford, S. et al. J. Exp. Med. 154, 1134-1139, 1981.
36. Hutchcraft, C.L., Gewurz, H., Hansen, B. et al. J. Immunol. 126, 1217-1219, 1981.
37. Pepys, M.B., Dyck, R.F., DeBeer, F.C. et al. Clin. Exp. Immunol. 38, 284-293, 1979.
38. Hind, C.R.K., Collins, P.M., Renn, D. et al. J. Exp. Med. 159, 1058-1069, 1984.
39. Hind, C.R.K., Collins, P.M., Caspi, D. et al. Lancet ii, 376-378, 1984.
40. Hind, C.R.K., Collins, P.M., Baltz, M.L. & Pepys, M.B. Biochem. J. 225, 107-111, 1985.
41. Potempa, L.A., Kubak, B.M. & Gewurz, H. J. Biol. Chem. 260, 12142-12147, 1985.
42. Skinner, M., Talarico, L., Cohen, A.S. & St. John, A. In Amyloid and Amyloidosis. Glenner, G.G., Costa, P.P., Freitas, A.F., Eds. Excerpta Medica, Amsterdam, 361-365, 1980.
43. Rubinow, A., Skinner, M. & Cohen, A.S. Circulation 63, 1285-1288, 1981.
44. Gertz, M., Skinner, M., Connors, L.H. et al. Am. J. Cardiol. 55, 1646, 1985.
45. Skinner, M., Stone, P., Shirahama, T. et al. Proc. Soc. Exp. Biol. Med. 181, 211-214, 1986.
46. Pras, M., Schubert, M., Zucker-Franklin, D. et al. J. Clin. Invest. 47, 924-933, 1968.
47. Skinner, M. & Cohen, A.S. Methods in Enzymology, 1986, (In press).
48. Gertz, M.A., Skinner, M., Cohen, A.S. & Kyle, R.A. J. Lab. Clin. Med. 102, 773-778, 1983.
49. Laurell, C.B. Scand. J. Clin. Lab. Invest. 29 (suppl. 124), 21-37, 1972.
50. Shirahama, T., Skinner, M., Sipe, J.D. & Cohen, A.S. Virchows Archiv (Cell Path.) 48, 197-206, 1985.
51. Yood, R.A., Skinner, M., Cohen, A.S. & Lee, V.W. J. Rheumatol. 8, 760-766, 1981.

SECTION IV

PATHOGENESIS

sub-editor: Mark B. Pepys

IV.1 AMYLOID PROTEIN AA AND ITS PRECURSOR, THE ACUTE
PHASE PROTEIN(S) ApoSAA: A PERSPECTIVE

Earl P. Benditt

Department of Pathology,
University of Washington,
Seattle, Washington 98195, U.S.A.

1.Introduction

It was a privilege to have been a participant in the first International
Symposium on Amyloidosis held under Dr. Mandema's guidance in
Groningen in 1967, and I am pleased to contribute to this volume in
honor of Professor Mandema. It provides me with an opportunity to
praise Professor Mandema's very considerable foresight in organizing
the original Groningen Symposium and also to review some of the
developments in our ideas concerning the structure and derivation of
amyloid.
My first involvement with the study of amyloid began many years ago
at the University of Chicago with the autopsy of a young man, age 19,
who had chronic osteomyelitis since the age of 12 years and died of
amyloidosis affecting his kidneys. The history of amyloid protein AA
began with the autopsy on a young woman who died of renal failure associated with chronic ulcerative colitis. On frozen material obtained from
that case, my colleagues and I established the fact that the fibrillar
substance in the abundant splenic amyloid was soluble in a protein denaturing solvent, 6M urea (1). Spectral, histochemical and ultracentri-
fugal analysis of the extract provided evidence that we were dealing
largely with protein molecules. Immunologic analysis indicated the
presence of only traces of serum constituents including gamma globulin.
We concluded that amyloid does not consist of a simple antigen-antibody
precipitate, a popular concept in 1962, and suggested the possibility
that amyloid fibrils are the product of the polymerization of a small
protein with itself or with other entities.
In a subsequent paper in 1964 (2), we pursued the analysis of the
original case and several other cases using the original solubilization
procedures and analysis of the extracted proteins by starch gel electrophoresis in the denaturing urea solvent. This enabled us to report for
the first time the fact that associated with amyloid substance in six
cases of the secondary amyloidosis there appeared to be a single main
proteinaceous constituent. A similar constituent was found in the kidney
of a case of familial Mediterranean fever. On the other hand, several
hearts with primary amyloidosis yielded proteins of different electrophoretic mobility, some of which have turned out to be immunoglobulin-
-derived. From the amyloid-rich organs of inflammation-associated cases,
the main constituent was isolated using molecular sieve chromatography.

101

This constituent proved to be a protein since it was found essentially entirely of amino acids. We obtained an amino acid composition, estimated its size to be about 10 Kdalton and named it amyloid α-protein. No protein of similar electrophoretic and spectral properties was found in non-amyloidotic tissues (3).

At the time of the first Groningen Amyloid Symposium, Glenner and Bladen had described the double pentameric structures now called P-component (4). We had observed similar structures. The question then was, what is the relationship of these structures to fibrils and various speculations were proposed. It is now clear that P-component is an entity in its own right not directly related to fibril structures.

2. Structure and pathogenesis of amyloidosis

The nature of the interaction of amyloid fibrils with Congo red is a significant and interesting question. The invention by Pras et al (5) of the water extraction method for preparing partly purified amyloid fibril fragments provided material with which to study the properties of the interaction. We were able to show that Congo red, when it interacts with the fibrils, produces a complex spectral shift and associated anomalous optical rotatory dispersion and circular dichroism, known as a Cotton effect (6). Furthermore, we showed that poly-L-lysine in aqueous solution-suspension in its α-helical conformation and to a lesser extent in its beta conformation, but not in its random conformation, induced a similar Cotton effect with the Congo red dye. Glenner and colleagues (7) later used the poly-L-lysine dried on slides and showed that in the dry state there is cross-beta conformation of the polymer and that when stained with Congo red it exhibits dichroic birefringence. On this basis, they suggested that the β-pleated sheet conformation was the critical feature. This parallelism is compatible with but does not provide final proof that the cross-β conformation is the essential feature responsible for the binding of Congo red and exhibition of the birefringence. Recent structural evidence derived from our sequence data on apoSAA, the precursor of amyloid protein A, suggests that hydrophobic properties leading to self-aggregation is an important feature and the one determining the initial deposition of the A protein into ordered fibrillar structures.

The association of amyloidosis in humans with chronic inflammation, in animals with prolonged immunization, and with plasma cell myeloma provided the foundation of a strong belief that amyloid fibrils were related to antibodies and presumed to be an antigen-antibody precipitate. Thus when Glenner et al (8) presented evidence that the substance found in a case of myeloma-associated amyloid was a fragment of an immunoglobulin light chain, this was considered to be the answer to amyloid. The belief in the light chain theory of amyloidosis was so strong that it was difficult then to get a paper published entitled "Chemical Classes of Amyloid Substance" (9) in which we showed that in addition to amyloid of the AA variety there were several other types. One problem that many people had with amyloid protein AA was the fact that it had no known source or function. The observation that a protein immunologically related to protein AA circulated (10) was therefore an important fact and led us to examine the characteristics of the circulating entity and uncover the apoSAA family of acute phase proteins. In the remainder of this communication, we wish to present some new facts about the apoSAA proteins in regard to their source and to their relationship to amyloid formation.

3. Apo-SAA

3.1. Structure and synthesis

The apoSAA's comprise a family of amphipathic proteins having a size of approximately 12 Kdalton in the serums of men, mice and other mammals and circulating mainly as a part of the high density lipoprotein fraction. Two apoSAA isotypes (1 and 2) appear in the plasma during the acute phase response to injury. Very low circulating serum levels of apoSAA are observed in normal individuals but these rise dramatically following tissue injury and are elevated in chronic inflammatory conditions. ApoSAA was discovered because of its reactivity with antibodies made against protein A obtained from amyloid deposits in tissues of man and mouse. Amino acid sequence analysis, along with the specific immunologic reactivity with the anti-amyloid protein A (AA) antibodies, established the relationship between the circulating acute phase SAA and the amyloid deposits. These observations suggested that serum amyloid A (SAA) is the precursor for amyloid A protein, the main protein constituent found in the amyloid fibrils of reactive amyloidosis (9). Mouse SAA is encoded by a family of at least three genes (11). It is well established that SAA_1 and SAA_2 are synthesized in the liver by hepatocytes (12) and are found circulating in nearly equal quantities associated with high density lipoprotein (HDL) (13). We have found by amino acid sequence analysis that, of the three possible SAA gene products, SAA_2 is the only isotype related to and hence the only possible precursor of murine amyloid fibril protein AA (14).

3.2. SAA gene expression

In order to explore the mechanism of SAA isotype-specific amyloid protein AA deposition, the molecular kinetics of the serum amyloid proteins were examined in CBA mice during casein induction of amyloidosis using a cDNA probe capable of hybridizing with all three SAA messages (15). We searched for the presence of SAA mRNA in spleen. In addition, hepatic SAA_1 and SAA_2 mRNA levels, rates of specific protein synthesis and secretion by hepatocytes, as well as serum levels of SAA_1

and SAA_2 were measured during the 20-day period of amyloid induction by casein. Total serum SAA levels peaked one day after we began casein treatment and thereafter declined. This decline was accounted for entirely by a dramatic fall in SAA_2, while SAA_1 levels remained nearly constant throughout. The ratios of hepatic SAA_2/SAA_1 mRNA, as determined by in vitro translation, remained constant during the 20-day period, as did amounts of SAA_1 and SAA_2 synthesized and secreted by freshly isolated hepatocytes.

The data indicate that the deposition of amyloid protein A derived from SAA_2 is not due to local SAA production, since we found no evidence of SAA message in spleen with the cDNA probe, nor is it due to excessive SAA_2 production compared with SAA_1. The data establish that amyloid deposition does involve the selective and accelerated removal of SAA_2 from the circulating pool of SAA_2.

We further explored SAA gene expression using the same cDNA probe but with endotoxin (LPS) as the acute-phase stimulant. When RNA's from a variety of tissues were examined, it was found that LPS induced low to moderate levels of SAA mRNA in some extrahepatic tissues. Our studies using translation of RNA from livers of treated mice provided evidence for expression of genes for SAA_1 and SAA_2 but not for SAA_3 (15). To extend our analysis we constructed DNA probes from the most divergent portion of the three gene-encoded messages described by Yamamoto and Migita (11). Probes were chosen from the 3'-untranslated portion of each message where the sequence divergence permitted Northern blotting at relatively high stringencies. Using the separate probes, studies of message induction by casein and LPS in both CBA and Balb/c mice were made.

Expression of mRNA's for the three SAA's in liver after Lps or casein injections is as follows: SAA_1 and SAA_2 mRNA's exhibit essentially the same time course: They are both maximally elevated by 4 hours and remain elevated until the 28th hour when the levels begin to decline. At 48 hours after a single Lps injection, SAA_1 and SAA_2 mRNA are 10% of the maximum level. The SAA_3 mRNA increases at a slower rate than SAA_1 and SAA_2, 20% of maximum at 4 hours, reaching a maximum equal to SAA_2 by 16 hours; disappearance is slightly faster than that of SAA_2 mRNA. The rise of SAA_1 and SAA_2 mRNA's after casein injection is significantly slower than after LPS. They are only slightly elevated by 4 hours followed by a rapid rise to 60% of maximum by 9 hours and maximum by 16 hours where it remains through 30 hours. SAA_3 is minimally elevated by casein injection and reaches only 2-5% of the maximum SAA_1 and SAA_2 levels at 16 hours.

Different tissues express the three SAA genes quite differently. These differences fall roughly into three classes: 1. tissues expressing all three genes (liver, adrenal, kidney, lung), 2. tissues expressing SAA_1 and SAA_3 (ileum), 3. tissues expressing only SAA_3 (spleen, heart, brain, testis, pituitary, pancreas).

The nature of stimulus to the acute phase reponse influences the amount of tissue expression of the three SAA genes. In the liver, LPS elicits all three about equally, but after casein, SAA_3 is only 1% of SAA_1 or SAA_2 mRNA expression.

4. Discussion

The differences in tissue expression of the three SAA mRNA's and their translation products, the different response time course and the differing response to specific acute-phase stimulants raise a new set of questions about possible functions as well as about regulation at the molecular level of this system. Behaviour of SAA_3 is clearly different from that of SAA_1 and SAA_2. Could this be due to its expression in a special, dispersed set of cells? Ramadori et al (16) using a cDNA probe spanning the region common to all three SAA messages showed the presence of SAA mRNA in spleen and lung of Lps or interleukin-1--stimulated mice and suggested that local production of SAA might provide the precursor for amyloid protein A. Our evidence indicates that this is not the case for the formation of splenic amyloid.

The widespread tissue messenger RNA expression of the SAA_3 gene, when compared with SAA_1 and SAA_2, is reminiscent of some features of apolipoproteins A-1 and E. The SAA's share amphipathic helical structure and affinity for HDL with apoA-1 and apoE. Moreover, the tissue expression of $apoSAA_3$ resembles very much that of apoE (17). Differences in tissue distribution of SAA_3 gene expression and responses to acute-phase stimuli from that of the SAA_1 and SAA_2 genes suggest that SAA_3 may have a different function from the others. Of note is the fact that we have not yet found evidence of the SAA_3 protein in the circulation; perhaps the SAA_3 product remains cell bound. Since the structural evidence points to the SAA protein family having a selective affinity for certain lipids, as indicated by an affinity for lipoprotein subclasses (13), it seems reasonable to suggest that SAA_1 and SAA_2 could be involved in intercellular lipid and other lipophilic substance transport, whereas SAA_3 may deal with intracellular traffic.

The study of amyloidosis and the discovery of the proteins that are involved in it has provided new insights into several different diseases and into some hitherto unsuspected physiological entities. There is undoubtedly much more to come.

Acknowledgements

I wish to acknowledge the excellent technical assistance of Marlene Wambach and Virginia Wejak for her patient and superior assistance in preparing the manuscript. Dr. John Morrow was most generous in permitting us access to unpublished data. The work described was supported by U.S.P.H.S. grant HL-03174 from the National Heart, Lung and Blood Institute.

References

1. Benditt, E.P., Lagunoff, D., Eriksen, N. & Iseri, O.A. Arch. Pathol. 74, 323-330, 1962.
2. Benditt, E.P. & Eriksen, N. Arch. Pathol. 78, 325-330, 1964.
3. Benditt, E.P. & Eriksen, N. Proc. Natl. Acad. Sci. USA 55, 308-316, 1966.
4. Glenner, G.G. & Bladen, H.A. Science 154, 271-272, 1966.
5. Pras, M., Schubert, M., Zucker-Franklin, D. et al. J. Clin. Invest. 47, 924-933, 1968.
6. Benditt, E.P., Eriksen, N. & Berglund, C. Proc. Natl. Acad. Sci. USA 66, 1044-1051, 1970.
7. Glenner, G.G., Eanes, E.D. & Page, D.L. J. Histochem. Cytochem. 20, 821-826, 1972.
8. Glenner, G.G., Harbaugh, J., Ohms, J.I. et al. Biochem. Biophys. Res. Commun. 41, 1287-1289, 1970.
9. Benditt, E.P. & Eriksen, N. Am. J. Pathol. 65, 231-252, 1971.
10. Levin, M., Pras, M. & Franklin, E.C. J. Exp. Med. 138, 373-380, 1973.
11. Yamamoto, K. & Migita, S. Proc. Natl. Acad. Sci. USA 82, 2915-2919, 1985.
12. Hoffman, J.S. & Benditt, E.P. J. Biol. Chem. 257, 10510-10517, 1982.
13. Hoffman, J.S. & Benditt, E.P. J. Biol. Chem. 257, 10518-10522, 1982.
14. Hoffman, J.S., Ericsson, L.H., Eriksen, N. et al. J. Exp. Med. 159, 641-646, 1984.
15. Meek, R.L., Hoffman, J.S. & Benditt, E.P. J. Exp. Med. 163, 499-510, 1986.
16. Ramadori, G., Sipe, J.D. & Colten, H.R. J. Immunol. 135, 3645-3647, 1985.
17. Elshourbagy, N.A., Liao, W.S., Mahley, R.W. & Taylor, J.M. Proc. Natl. Acad. Sci. USA 82, 203-207, 1985.

IV.2 SITES AND REGULATION OF BIOSYNTHESIS OF SAA

S. Bruce Dowton and Harvey R. Colten

Department of Pediatrics,
Washington University School of Medicine,
400 S Kingshighway Blvd., St. Louis, Missouri, U.S.A.

1. Introduction

Serum amyloid A (SAA) is a 12.5 Kdalton protein usually isolated in association with the HDL_3 subclass of serum lipoproteins (1). SAA is one of the plasma proteins which increase during inflammation or tissue injury (the positive acute phase reactants). Among these positive acute phase proteins SAA and C-reactive protein (CRP) are quantitatively the most impressive (100-1000 fold) (2). Hence the regulation of SAA synthesis has been a subject of general interest as well as a subject of importance to students of the biochemical basis of amyloidosis. The increase in SAA is detectable within four hours and usually peaks approximately 18 hours following initiation of tissue injury (3). SAA and the β-pleated sheet fibril protein amyloid A (AA) share considerable amino acid homology except that the 28 carboxy-terminal amino acids present in SAA are not represented in AA (4). Hence it is likely that SAA is the precursor of AA. The existing data suggest that cleavage by serine proteases, perhaps at the surface of monocytes and macrophages, may be responsible for the conversion of SAA to AA (5). Delineation of the exact mechanism of this potential precursor-product relationship awaits determination of the amino acid sequence of the peptides resulting from cleavage of purified SAA by specific neutral proteases plus studies of amyloid generation in tissue culture.

The development of methods for studying gene regulation, protein biosynthesis, secretion and assembly now permit the direct examination of several important questions regarding the relationship between SAA and post-inflammatory amyloid fibril formation. In this regard studies of the regulation of SAA biosynthesis as well as the identification of synthetic sites (cell-types) assumes pivotal importance. In this paper, the pertinent data concerning SAA gene structure, biosynthesis, post-synthetic modification and secretion are briefly reviewed in the context of current understanding of the regulatory mechanisms and mediators involved. The importance of integrating these findings with studies of tissue and organ specific SAA synthesis and AA deposition is emphasized.

2.SAA synthesis

An understanding of SAA gene structure, transcription, translation, post-translational modification and secretion is important for elucidating the mechanisms of action of specific mediators of SAA gene expression.

Initial analyses of human and murine cDNA and genomic clones for SAA indicate that SAA is encoded by multiple genes although the possibility of differential post-transcriptional processing or allotypic variation has not been definitively ruled out as an additional mechanism. For example, Sipe et al (6) have shown two different restriction digestion patterns from human SAA cDNA clones and similar findings for human genomic clones have been described (7). Similarly in the mouse, restriction maps of genomic clones indicate that murine SAA is probably encoded by at least three genes (8).

The mechanisms for control of expression of the different SAA genes is unknown but may be important in the pathogenesis of amyloidosis, as indicated below. The availability of cloned genomic SAA fragments which have been characterized by nucleotide sequence analysis will permit an examination of the differential expression of the various SAA genes under the influence of a variety of inflammatory mediators and in different control and amyloidotic cell populations.

Corresponding mRNA's have been isolated from strain-specific cDNA libraries, and characterized by nucleotide sequence analysis (9). The possibility that these represent allotypic variation has not been adequately excluded however. These clones have been utilized to examine the SAA specific mRNA populations in the liver in the first studies of this question. One murine SAA mRNA species (SAA_3) is less abundant in the liver than those for the other two major forms (8). The importance of extending these studies is exemplified by the suggestion that resistance to amyloid deposition in SJL mice may arise from the low level of production of SAA_2 specific mRNA, the putative precursor for AA in amyloid fibrils (8).

Data obtained thus far indicate that the transcriptional rate for SAA is an important control point in the regulation of SAA biosynthesis. Initial studies of murine and hamster hepatic SAA expression demonstrated a substantial increase in SAA specific mRNA following induction of an acute phase response (10, S.B.Dowton, unpublished data). These data established that pre-translational regulation and perhaps an increased transcription rate accounted for the observed increase in SAA synthesis. To directly test this question, in vitro transcription assays have been performed in isolated rabbit hepatic nuclei following administration of an inflammatory stimulus (G. Goldberger - personal communication). In similar experiments hamster hepatic nuclei were isolated by ultracentrifugation through 2.1M sucrose (in Hepes 1mM, $MgCl_2$ 3mM) following Dounce homogenization (sucrose 0.32M, Hepes 1mM, $MgCl_2$ 3mM). Suspensions of nuclei were incubated at $37^{\circ}C$ with transcription buffer (Tris 10mM, $MgCl_2$ 5mM, $MnCl_2$ 1mM, β-mercaptoethanol 0.1%, ATP 0.4mM, GTP 0.4mM, CTP 0.4mM, glycerol 18%) in the presence of ^{32}P UTP (100 μCi, 3000 Ci/mmole). Total nuclear RNA transcripts were isolated and hybridized with a denatured hamster SAA specific cDNA probe (S.B.Dowton, unpublished data) immobilized by dot blotting and baking onto nitrocellulose. Autoradiography revealed an increase in the elongation rate of nascent SAA transcripts (Fig. 1). These data cannot, however, address the rate of initiation of new transcription of the SAA genes.

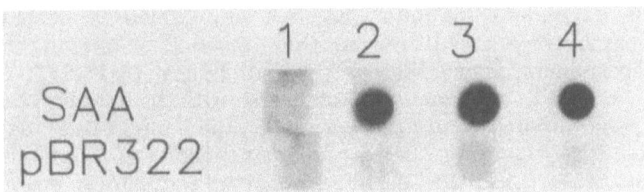

Figure 1: Nuclear run-off assay. Autoradiogram of total nuclear transcript mixture hybridized with hamster SAA-specific cDNA and pBR322. Lane 1: control (T=0); lanes 2, 3 and 4 are at 12, 24 and 48 hours following the induction of a sterile abscess using turpentine.

Although transcriptional rate is therefore important in the regulation of SAA gene expression, other levels of modulation must also be considered. The relative importance of post-transcriptional processing of mRNAs, their transport to cytoplasm and stability of specific mRNA cannot yet be assessed because of the paucity of available studies. An approach to these questions is feasible since it has been shown that cell free systems primed with mRNA from acute phase liver generate the pre-apoSAA primary translation product. In Xenopus oocytes or cell free translation systems containing microsomes cleavage of the signal peptide from pre-apoSAA occurs (6,11). In the intact cell monomeric SAA is then rapidly secreted after which it is assembled in the HDL$_3$ of plasma (12,13).

3. Mediators of the induction of SAA synthesis

Several mediators have been implicated in the regulation of expression of acute phase plasma protein genes. Attention was focused on monokines in 1980 when Selinger et al (12) demonstrated the induction of SAA production in murine hepatocyte cultures following exposure to conditioned macrophage supernatants. Initial studies of induction of SAA in culture were limited by relatively high levels of SAA expression in unstimulated cultures. Subsequent improvements in the methods for culture of murine hepatocytes permitted an accurate assessment of the response to various mediators (14). The availability of homogeneous preparations of peptide mediators, derived by cloning the relevant cDNA or genomic fragments into expression vectors for bacterial transformation has allowed early studies of the molecular modulation of SAA gene expression. One of the monokines capable of stimulating acute phase plasma protein synthesis in vivo and in isolated hepatocytes has been identified as interleukin-1 (IL-1) (15). IL-1, a 12.5 Kdalton polypeptide is elaborated by macrophages in response to several stimuli and is responsible for many of the physiologic and cellular sequelae of inflammation, including the increase in expression of some genes (e.g. SAA) and the decreased expression of others (e.g. albumin) (16).

The regulation of synthesis of SAA by IL-1 is primarily transcriptional. A dose dependent induction of SAA expression is observed when murine hepatocytes are cultured in the presence of varying concentrations of recombinant mouse IL-1 or purified human IL-1 (15). Studies of the action of IL-1 on L-cells transfected with a human SAA genomic clone suggest that at least some of the nucleotide sequence(s) responsible for mediating IL-1 responsiveness are contained in the transfected DNA; i.e. the IL-1 responsive regulatory sequences are within or flanking the SAA gene (17). Transcription activating factors have not been evaluated. Transfection of cloned fragments and site directed mutagenesis methods may permit more detailed analysis of the IL-1 responsive regions once the gene structure and sequence for SAA has been determined in greater detail. Comparison of SAA sequence data with that of other IL-1 responsive genes should narrow the focus of these studies and indicate the directions for further experimentation.

In human hepatoma cell lines, the biosynthesis of several acute phase proteins is also regulated by IL-1 and in addition, by another macrophage derived mediator, tumor necrosis factor (TNF) (18). Unfortunately even when maximally stimulated with IL-1 or TNF these well differentiated hepatoma cell lines, HepG2 and Hep3b fail to express SAA protein (Perlmutter et al, unpublished data). Hence, the effects of TNF on SAA gene expression can only be assessed in transfected L-cells. These studies are in progress.

Several other mediators induce the production of SAA. These include epidermal cell derived thymocyte activating factor (ETAF) and amyloid enhancing factor (19,20). The relationship of these to other more well defined mediators and their importance in the acute phase response awaits their purification to homogeneity and biochemical characterization. Similarly the mechanism of action of prostaglandin E_1 in increasing SAA concentration remains to be elucidated (21).

4. Sites of SAA synthesis

The liver is the main site for SAA synthesis. While amyloid protein is detectable in the Kupffer cells with the use of immunofluorescent labelling, hepatocytes are believed to be the major source of SAA (22). Heterogeneous participation of the hepatocyte population in SAA synthesis has been recognized using immunochemical methods which demonstrate non-uniform distribution of SAA in hepatic lobules following an amyloidogenic stimulus. Positively staining hepatocytes were initially randomly distributed throughout the lobules. Following longer exposure to the inflammatory agent anti-AA positive material was detected primarily on the surface of the hepatic cords delineating the space of Disse (23). Interestingly, these observations contrast with the distribution of another prominent acute phase reactant, C-reactive protein (CRP). Positive immunochemical anti-CRP reactions are seen initially in the periportal and perilobular regions (24). A centripetal progression of fluorescence is detected with advancing time following the acute phase stimulus.

Several early studies which suggested extrahepatic sites for SAA synthesis were based on radioimmunochemical or immunohistologic techniques. One study showed elevated SAA concentration in liver and kidney homogenates following administration of LPS using a sensitive radioimmunoassay but no difference in SAA concentration was detected in homogenates of spleen, lung or heart from control or stimulated mice (3). Immunofluorescent studies of extrahepatic SAA synthesis showed staining of adult dermal fibroblasts and vascular walls. These however, failed to distinguish between passive uptake and local synthesis (25). Nevertheless SAA has been demonstrated immunohistologically in fetal endothelial cells and embryonal fibroblasts in culture so that it is likely that, at least under certain conditions, fibroblasts can express SAA (25-27). On the other hand L cells, another fibroblast cell line, fail to express the SAA gene even when stimulated with IL-1. These data were derived during studies of SAA gene expression in L-cells transfected with a human SAA gene described above (17).

Messenger RNA specific for murine SAA has recently been detected in several organs representing different cell types (liver, heart, spleen, lung, intestine, kidney and peritoneal macrophages) following in vivo administration of endotoxin or recombinant IL-1 (rIL-1) (28). Preliminary data from similar experiments in the golden Syrian hamster support these findings (S.B. Dowton, unpublished observation). Extrahepatic SAA gene induction was detected in many tissues. These data indicate that at least transcription of SAA genes at extra-hepatic sites does follow an acute phase stimulus but do not yet establish synthesis of pre-apoSAA protein at extrahepatic sites.

Of particular interest is the fact that SAA specific mRNA was found abundantly at the site of inflammation indicating enhanced local SAA synthesis by recruited cells (monocytes, macrophages or polymorphonuclear leukocytes) or by resident cells in the inflammatory microenvironment. The observation that SAA is expressed in murine and hamster macrophages provides a model for examination of the regulation of SAA synthesis in culture in a cell which may be critical in local SAA production and its conversion to amyloid A fibrils.

Previous studies have shown deposits of fibrillar material in the brains of scrapie affected animals (29). This observation, coupled with the evidence that microglial cells are related to macrophages (30) prompted us to search for the presence of SAA specific mRNA in brains of hamsters affected by scrapie. No SAA specific mRNA was detected in the brains of these hamsters, nor those following induction of inflammation at a remote site (data not shown).

In another study, the absence of SAA specific mRNA in spleens of mice 7, 14 and 21 days following administration of casein would seem to conflict with the other findings (11). However, control data for hepatic SAA mRNA production were not provided at the same time points and the kinetics of SAA specific mRNA induction and degradation are yet to be evaluated. In addition, the comparison of casein with other inducers of acute inflammation is limited by the absence of information about the mechanisms involved. Therefore these studies are not comparable. Morrow et al (31) also failed to detect immunoprecipitable SAA primary translation products when kidney mRNA was translated in a cell free system. Technical considerations limit the certainty with which one can conclude whether or not the SAA gene(s) are not expressed in the kidney. Additional studies of in vitro translation are needed using RNA isolated from extrahepatic sites where SAA specific mRNA is abundant. Primary cultures of cells from organs besides the liver will also be useful in studying extrahepatic SAA synthesis and regulation. Further studies of this problem and the distribution of cells that synthesize SAA will be facilitated by the availability of in situ hybridization methods and SAA-cDNA and genomic clones from several species. These studies will permit analysis of the topography of SAA gene expression and its role in amyloid deposition.

5. SAA and amyloidosis

The ultimate significance of the regulation and sites of SAA biosynthesis in the pathogenesis of amyloidosis is unknown. While it seems likely that AA fibrils are cleavage products of SAA, several important questions remain. These include considerations of systemic or local origin of SAA ultimately deposited as AA, the cell type responsible for synthesis of SAA at extrahepatic sites and the possibility of differential regulation of SAA genes in the liver, at sites of tissue injury and in extrahepatic organs remote from an inflammatory focus.

Consideration of the role of other serum and tissue proteins and their interaction with SAA and AA during acute inflammation and amyloid deposition is of equal importance. One such protein is serum amyloid P (SAP) component. SAP, like CRP and the female protein (FP) of the golden Syrian hamster is a pentraxin (32,33). Human SAP concentrations do not alter appreciably during the acute phase response but SAP is an integral component of amyloid deposits. SAP may be involved in the modulation of the action of proteolytic enzymes and hence the cleavage of SAA to AA. The hamster female protein is probably the homologue of human SAP but has unusual characteristics in that expression of the FP gene is regulated not only by the mediators of acute inflammation but also by sex steroids. Unstimulated female hamsters have high serum FP concentrations which decrease with inflammation while in males the serum concentrations in the resting state are low and increase with acute phase stimuli (33). In the absence of chronic inflammatory conditions there is an extraordinarily high incidence of amyloidosis in female golden Syrian hamsters. Amyloidosis usually occurs in male hamsters in association with chronic inflammatory conditions (34). These observations suggest a critical role for SAP in the pathogenesis of amyloid deposition. Future areas of investigation of amyloidosis must therefore include not only study of SAA and AA but also expression of the other proteins involved, including SAP and the proteolytic enzymes involved in SAA to AA cleavage reactions.

References

1. Benditt, E.P. & Eriksen, N. Proc. Natl. Acad. Sci. USA 74, 4025-4028, 1977.
2. Kushner, I., Volanakis, J.E. & Gewurz, H. Ann. N.Y. Acad. Sci. 389, 39-48, 1982.
3. McAdam, K.P.W.J. & Sipe, J.D. J. Exp. Med. 144, 1121-1127, 1976.
4. Parmelee, D.C., Titani, K., Ericsson, N. et al. Biochemistry 21, 3298-3303, 1982.
5. Lavie, G., Zucker-Franklin, D. & Franklin, E.C. J. Immunol. 125, 175-180, 1980.
6. Sipe, J.D., Colten, H.R., Goldberger, G. et al. Biochemistry 24, 2931-2936, 1985.
7. Sack, G.H. Gene 21, 19-24, 1983.
8. Yamamoto, K., Shiroo, M. & Migita, S. Science 232, 227-229, 1986.
9. Yamamoto, K. & Migita, S. Proc. Natl. Acad. Sci. USA 82, 2915-2919, 1985.
10. Baumann, H., Held, W.A. & Berger, F.G. J. Biol. Chem. 259, 566-573, 1984.
11. Meek, R.L., Hoffman, J.S. & Benditt, E.P. J. Exp. Med. 163, 499-510, 1986.
12. Selinger, M.J., McAdam, K.P.W.J., Kaplan, M.M., et al. Nature 285, 498-500, 1980.
13. Hoffman, J.S. & Benditt, E.P. J. Biol. Chem. 257, 10518-10522, 1982.
14. Baumann, H., Jahreis, G.P. & Gaines, K.C. J. Cell. Biol. 97, 866-876, 1983.
15. Ramadori, G., Sipe, J.D., Dinarello, C.A. et al. J. Exp. Med. 162, 930-942, 1985.
16. Dinarello, C.A. Rev. Infect. Dis. 6, 51-95, 1984.
17. Woo, P., Sipe, J.D. & Colten H.R. In Proc. XXXIV Colloquium Protides of the Biolological Fluids (In press).
18. Perlmutter, D.H., Dinarello, C.A., Punsal, P.T. & Colten, H.R. (1986, submitted).
19. Sztein, M.B., Luger T.A. & Oppenheim, J.J. J. Immunol. 129, 87-90, 1982.
20. Cohen, A.S. Lab. Invest. 52, 319-325, 1985.
21. Brandwein, S.R., Sipe, J.D., Skinner, M. & Cohen, A.S. J. Rheumatol. 12, 418-426, 1985.
22. Benson, M.D. & Kleiner, E. J. Immunol. 124, 495-499, 1980.
23. Shirahama, T., Skinner, M. & Cohen A.S. Cell. Biol. Int. Rep. 8, 849-856, 1984.
24. Kushner, I. & Feldman, G. J. Exp. Med. 148, 466-477, 1978.
25. Linder, E., Anders, R.F. & Natvig, J.B. J. Exp. Med. 144, 1336-1346, 1976.
26. Linder, E., Lehto, V.P., Virtanen, I. et al. J. Exp. Med. 146, 1158-1163, 1977.
27. Bjerve, O. & Natvig, J.B. Scand. J. Immunol. 19, 287-292, 1984.
28. Ramadori, G., Sipe, J.D. & Colten, H.R. J. Immunol. 135, 3645-3647, 1985.
29. Marsh, R.F. & Kimberlin, R.H. J. Infect. Dis. 131, 104-110, 1975.
30. Hume, D.A. & Gordon, S. In Mononuclear Phagocytes, R. van Furth, Ed. Martinus Nijhoff/Dr W. Junk Publishers, Boston, 9-18, 1985.
31. Morrow, J.F. Stearman, R.S., Peltzman, C.G. & Potter, D.A. Proc. Natl. Acad. Sci. USA 78, 4718-4722, 1981.
32. Osmand, A.P., Friedenson, B., Gewurz, H., et al. Proc. Natl. Acad. Sci. USA 74, 739-743, 1977.
33. Coe, J.E., Margossian, S.S., Slayter, H.S. & Sogn, J.A. J. Exp. Med. 153, 977-991, 1981.
34. Parviz Pour, N., Moch, K., Greiser, E. et al. J. Natl. Cancer Inst. 56, 931-935, 1976.

IV.3   SERUM AMYLOID A PROTEIN IN PLASMA: CHARACTERISTICS OF
ACUTE PHASE HDL

D.R. van der Westhuyzen[1], G.A. Coetzee[1],
and F.C. de Beer[2]

UCT/MRC Muscle Research Unit,
Department of Medical Biochemistry,
University of Cape Town, Cape Town,
South Africa[1].

Department of Internal Medicine,
University of Stellenbosch, Tygerberg,
South Africa[2].

1. Introduction

The changes in plasma protein levels that constitute the acute phase response are the result of selectively altered hepatic protein synthesis. Macrophage-derived interleukin-1 (IL-1) affects gene expression, possibly through a dual signal system, decreasing mRNA for negative acute phase reactants like albumin and increasing mRNA for positive acute phase reactants (1). In the mouse, mRNA for serum amyloid A increases up to 500 fold to constitute up to 2.5% of total hepatic protein synthesis (2).

Serum Amyloid A (SAA) protein is one of the most dramatic positive acute phase proteins with levels increasing up to a thousand fold following infarction, inflammation or infection (3). The bulk of SAA (apo-SAA) exists as an apolipoprotein of HDL_3 in the plasma. Although HDL (expressed as HDL cholesterol) is a significant negative acute phase reactant, the lipoprotein may still play a significant role in the inflammatory response. HDL has been reported to function as a vehicle for transfer of non-polar toxins and damaged cellular constituents to the liver (4). In addition, the binding to HDL of bacterial lipopolysaccharides and of neutrophil elastase has been reported (5,6). Little, however, is known about the function of apo-SAA or apo-SAA rich HDL in the response to injury.

Amyloidosis is a rare complication where chronic elevation of SAA levels seems to be a prerequisite. Severe inflammatory conditions, like systemic lupus erythematosus or ulcerative colitis, where the acute phase response is blunted with lower SAA levels, are seldom complicated by amyloidosis (3). It is generally accepted that in the pathogenesis of amyloidosis the 11,500 dalton apo-SAA is cleaved by a protease to form the 76 amino-terminal fragment amyloid A protein, AA, which constitutes the bulk of the fibrils in reactive systemic amyloidosis (7). When human apo-SAA was introduced into amyloidotic mice, human AA was shown to be present in murine amyloid fibrils (8).

Where it has been shown in the mouse that only one of the major apo-SAA isoforms, SAA_2, is selectively removed from the circulation and found in murine amyloid, the situation in humans is unresolved (9): no specific amyloidogenic isoform has been identified amongst the two major and 4 minor SAA isoforms. Proteolytic enzymes may play a key role in the pathogenesis of amyloidosis. In this regard it is interesting to note that peripheral blood monocytes have membrane-associated proteases that have been shown to degrade apo-SAA to AA in certain individuals only (10).

In order to resolve the pathogenesis of AA amyloidosis, the exact physical nature of the acute phase HDL particle needs to be defined as this entity represents the bulk of plasma apo-SAA. Biological experiments using purified apo-SAA are more difficult to interpret due to problems of solubility and aggregation of the various isoforms. We have therefore concentrated here on recent studies describing the altered structure of HDL arising from association with apo-SAA during the acute phase.

2. Structure of SAA

Up to six isoforms of apo-SAA have been identified with different solubilities and isoelectric points (11). The amino acid sequence of one of the major isoforms has been determined and corresponds to a polypeptide of 104 amino acids (7). This is 28 amino acids longer than AA, whose sequence is identical with the 76 amino-terminal residues of apo-SAA (a serine-leucine bond at residues 76-77 of apo-SAA represents the site presumably vulnerable to cleavage). The six apo-SAA polymorphs are structurally similar. The molecular weight of each is about 11,500 dalton and they are indistinguishable by cationic and sodium dodecyl sulphate gel electrophoresis. Each form possesses a carboxy-terminal tyrosine residue and charge differences are apparently not due to differences in carbohydrate content. One of the other major isoforms shows a 30 residue sequence at the amino-terminal end identical to the fully-sequenced form, except for the absence of the amino--terminal arginine residue (7). More recent work, however, supports the notion that the human apo-SAA isoforms may be the products of different genes. The presence of at least two genes for human apo-SAA has been reported (12). In the mouse, 3 non-allelic apo-SAA genes exist (13,14).

One of the most interesting features of the SAA polypeptide is the presence of two regions (residues 1-24 and 50-74), which appear to be capable of forming amphiphilic (amphipathic) α-helices (about 7 turns each). An amphiphilic helix has been proposed as the basic structural element of the lipid-associating domain of the normal apolipoproteins of VLDL and HDL. The amphiphilic helix is characterized by its surface topography that consists of opposing polar and non-polar faces. This

116

structural property appears to underlie the apolipoprotein character of apo-SAA (7).

Segrest et al first noted that a 45-residue fragment of AA formed stable complexes with phospholipid, a finding that preceded the discovery that apo-SAA existed as an apolipoprotein of HDL (15). Subsequent studies by Bausserman et al showed that SAA itself is capable of independently forming complexes with phospholipid that are morphologically similar to those formed by the other common apoproteins of HDL (16). Like other apolipoproteins, apo-SAA exists in an aggregated form at slightly alkaline pH and characteristically increases its α-helical content on association with phospholipid (16).

3.Plasma distribution of SAA

Benditt and Eriksen were the first to recognize that serum amyloid A is transported in human plasma mainly in association with HDL (17) and this finding was confirmed for all other animals in which SAA could be identified, such as the rabbit (18), mouse (19), monkey (20) and mink (21).

The association of SAA with HDL is relatively specific with only small amounts (<10%) being generally associated with either very low density lipoprotein (VLDL), intermediate density lipoprotein (IDL) or low density lipoprotein (LDL) (17-19,22). In a non-human primate, the vervet monkey, apo-SAA was found to occur to a significant extent (about 20% of total protein) also in lymph chylomicrons (20). A small proportion of apo-SAA does appear to circulate in a lipoprotein-free form in human plasma. Such apo-SAA can be identified in lipoprotein-deficient serum following the removal of all lipoproteins by ultracentrifugation in solutions of high densities (p>1.25). In this respect, apo-SAA is not unlike the other apoproteins of HDL that also exist partially in the free form in the plasma.

The isoform make-up of acute phase HDL shows little apparent variability between subjects undergoing an acute phase response and no association between isoform pattern and disease type has been identified (23,24). The relative percentage of the major (pI 6.0 and 6.4) and minor (pI 5.6 and 7.7) apo-SAA isoforms and the ratio of the major isoforms to each other in different acute phase HDL_3 preparations is shown in Table I.

In the absence of any known functional assay for apo-SAA, quantitation has often been based on immunochemical techniques with their many accompanying difficulties. Recent studies have relied mostly on the quantitation through the staining of apo-SAA separated by polyacrylamide gel electrophoresis. Immunoassays of plasma SAA levels are improved through the use of apo-SAA-containing HDL_3, with known apo-SAA content, as a standard (25).

117

TABLE I: APO-SAA ISOFORMS IN ACUTE PHASE HDL$_3$

Plasma sample	Apo-SAA isoforms (% of total apo-SAA)				Apo-SAA 6.4/ apo-SAA 6.0
	pI 5.6	6.0	6.4	7.7	
Pool 1	5	40	50	5	1.3
Pool 2	3	36	34	26	1.0
Pneumonia 1	3	39	57	4	1.5
Pneumonia 2	3	32	60	5	1.9
Pneumonia 3	4	59	33	4	0.6
RA	5	42	47	7	1.1
Pancreatitis	2	47	44	7	0.9
Post surgery	2	33	50	16	1.5

Adapted from reference (24).

4.HDL structure

4.1.Structure of normal HDL

High density lipoproteins and the other major lipoprotein classes found in plasma are water-soluble complexes containing specific proteins and lipids (reviewed in ref.26). These lipoproteins are spherical particles whose structure is characterized by a hydrophobic core, composed mainly of cholesteryl esters and triglycerides, surrounded by a relatively hydrophilic shell composed of apolipoproteins, unesterified cholesterol and phospholipids. The components of the shell are able to project their hydrophobic domains towards the particle core and their hydrophilic domains towards the aqueous environment. A model for HDL structure is shown in Figure 1.

HDL are defined by flotation in the ultracentrifuge between density 1.063 and 1.21 g per ml, by their content of specific major apolipoproteins (apoproteins A-I and A-II) and by their alpha mobility on electrophoresis. Nevertheless, HDL represents a heterogeneous mixture of particles, and subclasses can be identified by a variety of techniques. The two major subclasses of HDL are HDL$_2$ (density 1.063-1.125 g/ml) and HDL$_3$ (density 1.125-1.21 g/ml). These two particles also differ in size (HDL$_2 \approx 100$ Å, HDL$_3 \approx 80$ Å) and in lipid and protein composition. Heterogeneity within both subclasses has also been recognized on the basis of density gradient or rate zonal ultracentrifugation (27) as well as by gradient polyacrylamide gel electrophoresis (28). The use of immunoaffinity chromatography has also demonstrated discrete types of HDL particles that differ in their relative content of the major apolipoproteins (29). A third and minor subclass of HDL, HDL$_1$, is less dense (density 1.03-1.10 g/ml) and larger (130-250 Å) than HDL$_2$ and in addition is rich in apolipoprotein E. The metabolic interrelationships between the different HDL subclasses is poorly understood although it appears that the subclasses represent particles at different stages of assembly and remodelling.

118

Structural model of human HDL$_3$

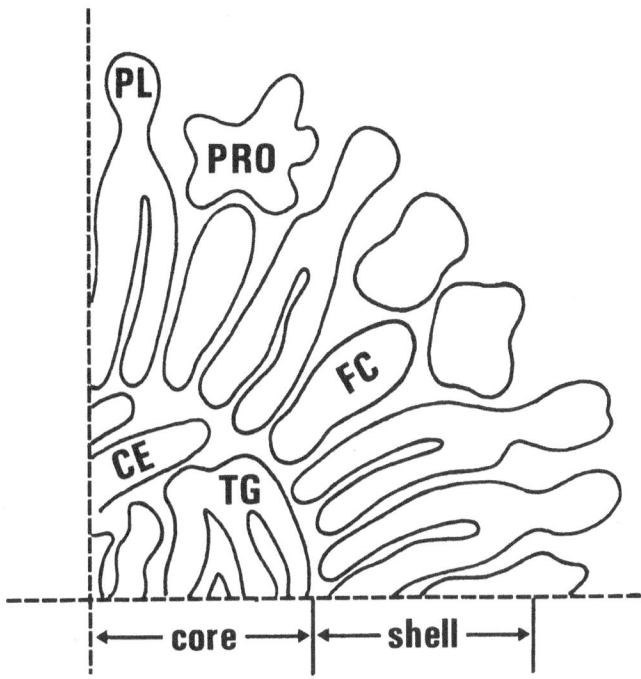

Figure 1: Adapted from Shen et al (35). PL = phospholipids; PRO = protein; FC = free cholesterol; CE = cholesterol ester; TG = triglyceride. Normal major apolipoproteins, apo-A-I, apo-A-II. Acute phase apolipoproteins, apo-SAA, apo-A-I, apo-A-II.

4.2. Distribution of SAA in HDL

As mentioned, the bulk of apo-SAA is found associated with HDL. More specifically, the majority of apo-SAA (>75%) is present in the HDL$_3$ subclass (17) where it tends to associate preferentially with the denser particles. It is now well-recognized that during an acute phase period SAA often becomes a significant apolipoprotein of HDL and in terms of protein mass per particle, SAA is sometimes even the major apoprotein. Typical values for the relative content of apo-SAA in acute phase HDL$_3$ range from 20-50% or more of total protein (22,30-32). This corresponds to plasma levels of apo-SAA which can reach more than 500 mg/l (25). Some reports have indicated smaller proportions of the total apo-SAA in HDL_3. For example, in trauma patients the proportion of total apo-SAA in HDL_3 ranged from 15% to more than 50% (31). Bausserman et al (11) reported that 40-60% of apo-SAA was recovered in the HDL density range. The explanation for this variability is not clear. The other most significant apo-SAA-containing fraction recovered following density gradient ultracentrifugation is the density >1.21 layer. The possibilities are that apo-SAA could exist as a free protein in this fraction or as a component of a very high density lipoprotein fraction.

It is well established that a variety of pathological conditions result in reduced HDL cholesterol and total apolipoprotein levels giving rise to the so-called negative acute phase response. In general, reduced HDL_2 and HDL_3 levels have been found in situations where apo-SAA levels are markedly increased, for example, in patients suffering from trauma (31) or bacterial infection (22). The most marked effect is generally seen in the HDL_2 subclass. In the detailed study of apo-SAA-enriched HDL from subjects with myocardial infarction, Barter and co-workers reported the virtual absence of any HDL_2 as judged by density. SAA-enriched HDL had a density comparable to that of normal HDL_3, whereas the size of these particles was much larger than HDL_3, extending well into the size range of HDL_2 (see below). Given the complexity of factors known to effect changes in HDL levels, large variations in the response of HDL subclasses can be expected during the acute phase response. It should be emphasized that our understanding of the factors that regulate HDL levels in humans is limited and there is a lack of evidence for the operation of homeostatic mechanisms regulating the concentrations of either HDL or its subclasses.

4.3. Acute phase HDL_2

While the bulk of apo-SAA is in the HDL_3 subclass, apo-SAA can nevertheless also become a very significant apoprotein in HDL_2. Typical values in trauma patients and in patients suffering acute bacterial infection reach about 20% of total HDL apoproteins (22,31). In these studies, the increased apo-SAA levels appeared to be matched by reduced apo-A-I levels, whereas another major HDL apoprotein, apo-A-II, seemed to remain unchanged. Other apolipoproteins were found in only small amounts, the most significant being apo-E that was preferentially associated with HDL_2 as in the case with normal HDL.

4.4. Acute phase HDL_3

Surprisingly few studies on the composition and structure of acute phase HDL_3 are available (Table II). Nevertheless, certain essential features of apo-SAA-enriched HDL_3 have become available from recent investigations of murine (33), primate (34) and human acute phase HDL_3 (22,30); the acquisition of apo-SAA results in the displacement of normal apolipoproteins from HDL particles, apo-SAA associates preferentially with denser HDL particles, apo-SAA-enriched HDL_3 is significantly larger than its normal counterpart, and apo-SAA-enriched HDL_3 represents a polydisperse mixture of particles differing in apolipoprotein composition and SAA content.

TABLE II: COMPOSITION AND SIZE OF NORMAL AND ACUTE PHASE HDL_3

	Normal HDL_3	Acute phase HDL_3[a]
Size[b,c] (nm)		
diameter	8.2 - 9.0	9.2 - 10.4
Composition[c] (%)		
protein	53 ± 5	59 ± 8
phospholipids	23 ± 4	23 ± 5
cholesterol esters	13 ± 4	9 ± 5
free cholesterol	2 ± 1	3 ± 2
triglycerides	9 ± 4	6 ± 4
Apolipoproteins[c] (%)		
apo-A-I	86 ± 3	67 ± 8
apo-A-II	14 ± 3	8 ± 6
apo-SAA	-	25 ± 11

a. typical values in subjects with large amounts of apo-SAA;
b. values from ref. (30);
c. values from ref. (22), not including minor apolipoproteins.

In particles in which apo-SAA may comprise up to 80% of the total apoproteins, particle density and protein-lipid composition have been reported to be changed relatively little compared to normal (22,30,34). The displacement is primarily of apo-A-I whereas the A-II and C apolipoproteins are relatively less affected.

A possibility remains that the incorporation of apo-SAA into HDL partly involves the displacement of some lipid from the particle shell. Studies in man and monkeys have not produced evidence for significant changes in protein and lipid compositions of HDL_3 (22,34). SAA may therefore be accommodated on HDL particles in the place of other apoproteins without altering the overall lipid and protein content. Studies in vitro have clearly demonstrated the ability of purified apo-SAA to associate avidly with normal HDL_3 particles (22,30). It seems possible that depending on the molar amounts of apo-SAA that are incorporated and the molar amounts of apo-A-I that are displaced, some particles will be richer in total apoprotein and will thus be slightly denser. For example, a 30% content of apo-SAA in acute phase HDL_3 (a typical level in denser particles) would be consistent with the replacement of one apo-A-I molecule per particle by apo-SAA. Given the relative molecular weights of the two apolipoproteins (apo-A-I, 28,000 and apo-SAA, 11,500 dalton) the replacement of one apo-A-I (of the probable 3 apo-A-I molecules per particle) by three apo-SAA molecules would lead to a slight increase in the relative protein content and hence density of the particle.

The noteworthy study on subjects suffering from myocardial infarction (30) as well as a study of the mouse (33), have indicated that some displacement of phospholipid by protein can occur and that apo-SAA may therefore take over part of the role played by phospholipids in the particle shell.

The interpretation of the compositional data is complicated by the fact that, like normal HDL$_3$, the corresponding acute phase lipoprotein fraction is heterogeneous in structure and represents a mixture of particles differing in density, size and composition (Fig. 2).

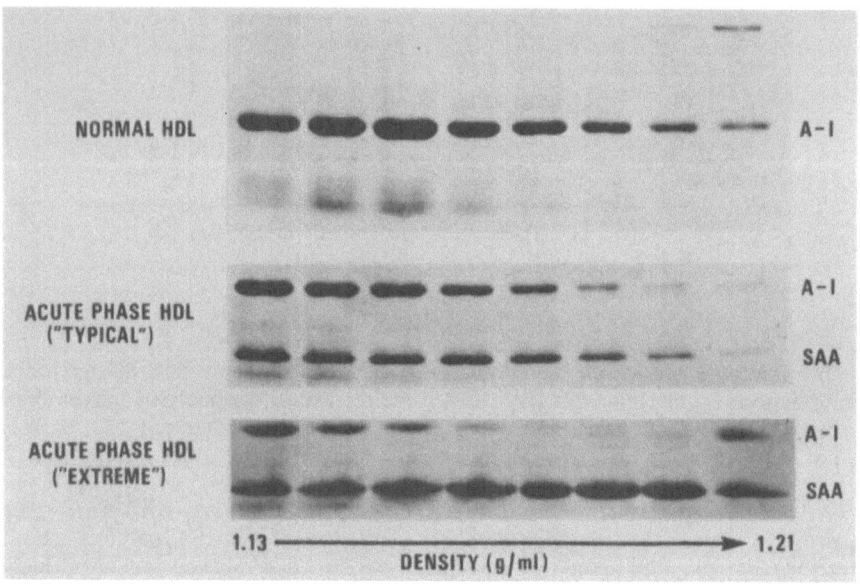

Figure 2: Distribution of apolipoproteins in normal and acute phase HDL. Analysis of the apolipoprotein composition of HDL performed by fractionation of a total HDL gradient (d 1.11-1.21 g/ml) following ultracentrifugation and SDS-polyacrylamide gel electrophoresis.

Nevertheless, in humans a consistent finding is that apo-SAA content increases progressively with increasing particle density (22) and a similar situation occurs in non-human primates (34) and the mouse (31). At least two discernible subspecies of acute phase HDL$_3$ can often be distinguished by apolipoprotein composition, with mean densities of about 1.14 and 1.165 g/ml, respectively. Both of these subspecies have apo--A-I as a major apoprotein and the less dense subspecies contains the bulk of the HDL apo-A-II, whereas apo-SAA was associated preferentially with the denser fraction (22).

The polydispersity of acute phase HDL$_3$ with respect to apolipoprotein content has also been demonstrated (as in the case of normal HDL_3) by immunoabsorption techniques. Cheung and Albers (29) demonstrated that in the normal HDL_3 subfraction, some particles contain both apo-A-I and A-II, whereas others contain only apo-A-I. Similarly, in acute phase HDL_3, some particles contain, together with apo-SAA, both of these apolipoproteins while others contain only apo-A-I (22).

Heterogeneity in particle size, based on the technique of gradient gel electrophoresis, has also been found in normal HDL_3 (28) and similarly in acute phase particles (22,30). The more suprising finding in the acute phase studies has been that the average SAA-enriched particle is larger than its normal HDL_3 counterpart of comparable density. The alternative technique of gel filtration yields the same conclusion that acute phase particles are inappropriately large for their density in comparison to the normal lipoprotein classes. It has been suggested that the acute phase particle may represent HDL_2-like lipoproteins that have gained sufficient protein to appear as dense as normal HDL_3 while still retaining their larger size (30). Alternatively, the presence of SAA in HDL_3 may result in changes in the physical properties of particles (for example, acute phase HDL_3 exhibits a retarded mobility on agarose electrophoresis compared to normal HDL_3 (24). Considerations have been formulated by which the core radii of lipoprotein particles can be determined from their surface to volume ratios (35). When such calculations were applied to acute phase HDL_3 , results suggested that an increase in the width of the shell of the particle may be responsible for the increase in particle size (22). Considering the smallness of HDL particles, in which the shell domain comprises about 80% of the particle volume, even small changes in shell structure and width would be expected to exert significant effects on overall particle size.

Further studies of the interaction of apo-SAA and HDL wil be useful in understanding how acute phase HDL particles are assembled and metabolized. Studies of the structure of apo-SAA-enriched HDL_3 that have been reconstituted in vitro have indicated that apo-SAA exhibits a high-affinity for HDL and is able to displace the bulk of apo-A-I from particles (22,30). Since apo-SAA is apparently secreted by hepatocytes in a monomeric and lipid-free form (36), it is possible that newly--synthesized apo-SAA associates with existing HDL in the circulation, resulting in a remodelling of the surface of such particles to yield HDL which are relatively large, dense and depleted of apo-A-I.

5. Concluding remarks

The formation of apo-SAA-HDL is probably of functional importance in inflammatory processes of different kinds. Although apolipoproteins have been shown to act as targeting devices for receptor-mediated uptake processes and also as enzymatic co-factors, functions of this type that may be fulfilled by apo-SAA are unknown. Studies in cynomolgus monkeys (36), vervet monkeys (20) and BALB/o mice (37) have all shown a greater catabolic rate for apo-SAA than for any other HDL apoprotein. This suggests either that apo-SAA is associated with an HDL population that turns over more rapidly than the bulk of HDL, or that apo-SAA dissociates from HDL before clearance from plasma. Differing rates of synthesis rather than of catabolism are likely to be responsible for the differing steady-state concentrations of apo-SAA isoforms, since the die-away curves for a major and a minor isoform in cynomolgus monkeys are similar (36).

Further studies on the cellular interaction and metabolism of apo-SAA are essential to elucidate its function. Such studies would be necessarily complex given the dynamic state and differing half-lives of the individual HDL components and the polydispersity of HDL particles. Special attention needs to be given to potential apo-SAA damage caused by harsh isolation techniques and radioiodination. For example, it has been shown that the property of rapid clearance of apo-SAA in BALB/c mice is lost when reconstituted ^{125}I-apo-SAA-HDL is used (37).

There is no question that expansion of our knowledge of the metabolism and function of apo-SAA would assist materially in clarifying the mechanism(s) of amyloidogenesis. Progress which has been made in defining the physical/chemical nature of apo-SAA in plasma has already helped in setting the stage for further investigations.

References

1. Ramadori, G., Sipe, J.D., Dinarello, C.A. et al. J. Exp. Med. 162, 930-942, 1985.
2. Morrow, J.F., Stearman, R.S., Peltzman, C.G. & Potter, D.A. Proc. Natl. Acad. Sci. USA 78, 4718-4722, 1981.
3. De Beer, F.C., Mallya, R.K., Fagan, E.A. et al. Lancet ii, 231-232, 1982.
4. Benditt, E.P., Eriksen, N. & Hoffman, J.S. In Amyloid and Amyloidosis, Glenner, G.G., Costa, P.P. & Freitas, A.F., Eds. Excerpta Medica, Amsterdam, 397-405, 1980.
5. Ulevitch, R.J., Johnston, A.R. & Weinstein, D.B. J. Clin. Invest. 67, 827-837, 1981.
6. Jacob, M.P., Bellon, G., Robert, L. et al. Biochem. Biophys. Res. Commun. 103, 311-318, 1981.
7. Parmalee, D.C., Titani, K., Ericsson, L.H. et al. Biochemistry 21, 3298-3303, 1982.
8. Husebekk, A., Skogen, B., Husby, G. & Marhaug, G. Scand. J. Immunol. 21, 283-287, 1985.
9. Meek, R.L., Hoffman, J.S. & Benditt, E.P. J. Exp. Med. 163, 499-510, 1986.
10. Lavie, G., Zucker-Franklin, D. & Franklin, E.C. J.Exp. Med. 148, 1020-1031, 1978.
11. Bausserman, L.L., Herbert, P.N. & McAdam, K.P.W.J. J. Exp. Med. 152, 641-656, 1980.
12. Sipe, J.D., Colten, H.R., Goldberger, G. et al. Biochemistry 24, 2931-2936, 1985.
13. Yamamoto, K. & Migita, S. Proc. Natl. Acad. Sci. USA 82, 2915-2929, 1985.
14. Stearman, R.S., Lowell, C.A., Peltzman, C.G. & Morrow, J.F. Nucleic Acids Res. 14, 797-809, 1986.
15. Segrest, J.P., Pownall, H.J., Jackson, R.L. et al. Biochemistry 15, 3187-3191, 1976.
16. Bausserman, L.L., Herbert, P.N., Forte, T. et al. J. Biol. Chem. 258, 10681-10688, 1983.
17. Benditt, E.P. & Eriksen, N. Proc. Natl. Acad. Sci. USA 74, 4025-4028, 1977.
18. Skogen, B., Borresen, A.L., Natvig, J.B. et al. Scand. J. Immunol. 10, 39-45, 1979.
19. Benditt, E.P., Eriksen, N. & Hanson, R. Proc. Natl. Acad. Sci. USA 76, 4092-4096, 1979.
20. Parks, J.S. & Rudel, L.L. Am. J. Pathol. 112, 243-249, 1983.
21. Marhaug, G., Borresen, A.L., Husby, G. & Nordstoga, K. Comp. Biochem. Physiol. 78B, 401-406, 1984.
22. Coetzee, G.A., Strachan, A.F., Van der Westhuyzen, D.R. et al. J. Biol. Chem. (In Press).
23. Maury, C.P.J., Enholm, C. & Lukka, M. Ann. Rheum. Dis. 44, 711-715, 1985.
24. Strachan, A.F., De Beer, F.C., Coetzee, G.A. et al. In XXXIVth Colloquium Protides of the Biological Fluids, Peeters, H., Ed. Pergamon Press, Brussels (In Press).
25. Godenir, N.L., Jeenah, M.S., Coetzee, G.A. et al. J. Immunol. Methods 83, 217-225, 1985.
26. Eisenberg, S. J. Lipid Res. 25, 1017-1058, 1984.

27. Patsch, W., Schonfeld, G., Gotto, A.M., Jr. & Patsch, J.R. J. Biol. Chem. 255, 3178-3185, 1980.
28. Blanche, P.J., Gong, E.L., Forte, T.M. & Nichols, A.V. Biochim. Biophys. Acta 665, 408-419, 1981.
29. Cheung, M.C. & Albers, J.J. J. Biol. Chem. 259, 12201-12209, 1984.
30. Clifton, P.M., Mackinnon, A.M., & Barter, P.J. J. Lipid Res. 26, 1389-1398, 1985.
31. Eriksen, N. & Benditt, E.P. Clin. Chim. Acta 140, 139-149, 1984.
32. Bausserman, L.L., Herbert, P.N. & McAdam, K.P.W.J. Clin. Chim. Acta 118, 201-207, 1982.
33. Hoffman, J.S. & Benditt, E.P. J. Biol. Chem. 257, 10510-10517, 1982.
34. Parks, J.S. & Rudel, L.L. J. Lipid. Res. 26, 82-91, 1985.
35. Shen, B.W., Scanu, A.M. & Kezdy, F.J. Proc. Natl. Acad. Sci. USA 74, 837-841, 1977.
36. Hoffman, J.S. & Benditt, E.P. J. Biol. Chem. 257, 10518-10522, 1982.
37. Bausserman, L.L., Herbert, P., Rodger, R. & Nicolosi, R.J. Biochim. Biophys. Acta 792, 186-191, 1984.
38. Hoffman, J.S. & Benditt, E.P. J. Clin. Invest. 71, 926-934, 1983.

IV.4 CORRELATION BETWEEN SEQUENCE VARIABILITY AND STRUCTURE PREDICTION IN AA PROTEINS

William G. Turnell and Mark B. Pepys

MRC Acute Phase Protein Research Group,
Immunological Medicine Unit, Department of Medicine,
Royal Postgraduate Medical School,
Hammersmith Hospital, Ducane Road, London, W12 OHS, U.K.

1. Introduction

Reactive systemic amyloidosis is a serious clinical disorder character-ized by the extracellular accumulation of fibrils of protein AA (1,2). Recent studies of experimentally induced systemic amyloidosis in mice have shown that despite equal expression of the major murine gene pro-ducts under experimental conditions, only one isotype is deposited as AA fibrils in vivo (3,4). This may also be the situation in the genetic amyloidosis associated with familial Mediterranean fever (FMF) in humans (5). Important questions thus arise as to how the chemistry and meta-bolism of different AA proteins might be related to particular dif-ferences in their sequences.

All AA sequences reported to date form a highly homologous set and presumably, therefore, code for common structural constraints. As a basis for the subsequent estimation of the relative importance of partic-ular variations between AA sequences we have mapped the sites of con-servation or change against our previously determined secondary struc-ture prediction of human $SAA_1(\alpha)$ (6).

Residues are numbered with respect to the sequence of AA that is identical to the first 76 residues of the human sequence $SAA_1(\alpha)$ (7). Serum amyloid A (SAA) is an apolipoprotein of high density lipoprotein (HDL) (8) and is the precursor of AA protein (9).

Throughout this article the term sequence "homology" (as opposed to "identity") refers to pairs of residues that belong to one of the follow-ing groups: FLIMV; FYW; EDY; CST; SAG; VA; CV; QE; QN; DN; RH; RK. These groups take into account the hydrophobicity, size and electronic structure of the amino acid side-chains, as well as the dual nature of residues such as tyrosine, cysteine and phenylalanine.

References to sequences are given in ref. (6).

2. Analysis

Residues 1-11. On the basis of the distribution of hydrophobic resi-dues this region is predicted to provide an NH_2-terminal transmembrane lipid-binding structure. Such a localized site at a terminus of an otherwise water-soluble globular protein is compatible with the reported experimental data on SAA/AA lipid-binding (10).

With the exception of position nine, the first eleven residues of mouse SAA_2/AA_2 are homologous with the eleven residues of the extra-cytosolic portion (residues 29 to 39) of the transmembrane NH_2-terminal anchor region of neuraminidase from human influenza virus A/PR/8/34 (11) (data not shown). Position nine is an acidic group in all SAA and AA sequences but is positively charged in the neuraminidase sequence. The pattern of hydropathicities is closely similar in both sequences. This pattern, which is preserved in all SAA and AA sequences despite considerable sequence variability in this region, is common to NH_2- -terminal membrane anchor sequences from diverse origins (Fig. 1). The NH_2-terminal regions of SAA/AA sequences all exhibit three distinct segments that are also characteristic of transmembrane signal peptides (12):

a. A short, often positively charged, NH_2-terminal segment. This is six residues long in duck AA, two residues in human SAA_1 and monkey AA, but is only one residue in other SAA/AA sequences. In duck this segment is only weakly homologous with the cytosolic protein of NH_2- -terminal transmembrane sequences (Fig. 1) as might be expected from a comparison of the lipid monolayer structure of the HDL outer-coat (13) with the lipid bilayer of most cellular and viral membranes.

b. A central hydrophobic segment of seven to fifteen residues spans a lipid monolayer or bilayer as a weakly amphipathic α-helix (14). In SAA/AA all of the polar residues in this segment are neutral except for Arg^5 of duck AA (i.e. the ninth residue of the duck sequence) (Fig. 1). Arginines are rare but not unknown within the first two turns of transmembrane helices (see, for example, vesicular stomatitis virus glycoprotein (12,15). The hydrophobic/amphipathic segment of residues 2 to 8 found in all SAA/AA sequences is sufficient to span the lipid monolayer of the HDL outer-coat as two turns of an α-helix (Fig. 1).

c. A more polar segment spanning the extra-cytosolic side of the lipid membrane and containing the cleavage site of a signal peptide. The equivalent site in human $SAA_1(\alpha)$ is the second splice junction (16,17). The first exon lies in the five prime untranslated region. Most of the second exon is lost post-translationally as a signal peptide (18) and so this putative lipid-binding segment may be an adaptive remnant of the latter.

Residues 12-27. This region is predicted by Fourier analysis of $SAA_1(\alpha)$ to form four turns of an amphipathic helix typical of small globular proteins. In view of the statistical analysis of hydropathicity distributions around relatively short α-helices by Flinta et al (19) it is important to verify that a strong correlation exists between the spatial distribution of sequence variability and of hydrophobicity. Figure 2 demonstrates this relationship, confirming that residues 14, 25, 18, 22, 15, 26, 19, 12 and 23 could form a surface that is both variable between species and isotypes and is of a mixed polar and non-polar character which is typical of surfaces of water-soluble globular proteins. The correlation

shown in Fig. 2 adds powerful support to the secondary structure prediction.

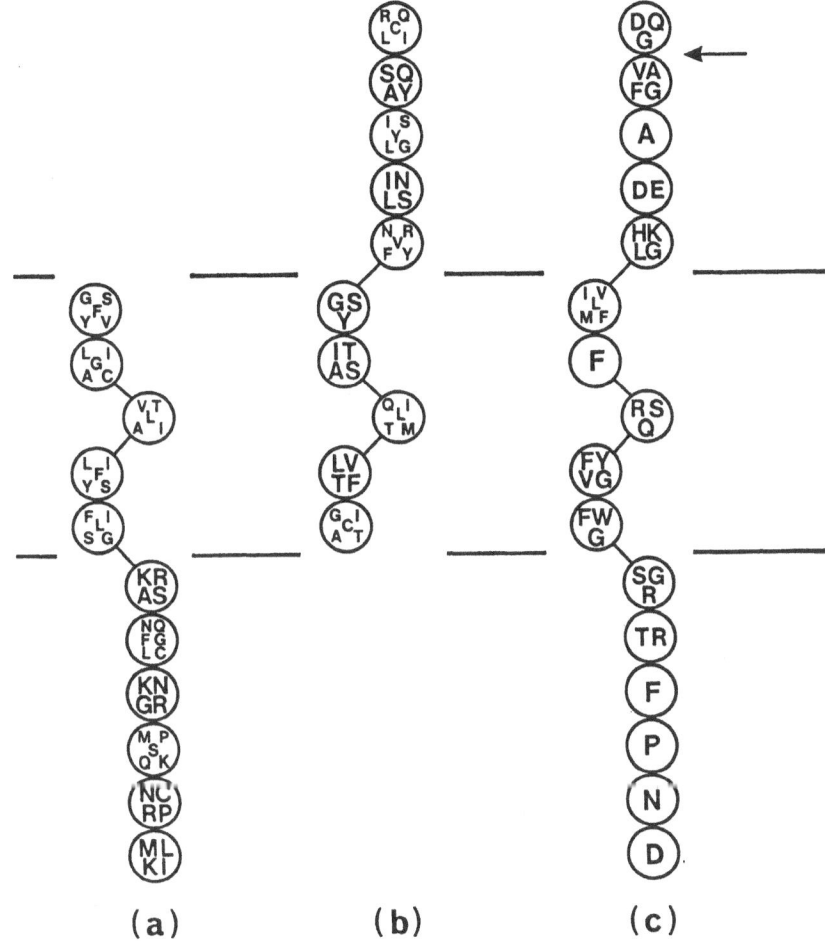

Figure 1: Compilation of NH₂-terminal transmembrane anchor segments (in the single letter
amino acid code, see Table 1) from six independent extra-cytosolic proteins listed by von
Heyne (12). a. The cytosolic segments and first third of the transmembrane segments; b.
The last third of the transmembrane segments together with the extra-cytosolic segments;
c. Compilation of the NH₂-terminal region from fifteen SAA/AA sequences. The first four
residues are from duck AA alone. The polypeptide chains run from bottom to top. The pair
of horizontal lines respresents the depth of the hydrophobic segment of a lipid monolayer
and the arrow points to the second splice junction of human SAA₁(α) (16).

Situated along edges of the mixed/hydrophobic interface, residues 16
and 21 are invariant in all SAA/AA sequences (Fig. 2) and are not positively charged as in equivalent positions on some amphipathic α-helices
that are thought to form the lipid-binding structures of human apoA-1,

murine apoA-IV, and related apolipoproteins (20,21).

The strict conservation of the hydrophobic surface formed by residues 27, 20, 13, 24 and 17 is typical of the constraints upon the sizes
of side-chains, in addition to those upon their hydrophobicities, that
are found within the close-packed interiors of globular protein domains
(22).

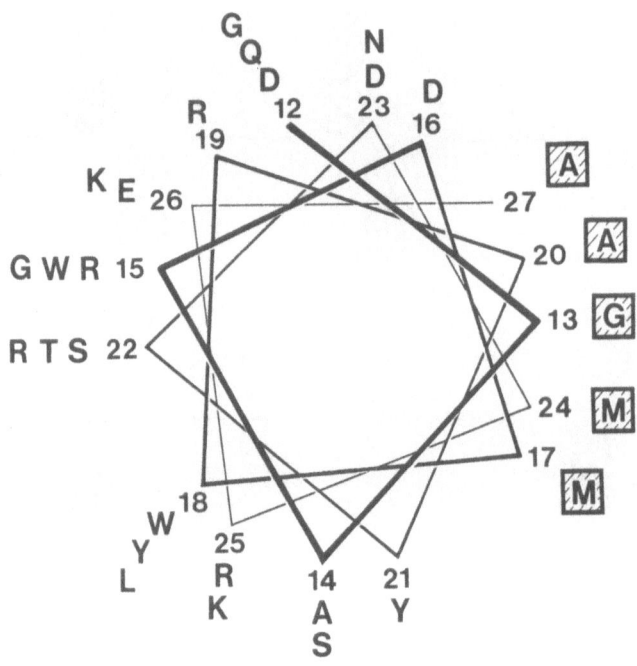

<u>Figure 2</u>: Helical wheel presentation (26) of the predicted α-helix 12-27 of human SAA₁(α)
together with the equivalent side-chains from fourteen other SAA/AA sequences. Conserved
hydrophobic residues (including glycines) are boxed.

<u>Residues 28-34</u>. These form a linking region between predicted secon-
dary structural motifs which is therefore likely to be on the surface of
the SAA/AA protein fold. Positions 28 to 31 show non-homologous
subtitutions between sequences and position 32 homologous substitutions.

<u>Residues 35-46</u>. A β-hairpin is predicted for these residues which are
identical at all the equivalent positions in SAA/AA except 46. Position
46 is always polar and as it occurs at the end of a predicted
amphipathic β-strand (Fig. 3) is expected to be on the surface of the
protein structure.

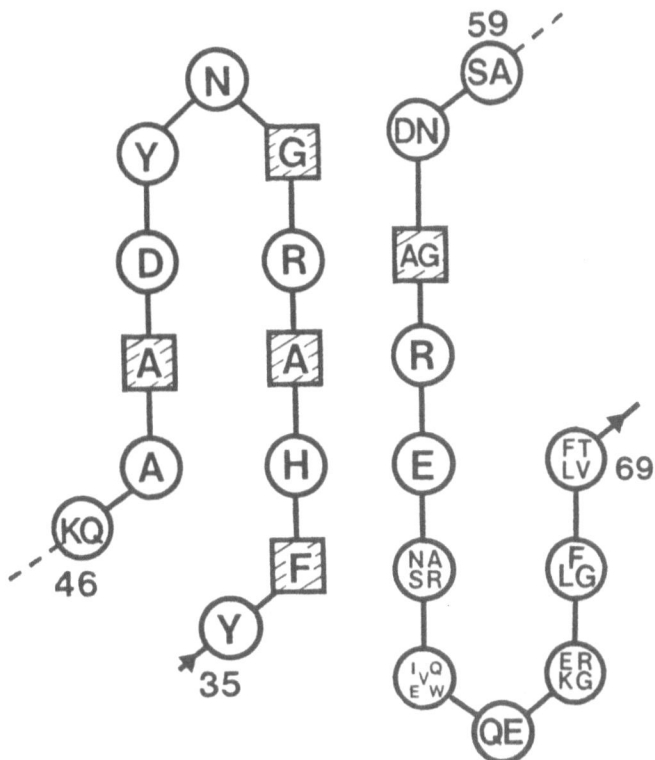

Figure 2: A schematic drawing of the predicted β-hairpins of human SAA₁ arranged so as to form one of several possible hydrophobic patches. The side-chains that form the hydrophobic surface in this arrangement are boxed (see text). Residues from fourteen additional SAA/AA sequences are plotted at equivalent positions.

Residues 47-55. These are identical in all known sequences of SAA/AA except for homologous substitutions (Val/Ala) at position 52. The region is predicted to be a functionally important calcium-binding loop.

Residues 56-59. Position 56 is variable between sequences but is always charged, 57 shows non-homologous changes. Position 59 is the C-terminus of exon three in human $SAA_1(\alpha)$ (16). The region lies immediately before a predicted β-strand. All these data suggest that the residues form a surface loop in the protein fold.

Residues 60-69. The region encompasses a predicted β-hairpin which shows, however, considerable sequence variability, in contrast to the predicted hairpin 35-45. X-ray diffraction intensities from wet human AA fibrils can be simulated with a β content for the fibre of one sheet of 4 ± 1 strands per AA molecule (23). The order of the strands remains unknown, but Fig. 3 shows how both predicted hairpins could be aligned to form a four-stranded β-sheet with the conserved residues at positions 36, 38, 40, 44 and 61 forming a hydrophobic "slipper" typical of β structures in small globular proteins (24). Other strand arrangements, not shown in Fig. 3 are equally likely.

Position 65, predicted to form part of a surface β-bend at the end of the strand 60-63 (Fig. 3) is highly variable between sequences and forms the C-terminus of an AA protein of human origin (25) and of AA from mink.

Residues 70-76. Predicted to provide a connecting loop followed by the beginning turn of the second α-helix of SAA, this peptide forms the last seven residues of most AA sequences. The connecting loop (70-73) is made up of conserved glycines or positions of sequence variation. As it is near the terminus of a predicted helix it is likely to contribute to the surface of the tertiary fold of SAA. In AA however, the whole of this C-terminal "tail" may well adopt a different, less well defined, structure.

3. Conclusions

There is a clear correlation between the previously predicted surface groups of $SAA_1(\alpha)$ (6) and sites of variation between AA sequences. As more SAA and AA sequences are reported they will either reinforce or weaken this correlation, so testing the accuracy of the structure prediction. If the correlation holds it should provide a rationale for the estimation of the relative importance of particular variations between AA sequences.

TABLE I: SINGLE LETTER AMINO ACID CODE

Ala = A	Arg = R	Asn = N	Asp = D	Asx = B	Cys = C	Gln = Q	Glu = E	Glx = Z
Gly = G	His = H	Ile = I	Leu = L	Lys = K	Met = M	Phe = F	Pro = P	Ser = S
Thr = T	Trp = W	Tyr = Y	Val = V					

References

1. Glenner, G.G. N. Engl. J. Med. 302, 1283-1292, 1980.
2. Pepys, M.B. In Samter, M. et al. eds Immunological Diseases, 4th edn., Little Brown & Co., Boston (In press).
3. Hoffman, J.S., Ericsson, L.H., Eriksen, N. et al. J. Exp. Med. 159, 641-646, 1984.
4. Meek, R.L., Hoffman, J.S. & Benditt, E.P. J. Exp. Med. 163, 499-510, 1986.
5. Woo, P. This Volume, IV.5.
6. Turnell, W., Sarra, R., Glover, I.D. et al. Mol. Biol. Med., 1986 (In press).
7. Parmelee, D.C., Titani, K., Ericsson, L.H. et al. Biochemistry 21, 3298-3303, 1982.
8. Benditt, E.P., Eriksen, N. & Hanson, R.H. Proc. Natl. Acad. Sci. USA 76, 4092-4096, 1979.
9. Husebekk, A., Skogen, G., Husby, G. & Marhaugh, G. Scand. J. Immunol. 21, 283-287, 1985.
10. Turnell, W., Sarra, R., Baum, J.O. & Pepys, M.B. In XXXIV Colloquium Protides of the Biological Fluids. Peeters, H., Ed. Pergamon Press, Oxford, England (In press).
11. Fields, S., Winter, G. & Brownlee, G.G. Nature, 290, 213-217, 1981.

12. Von Heyne, G. J. Mol. Biol. 189, 239-242, 1986.
13. Eisenberg, S. J. Lipid Res. 25, 1017-1058, 1984.
14. Eisenberg, D., Schwarz, E., Komaromy, M. & Wall, R. J. Mol. Biol. 179, 125-142, 1984.
15. Rose, J.K., Welch, W.J., Sefton, B.M., et al. Proc. Natl. Acad. Sci. USA 77, 3884-3888, 1980.
16. Sack Jr, G.H., Lease, J.J. & De Berry, C.S. In XXXIVth Colloquium Protides of the Biological Fluids. Peeters, H., Ed. Pergamon Press, Oxford, England (In press).
17. Woo, P. In XXXIVth Colloquium Protides of the Biological Fluids. Peeters, H., Ed. Pergamon Press, Oxford, England (In press).
18. Sipe, J.D., Colten, H.R., Goldberger, G. et al. Biochemistry 24, 2931-2936, 1985.
19. Flinta, C., von Heyne, G. & Johansson, J. J. Mol. Biol. 168, 193-196, 1983.
20. Boguski, M.S., Elshourbagy, N., Taylor, J.M. & Jeffrey, G.I. Proc. Natl. Acad. Sci. USA 81, 5021-5025, 1984.
21. Anantharamaiah, G.M., Gawish, A., Brouillette, C.G. et al. In XXXIV Colloquium Protides of the Biological Fluids. Peeters, H., Ed. Pergamon Press, Oxford, England (In press).
22. Richards, F.M. J. Mol. Biol. 82, 1-14, 1974.
23. Turnell, W., Sarra, R., Baum, J.O. et al. Mol. Biol. Med. (In press).
24. Chothia, C. & Janin, J. Proc. Natl. Acad. Sci. USA 78, 4146-4150, 1981.
25. Sletten, K., Husby, G. & Natvig, J.B. Biochem. Biophys. Res. Commun. 69, 19-25, 1976.
26. Schiffer, M. & Edmundson, A.B. Biophys. J. 7, 121-135, 1967.

IV.5 GENE STRUCTURE OF A HUMAN SERUM AMYLOID A PROTEIN AND COMPARISON WITH AMYLOID A

Patricia Woo

Clinical Research Centre,
Watford Road, Harrow.
Middlesex HA1 3UJ, U.K.

1. Introduction

The protein in deposits of reactive amyloidosis is amyloid A (AA) protein (1,2). Isolates of AA protein from human and various animals have similar molecular weights of about 8,000 dalton and similar amino acid sequences of 76 residues (3-5). The only serum protein which bears close biochemical and immunochemical identity with AA is serum amyloid A (SAA) protein, found mainly in the HDL fraction of plasma (6). It is a major acute phase reactant in man, rabbit, mice and other mammals (7). Its molecular weight is about 12-14,000 dalton when dissociated from HDL and is not glycosylated. Since SAA can be cleaved at the carboxy-terminus by proteolytic enzymes, it has been presumed to be the precursor for AA. Precursor-product relationship was recently demonstrated by Husebekk and colleagues (8): human SAA was shown to be incorporated into mouse AA by immunochemical methods.

Murine SAA is encoded by a family of 3 genes (9). SAA1 and SAA2 are found in equal quantities associated with HDL (10), but no polypeptide corresponding to SAA3 has been isolated. SAA3 mRNA has been detected but is apparently unstable (11). Of the two gene products, SAA2 is the sole precursor of murine AA, despite equal expression of SAA1 and SAA2 (12).

There is also a gene family for human SAA. There are two major and four minor isotypes in serum (13,14). Their molecular weights are the same, so that the differences are unlikely to be due to glycosylation. Structural studies at the amino acid, genomic DNA and mRNA levels are still incomplete. The amino acid sequence of SAA1 has been determined (15). It has two allelic forms, α and β, with double substitution of valine for alanine at residues 52 and 57. Incomplete sequence of SAA2 shows that it lacks the N-terminal arginine, but the following 30 residues are identical to SAA1 (14). Limited N-terminal analysis by Bausserman and colleagues (16) suggests that SAA4 is homologous to SAA1 and SAA5 to SAA2. Therefore these isotypes should be products of at least 3 genes. Three human SAA genomic clones have been isolated from a λ genomic library, using a cross-hybridizing mouse SAA cDNA clone, pRS48 (17). Two of these clones bear close homology to each other and the third is homologous to SAA1β. Two human SAA cDNA clones have been identified so far (18,19) and one of these (pA1) has been completely sequenced: the derived amino acid sequence is

135

identical to that of SAA1α (15). The total number of human SAA genes and mRNA is still unclear at present.

2. Gene structure of a human SAA genomic clone

To study the structural variants of SAA, 2 human SAA genomic clones were isolated from λ L47-1 genomic library (kindly donated by S. Karathanasis) using the human specific, variable portion of the cDNA pA1: i.e. corresponding to amino acid residues 55-104 + 3' untranslated region. DNA sequence was obtained using the dideoxy chain termination method (10). The restriction maps of these two clones were identical and the gene structure of one is shown in Fig. 1.

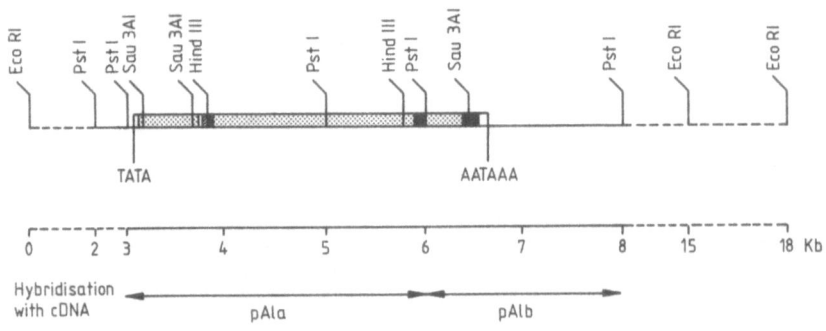

Figure 1: Gene structure of a SAA genomic clone, SAAg9.

■ — Coding regions in exons 2, 3 and 4; ▨ — Leader sequence in exon 2;

▨ — Intron; ☐ — Untranslated region.

TATA — Hogness box.
AATAAA — Polyadenylation signal.
pA1a — portion of the cDNA for SAA1 (pA1) that contains the conserved region.
pA1b — portion of the cDNA for SAA1 (pA1) that contains the variable region and is human-specific.

The organization of the gene is similar to that of other apolipoprotein genes. There are three introns, one in the 5' untranslated region, one near the N-terminus after amino acid residue 12, and one in the centre of the coding region, at residue 59. DNA sequence of exon 2 and 3 is identical to that of SAA1β. However, there are nucleotide differences in exon 4 (residues 60-104 + 3' untranslated region) leading to 6 amino acid substitutions (Table I): asparagine instead of aspartic acid at residue 60, leucine for phenylalanine at residue 68, threonine for phenylalanine at residue 69, arginine for histidine at residue 71, lysine for glutamic acid at residue 84 and arginine for lysine at residue 90. All except the substitution of threonine involve a single base change.

TABLE I: COMPARISON OF THE NUCLEOTIDE AND DERIVED AMINO ACID SEQUENCE OF THE cDNA FOR
apoSAAlα (18) AND THE CORRESPONDING CODING REGIONS OF THE GENOMIC CLONE SAAg9.
[Exon 4 begins at amino residue 60]

a		Ala	Val	Asn			Leu Thr
b SAAg9		C	T	A			C ACA
c ApoSAAlα	GGT GTC TGG GCT GCA GAA GCG ATC AGC GAT GCC AGA GAG AAT ATC CAG AGA TTC TTT GGC						
d	Gly Val Trp Ala Ala Glu Ala Ile Ser Asp Ala Arg Glu Asn Ile Gln Arg Phe Phe Gly				60		70

a	Arg			Lys		Arg
b SAAg9	G		C	A		G
c ApoSAAlα	CAT GGT GCG GAG GAC TCG CTG GCT GAT CAG GCT GCC AAT GAA TGG GGC AGG AGT GGC AAA					
d	His Gly Ala Glu Asp Ser Leu Ala Asp Gln Ala Ala Asn Glu Trp Gly Arg Ser Gly Lys		80			90

Line a Amino acid residues of the genomic clone SAAg9 that are different from apoSAAlα.
Line b Nucleotides of SAAg9 that are different from apoSAAlα.
Line c Nucleotide sequence of apoSAAlα from base 151 to 270.
Line d Corresponding derived amino acid sequence for apoSAAlα from residue 51 to 90.
[numbers are shown below line d]

3. Homology between SAA derived amino acid sequences and human AA proteins

The first 76 residues of SAA1 from the N-terminus are homologous
with AA from tissue amyloid deposits (15). However, there is heterogeneity near the C-terminus of AA (Table II). AA from RA and JRA patients are homologous to SAAlα, but AA from a familial Mediterranean
fever (FMF) patient is homologous to SAA1β with 4 additional amino acid
substitutions. The derived amino acid sequence of the coding regions of
the SAA gene from residues 1-76 is identical to that of FMF amyloid
protein.

Reactive amyloidosis secondary to chronic inflammatory arthritis develops after prolonged active disease. The overall incidence of amyloidosis
in JRA is about 1%, 4% in systemic Stills disease, with no clear genetic
pattern. However, amyloidosis associated with FMF in Sephardic Jews is
inherited in an autosomal recessive manner (21). Moreover, the development of amyloidosis is not necessarily related to the the severity or the
duration of FMF. Amino acid analysis of the AA proteins in different
diseases (4,5,22-24) shows that SAA1 is deposited. Its presence may be
related to accelerated intravascular clearance of this particular SAA
polymorph, analogous to murine SAA2 (25). In the hereditary
amyloidosis of FMF the sequence of AA shows an important amino acid
substitution at residue 69 involving changes in all 3 nucleotides. The
secondary structure of SAA1 has been predicted by mathematical analysis from its amino acid composition (26). There are two α amphipathic
helices (residues 12-27 and 72-87) which are also confirmed by the
model of Segrest et al (27), separated by two β hairpin turns. The
second turn ends at residue 68, so that the tripeptide 69-71 linking the

TABLE II: COMPARISON OF THE SEQUENCES OF VARIOUS HUMAN AMYLOID PROTEINS

```
              5                  10                 15                 20
a.  NH2-Arg-Ser-Phe-Phe-Ser-Phe-Leu-Gly-Glu-Ala-Phe-Asp-Gly-Ala-Arg-Asp-Met-Trp-Arg-Ala-
b.
c.
d.
e.

              25                 30                 35                 40
a.    Tyr-Ser-Asn-Met-Arg-Glu-Ala-Asn-Tyr-Ile-Gly-Ser-Asp-Lys-Tyr-Phe-His-Ala-Arg-Gly-
b.         Asp
c.
d.         Asp
e.

              45                 50                 55                 60
a.  Asn-Tyr-Asp-Ala-Ala-Lys-Arg-Gly-Pro-Gly-Gly-Val-Trp-Ala-Ala-Glu-Ala-Ile-Ser-Asp-
b.  Asx(Tyr-Asx-Ala)Ala-COOH
c.
                                           Trp
d.                                    Ala-     Arg          Val          Asn
                                      Ala-Arg
e.                                    Val-Arg

              65                 70                 75
a.  Ala-Arg-Glu-Asn-Ile-Gln-Arg-Phe-Phe-Gly-His-Gly-Ala-Glu-Asn-Ser-COOH

c.          -COOH
d.                    Leu-Thr       Arg          Asp
                                                     Lys        Ala
e.               Asp                                    -Glu-      -COOH
                                                     Ser        Val
                                                                Thr
                                                                Lys
```

a. the continuous sequence of 76 residues of protein AA from the liver of a patient with juvenile rheumatoid arthritis (5).
b. AA protein from the spleen of a patient with rheumatoid arthritis (22).
c. AA protein from the liver of a patient with ankylosing spondylitis (23).
d. AA protein from the spleen of a patient with familial Mediterranean fever (4).
e. AA protein from the liver of a patient with Waldenström's macroglobulinaemia (24).

β turn to the α helix is very likely to be on the surface of the protein, as is usual for peptides linking defined secondary structures in globular proteins. In FMF amyloid, a hydrophobic residue phenylalanine is replaced by a polar residue threonine in the region linking the β turn to the α helix on the surface of the protein and therefore will affect its quaternary structure. The effect could be changes in its ligand binding and cleavage properties. Since SAA is cleaved to form AA at around residue 76, these changes could be significant in the deposition of amyloid.

Variations described here in the DNA sequence of SAA1 may therefore play an important role in the pathogenesis of FMF amyloidosis.

References

1. Cohen, A.S. N. Engl. J. Med. 277, 522-530, 1967.
2. Benditt, E.P. & Eriksen, N. Am. J. Pathol. 65, 231-252, 1971.
3. Hermodson, M.A., Kuhn, R.W., Walsh, K.A. et al. Biochemistry 11, 2934-2938, 1972.
4. Levin, M., Franklin, E.C., Frangione, B. & Pras, M. J. Clin. Invest. 51, 2773-2776, 1972.
5. Sletten, K. & Husby, G. Eur. J. Biochem. 41, 117-125, 1974.
6. Benditt, E.P. & Eriksen, N. Proc. Natl. Acad. Sci. USA 74, 4025-4028, 1977.

7. Selinger, M.J., McAdam, K.P.W.J., Kaplan, M.M., et al. Nature 285, 498-500, 1980.
8. Husebekk, A., Skogen, B., Husby, G. & Marhaug, G. Scand. J. Immunol. 21, 283-287, 1985.
9. Yamamoto, K.I., Shiroo, M. & Migita, S. Science 232, 227-229, 1986.
10. Hoffman, J.S. & Benditt, E.P. J. Biol. Chem. 257, 10510-10517, 1982.
11. Lowell, C.A., Stearman, R.S. & Morrow, J.F. J. Biol. Chem. (In press).
12. Hoffman, J.S., Ericsson, L.H., Eriksen, N., et al. J. Exp. Med. 159, 641-646, 1984.
13. Eriksen, N. & Benditt, E.P. Proc. Natl. Acad. Sci. USA 77, 6860-6864, 1980.
14. Bausserman, L.L., Herbert, P.N., McAdam, K.P.W.J. J. Exp. Med. 152, 641-656, 1980.
15. Parmelee, D.C., Titani, K., Ericsson, L.H. et al. Biochemistry, 21, 3298-3303, 1982.
16. Bausserman, L.L., Saritelli, A.L., Herbert, P.N. & McAdam, K.P.W.J. Biochim. Biophys. Acta 704, 556-559, 1982.
17. Sack Jr, G.H., Lease, J.J. & DeBerry C.S. In XXXIV Colloquium Protides of the Biological Fluids, Pergamon Press, Oxford, (In press).
18. Sipe, J.D., Colten, H.R., Goldberger, G., et al. Biochemistry 24, 2931-2936, 1985.
19. Sipe, J.D., Woo, P., Goldberger, G. et al. In Amyloidosis. Glenner G.G., Osserman, E.F., Benditt, E.P., Calkins, E., Cohen, A.S., Zucker-Franklin, D., Eds. Plenum Press, 57-60, 1986.
20. Sanger, F., Nicklen, S. & Coulsen, A.R. Proc. Natl. Acad. Sci. USA 74, 5463-5467, 1977.
21. Glenner, G.G., Ignaczak, T.F. & Page, D.L. In Metabolic basis of inherited disease, 4th Edition. Stanbury, J.B., Wyngaarden, J.B., Fredrickson, D.S., Eds. Pub. McGraw Hill, New York, 1308-1339, 1978.
22. Ein, D., Kimura, S., Terry, W.D. et al. J. Biol. Chem. 247, 2653-2655, 1972.
23. Sletten, K., Husby, G. & Natvig, J.B. Biochem. Biophys. Res. Commun. 69, 19-25, 1976.
24. Møyner, K., Sletten, K., Husby, G. & Natvig, J.B. Scand. J. Immunol. 11, 549-554, 1980.
25. Meek, R.L., Hoffman, J.S. & Benditt, E.P. J. Exp. Med. 499-510, 1986.
26. Turnell, W., Sarra, R., Glover, I. et al., Mol. Biol. Med. (In press).
27. Segrest, J.P., Jackson, R.L., Morrisett, J.D. & Gotto Jr. A.M. FEBS Lett. 38, 247-253, 1974.

IV.6 STRUCTURE AND EXPRESSION OF MURINE SERUM AMYLOID A PROTEIN GENES: IMPLICATIONS FOR AMYLOIDOGENESIS

Ken-ichi Yamamoto

Department of Molecular Immunology
Cancer Research Institute
Kanazawa University, Kanazawa, Japan.

1. Introduction

Secondary amyloidosis associated with chronic inflammatory diseases such as rheumatoid arthritis is caused by deposition of amyloid fibrils in various tissues. The major component of amyloid fibrils (amyloid A component, AA) is derived from a serum protein termed serum amyloid A protein (SAA). Although SAA is normally a trace component of high density lipoproteins, its concentration is frequently increased several hundredfold in various inflammatory diseases. Increased SAA concentrations are believed to predispose to the formation of amyloid fibrils (1,2). In the mouse which is a most widely used animal for experimental amyloidosis, two electrophoretically distinct SAA isotypes, SAA1 (11.75 Kdalton, pI=6.35) and SAA2 (11.65 Kdalton, pI=6.20), have been identified (3). A comparison of the partial amino-terminal amino acid sequences of SAA1 and SAA2 from several mouse strains with those of several different mouse AA has shown that mouse AA contains only a single--type of amino-terminal sequence which is identical with that of SAA2, indicating that AA is derived from only one of the SAA isotypes in mice and that the other mouse SAA isotype does not deposit as AA (4). Recently, we have isolated cDNA clones encoding BALB/c mouse SAA1 and SAA2 and determined their base sequences (5). SAA1 and SAA2 are highly homologous and show a 91% homology in the deduced amino acid sequences (Table I and Table II).

TABLE I:
SEQUENCE HOMOLOGY BETWEEN MOUSE SAA1, SAA2 and SAA3

	Nucleotide sequence		Amino acid sequence
	coding region	3'-untranslated region	
SAA1 vs. SAA2	95%	90%	91%
SAA1 vs. SAA3	75%	-	70%
SAA2 vs. SAA3	72%	-	67%
	(54%)		(37%)

-: No significant homology.
Figures in parentheses indicate percentage homology in signal peptide sequences.

141

TABLE II: NUCLEOTIDE AND DEDUCED AMINO ACID SEQUENCES FOR MOUSE SAA1, -2, -3 cDNA CLONES

```
SAA2  ATA GAC CAC CAG ATC TGC CCA GGA GAC ACC AGC AGG ATG AAG CTA CTC ACC AGC CTG GTC   60
                                                    M   K   L   L   T   S   L   V
SAA3  CCT GGG GTC CCA GAA GGA GCT CGC AGC ACG AGC AGG ATG AAG CCT TCC ATT GCC ATC ATT
                                                    M   K   P   S   I   A   I   I
                                                   -19

SAA1  TTC TGC TCC CTG CTC CTG GGA GTC TGC CAT GGA GGG TTT TTT TCA TTT GTT CAC GAG GCT  120
       F   C   S   L   L   L   G   V   C   H   G   G   F   F   S   F   V   H   E   A
SAA2  TTC TGC TCC CTG CTC CTG GGA GTC TGC CAT GGA GGG TTT TTT TCA TTT ATT GGG GAG GCT
       F   C   S   L   L   L   G   V   C   H   G   G   F   F   S   F   I   G   E   A
SAA3  CTT TGC ATC TTG ATC CTG GGA GTT GAC AGC CAA AGA TGG GTC CAG TTC ATG AAA GAA GCT
       L   C   I   L   I   L   G   V   D   S   Q   R   W   V   Q   F   M   K   E   A
                                      -1  +1

SAA1  TTC CAA GGG GCT GGG GAC ATG TGG CGA GCC TAC ACT GAC ATG AAG GAA GCT AAC TGG AAA  180
       F   Q   G   A   G   D   M   W   R   A   Y   T   D   M   K   E   A   N   W   K
SAA2  TTC CAA GGG GCT GGA GAC ATG TGG CGA GCC TAC ACT GAC ATG AAG GAA GCT GGC TGG AAA
       F   Q   G   A   G   D   M   W   R   A   Y   T   D   M   K   E   A   G   W   K
SAA3  GGT CAA GGG TCT AGA GAC ATG TGG CGA GCC TAC TCT GAC ATG AAG AAA GCT AAC TGG AAA
       G   Q   G   S   R   D   M   W   R   A   Y   S   D   M   K   K   A   N   W   K
      10                          20

SAA1  AAC TCA GAC AAA TAC TTC CAT GCT CGG GGG AAC TAT GAT GCT GCT CAA AGG GGT CCC GGG  240
       N   S   D   K   Y   F   H   A   R   G   N   Y   D   A   A   Q   R   G   P   G
SAA2  GAT GGA GAC AAA TAC TTC CAT GCT CGG GGG AAC TAT GAT GCT GCC CAA AGG GGT CCC GGG
       D   G   D   K   Y   F   H   A   R   G   N   Y   D   A   A   Q   R   G   P   G
SAA3  AAC TCA GAC AAA TAC TTC CAT GCT CGG GGG AAC TAT GAT GCT GCC CGG AGG GGT CCC GGG
       N   S   D   K   Y   F   H   A   R   G   N   Y   D   A   A   R   R   G   P   G
      30                          40

SAA1  GGA GTC TGG GCT GCT GAG AAA ATC AGT GAT GGA AGA GAG GCC TTT CAG GAA TTC TTC GGC  300
       G   V   W   A   A   E   K   I   S   D   G   R   E   A   F   Q   E   F   F   G
SAA2  GGA GTC TGG GCT GCT GAG AAA ATC AGT GAT GCA AGA GAG AGC TTT CAG GAA TTC TTC GGC
       G   V   W   A   A   E   K   I   S   D   A   R   E   S   F   Q   E   F   F   G
SAA3  GGA GCC TGG GCT GCT AAA GTC ATC AGC GAT GCC AGA GAG GCT GTT CAG AAG TTC ACG GGA
       G   A   W   A   A   K   V   I   S   D   A   R   E   A   V   Q   K   F   T   G
      50                          60

SAA1  AGA GGA CAT GAG GAC ACC ATT GCT GAC CAG GAA GCC AAC AGA CAT GGC CGC AGT GGC AAA  360
       R   G   H   E   D   T   I   A   D   Q   E   A   N   R   H   G   R   S   G   K
SAA2  AGA GGA CAC GAG GAC ACC ATG GCT GAC CAG GAA GCC AAC AGA CAT GGC CGC AGT GGC AAA
       R   G   H   E   D   T   M   A   D   Q   E   A   N   R   H   G   R   S   G   K
SAA3  CAT GGA GCA GAG GAC TCA AGA GCT GAC CAG TTT GCC AAT GAG TGG GGC CGG AGT GGC AAA
       H   G   A   E   D   S   R   A   D   Q   F   A   N   E   W   G   R   S   G   K
      70                          80

SAA1  GAC CCC AAT TAC TAC AGA CCT CCT GGA CTG CCT GAC AAA TAC TGA GCG TCC TCC TAT TAG  420
       D   P   N   Y   Y   R   P   P   G   L   P   D   K   Y   *
SAA2  GAC CCC AAT TAC TAC AGA CCT CCT GGA CTG CCT GAC AAA TAC TGA GAG TCC TCC TAT TAG
       D   P   N   Y   Y   R   P   P   G   L   P   A   K   Y   *
SAA3  GAC CCC AAC CAC TTC CGA CCT GCT GGC CTG CCT AAA AGA TAC TGA GTT TTC TCT TCC TGT
       D   P   N   H   F   R   P   A   G   L   P   K   R   Y   *
      90                          100
```

The deduced amino acids are numbered sequentially from the known N-terminus of the mature SAA (the amino acids of the signal peptide are numbered -19 to -1).
Nucleotide and amino acid substitutions are indicated by underlines.

Other investigators have isolated a cDNA clone encoding the third SAA isotype (SAA3) (6), the sequence of which shows a considerable divergence from those of the SAA1 and SAA2 cDNAs (Fig. 1 and Table I). Therefore, there appear to be multiple SAA genes in mice. This is also consistent with the results of genomic Southern blot analysis (7). Here I present evidence that mouse SAA is encoded by four genes which show diverse expression during acute inflammation (8), and discuss a possible significance of the diversity in SAA gene expression to amyloidogenesis.

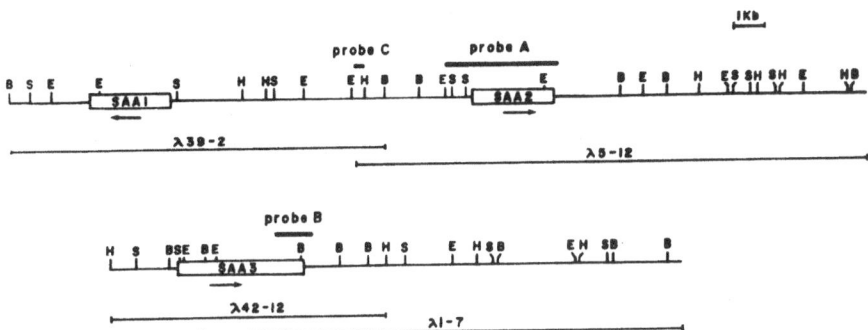

Figure 1: Restriction maps of the mouse genomic clones containing SAA1, -2 and -3 genes. The 5'- and 3'- ends for the SAA1, -2 and -3 genes were determined by DNA sequencing, primer extention and S1 mapping; the arrows indicate orientation of gene transcription. The regions covered by the probes are indicated by bars. Restriction enzymes: E, EcoRI; B, BamHI; H, HindIII; S, SacI.

2. The structure of SAA genes

Mouse SAA2 cDNA was used to screen the BALB/c mouse HaeIII and Sau3A genomic libraries in phage Charon 4A and 28 (9) and four positive phage clones were isolated. The two clones, λ5-12 and λ09-2, were identified as carrying the SAA2 and SAA1 genes, respectively, on the basis of their hybridization with the SAA2 and SAA1 specific synthetic oligonucleotide probes (Table III) and of the presence of unique restriction sites (5).

TABLE III: BASE SEQUENCES OF SYNTHETIC OLIGONUCLEOTIDE PROBES

SAA mRNA	5' ------ ATG ------------------------------ TGA ------------------ 3'
SAA probe 1	3' - A G T A A A C A A G T G C T C C G A - 5'
SAA probe 2	3' - A G T A A A T A A C C C C T C C G A - 5'
SAA probe 3	3' - G T C A A G T A C T T T C T T C G A - 5'

SAA probe 1, 2 and 3 are complementary to SAA1, SAA2 and SAA3 mRNA respectively (5).
Base differences are underlined.

To define a possible linkage of the SAA1 and SAA2 genes, a 300 bp probe (probe C in Fig. 1) was prepared from the 5'-end of the λ5-12 clone and was used in hybridization with the λ39-2 clone. The results indicate that the 5'-end of the λ5-12 clone hybridized to the 3'-end of the λ39-2 clone (not shown), establishing that the SAA1 and SAA2 genes are directly adjacent in divergent transcriptional orientation (Fig. 1). The other two overlapping clones, λ1-7 and λ42-12, hybridized with a SAA2 cDNA probe only under low stringency conditions, but were effectively hybridized with a SAA3 specific synthetic oligonucleotide probe (Table III): the clones gave single hybridizing fragments upon digestion with EcoRI (7.0 kb), BamHI (2.8 kb), XbaI (1.1 kb) and BglII (4.4 kb). Comparison of these data with the restriction map for the SAA3 gene and its flanking regions (10) confirms that these two clones contain the SAA3 gene (Fig. 1). To study further the organization of SAA gene in the mouse chromosomal DNA, we carried out Southern blot analysis of liver DNA from BALB/c mice with a 3.4 kb XbaI fragment from the SAA2 genomic clone (probe A in Fig. 1) and a 1.1 kb XbaI fragment from the SAA3 genomic clone (probe B in Fig. 1) as hybridization probes. As shown in Fig. 2, lane A, the probe A hybridized to two genomic fragments in Southern blots made with four different restriction enzymes.

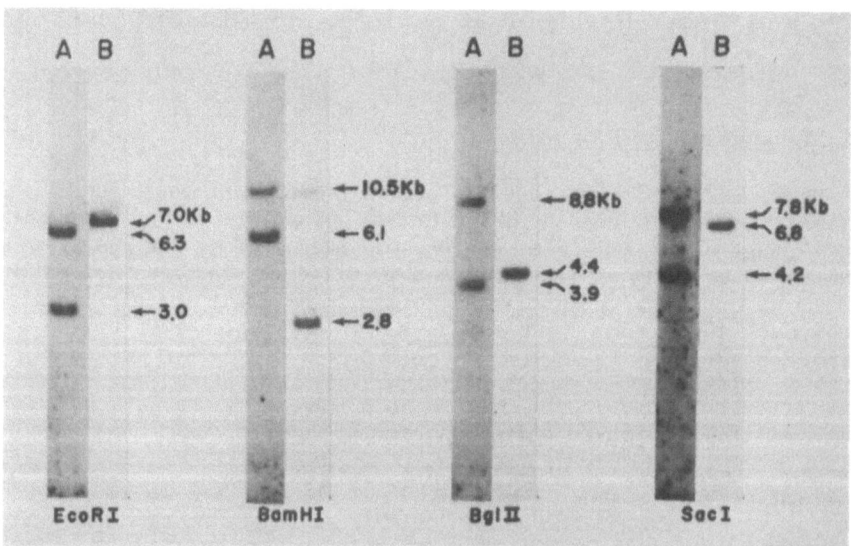

Figure 2: Southern blot analysis of BALB/c mouse genomic DNA with the SAA2 (probe A, Table III and SAA3 (probe B, Table III) genomic probes. Two µg of BALB/c mouse liver DNA (14) was digested to completion with restriction enzymes, sized on a 0.8% agarose gel, transferred to a nitrocellulose filter (15), and hybridized with radio-active probes.
The filters were washed two times at room temperature with 0.3 M NaCl/0.03 M sodium citrate (2x SSC) and three times at 65° C for 20 minutes with 0.1x SSC/0.1% SDS, and autoradiographed at -70° C. Blots hybridized with the probe A and B are indicated by A and B respectively.

In each case, one of two fragments hybridized with the probe A (3 kb EcoRI, 6.1 kb BamHI, 3.9 kb BglII and 7.8 kb SacI fragments) had the fragment length characteristic of the SAA2 gene, and the other fragments (6.3 kb EcoRI, 10.5 kb BamHI, 8.8 kb BglII and 4.2 kb SacI fragments) were thought to be derived from the SAA1 gene as seen in Table II (BglII sites are not shown in Fig. 1). The filters used above were boiled for 5 minutes in 10 mM Tris-1 mM EDTA (pH 8.0) and were rehybridized with the probe B. The resulting autoradiogram (Fig. 2, lane B) showed that only single fragments were visible in blots made with several restriction enzymes: the size of these fragments were as expected from the restriction map for the SAA3 gene shown in Fig. 1. Southern blot hybridization was also carried out in low stringency conditions (1xSSC at 50°C) to examine the possibility that other distantly related SAA genes might be present. The results showed that SAA probes hybridized to a 4.8 kb EcoRI fragment in addition to the 7.0 kb (SAA3 gene), 6.3 kb (SAA1 gene) and 3.0 kb (SAA2 gene) EcoRI fragments (not shown), indicating the presence of the fourth SAA gene (SAA4 gene). Recently, we have cloned a 79 kb region of mouse chromosome and have confirmed the presence of the SAA4 gene: the SAA4 gene is located approximately 5 Kb downstream from the 3'-end of the SAA1 gene, between the SAA1 and SAA3 genes (K. Yamamoto, et al, manuscript submitted). These results, therefore, indicate that mouse SAA is encoded by a family of four closely-linked genes.

The complete DNA sequence of the SAA2 gene has been determined by the dideoxy chain termination method (K. Yamamoto, et al, manuscript in preparation). Fig. 3 schematically illustrates the exon-intron structure of the SAA2 gene.

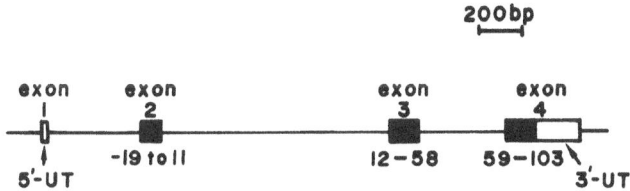

Figure 3: Exon-intron organization of the SAA2 gene. Numbers below the line indicate the amino acids at which intron/exon junctions occur: 5'- and 3'- UT, 5'- and 3'- untranslated regions in the mRNA transcripts respectively.

Comparison of the structure of the SAA2 gene with that of the SAA3 gene (10) revealed differences in the size of the first and fourth exons, and of the introns, though the exon-intron junctions were completely conserved in these genes. In addition, while the sequences of the exon 3 were highly conserved in these genes, the sequences of the exon 1 showed extensive divergence (K. Yamamoto, et al, manuscript in preparation).

3.The expression of SAA genes

We studied the expression of the SAA1, SAA2 and SAA3 genes by using 18 base-long synthetic oligonucleotide probes (11) complementary to the region where the SAA1, SAA2 and SAA3 cDNA sequences diverge (Table III) (5). The oligonucleotide probes were labeled at the 5'-end with T4 polynucleotide kinase in the presence of $[\gamma-^{32}P]ATP$ (12) for Northern blotting experiments. The SAA1 and SAA2 specific probes strongly hybridized to liver RNA from LPS-stimulated BALB/c and Swiss mice but not to RNA from normal mice, whereas the SAA3 specific probe hybridized only very weakly to RNA from LPS-stimulated mice. In SJL mice, the SAA2 specific probe showed only weak hybridization to LPS--induced RNA, though the SAA1 specific probe hybridized to LPS-induced RNA of SJL mice as strongly as to those of BALB/c and Swiss mice. These results were further confirmed by the results of in vitro translation of liver mRNA from LPS-stimulated mice (Fig.4).

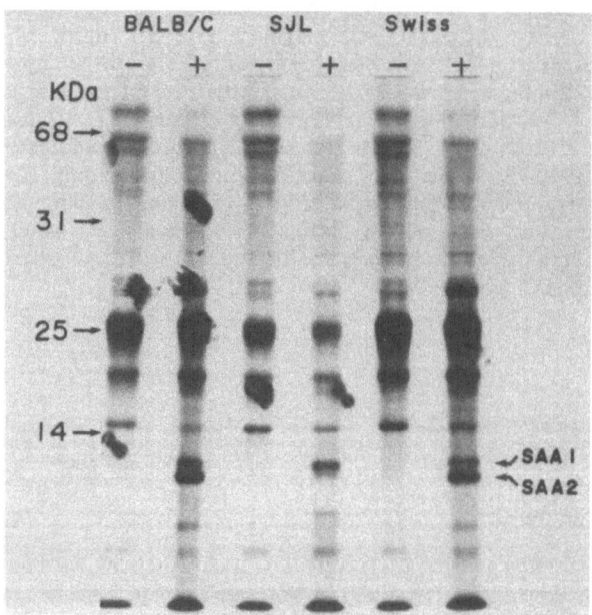

Figure 4: SDS-polyacrylamide gel electrophoretic analysis of cell-free translation products of liver mRNA from normal (-) and LPS-stimulated (+) mice. Poly(A) RNA was trans-lated in a wheat germ system (Bethesda Research Laboratories) in the presence of ^{35}S-methionine, and translation products were analyzed on 13% slab gels containing 6M urea (19).

mRNA from LPS-stimulated BALB/c and Swiss mice directed the synthesis of large quantities of two polypeptides with apparent m.w. of 12.8 Kdalton and 12.5 Kdalton corresponding to pre-SAA1 and pre-SAA2, respectively. However, in translation of mRNA from LPS-stimulated SJL mice, the intensity of the SAA2 band reduced substantially, though the intensity of the SAA1 band was comparable to those in BALB/c and Swiss mice. These results show that during acute phase reaction both of the SAA1 and SAA2 genes are expressed at high levels in BALB/c and Swiss mice, though the SAA3 gene expression is barely detectable, and that in SJL mice the SAA2 gene expression is very low. An implication of these results to amyloidogenesis is that the decreased expression of the SAA2 gene in SJL mice is related to resistance of these mice to azocasein-induced amyloidosis (13), since only SAA2 protein is amyloidogenic in mice (4). To define further SAA2 gene defects in SJL mice, Southern blots of restriction enzyme digested liver DNA from SJL as well as BALB/c mice were hybridized with the SAA2 gene probe (probe A in Fig. 1). As shown in Fig. 5, the resulting auto-radiograms reveal no visible deletion in the SAA2 gene and its flanking regions in SJL mice.

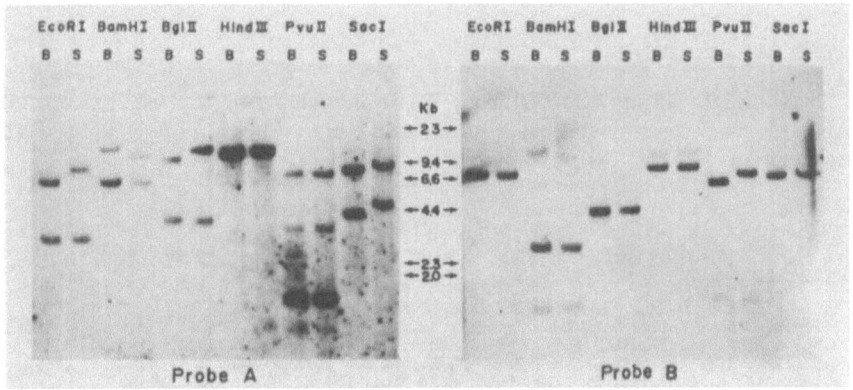

Figure 5: Southern blot analysis of SJL mouse genomic DNA. Two μg of BALB/c (B) and SJL (S) mouse liver DNA was digested with restriction enzymes, sized on 0.8% gels, transferred to a nitrocellulose filter, and hybridized with the probe A and B as described in the legend to Figure 2.

However, SAA genes show restriction site length polymorphism (Fig. 5) as reported previously by Taylor and Rowe (7). Interestingly, 129/J mice which show an identical restriction fragment pattern with SJL mice upon genomic Southern blot analysis with SAA probes (7) are also defective in the SAA gene expression (unpublished data). These results suggest that defective SAA2 gene expression in these mice is due to structural variations, possibly in the 5'-flanking promotor region or in the exon-intron junctions of the SAA2 gene. We have also studied the gene expression for SAA isotypes in another amyloidosis-resistant mice, A/J mice (13). It was found that A/J mice express both SAA2 and SAA1 genes at high levels during acute inflammation (unpublished data), indicating that resistance to amyloidosis of this mouse is not due to defective SAA gene expression.

4.Summary

The present study demonstrates that mouse SAA is encoded by four genes which are tightly clustering in the 79 kb region of mouse chromosome. During acute phase reaction these genes show diverse expression. While the genes for two major SAA isotypes of mouse (SAA1 and SAA2) are expressed at high levels in BALB/c and Swiss mice, the gene for a minor third SAA isotype (SAA3) is expressed only at a very low level. Furthermore, in amyloidosis-resistant SJL mice, the SAA2 gene expression is meager. The results of genomic Southern blot analysis suggest that the defective SAA2 gene expression in SJL mice is due to structural variations in the SAA2 gene. Since only SAA2 protein is amyloidogenic in mice, defective SAA2 gene expression is probably a primary cause for resistance to amyloidosis of this mouse. Thus, these results argue for the hypothesis that the structural diversity in SAA genes play a role in determining susceptibility to amyloidosis.

Acknowledgements

I thank S. Migita, M. Shiroo, K. Nakayama for the discussion, K. Aikoshi for technical assistance and H. Horita for typing the manuscript.

References

1.Glenner, G.G. N. Eng. J. Med. 302, 1283-1292, 1333-1343, 1980.
2.Pepys, M.B. & Baltz, M.L. Adv. Immunol. 34, 141-212, 1983.
3.Hoffman, J.S. & Benditt, E.P. J. Biol. Chem. 257, 10510-10517, 1982.
4.Hoffman, J.S., Ericsson, L.H., Eriksen, E., et al. J. Exp. Med. 159, 641-646, 1984.
5.Yamamoto, K. & Migita, S. Proc. Natl. Acad. Sci. USA 82, 2915-2919, 1985.
6.Morrow, J.F., Stearman, R.S., Peltzman, S.G. et al. Proc. Natl. Acad. Sci. USA 78, 4718-4722, 1981.
7.Taylor, B.A. & Rowe, R. Mol. Gen. Genet. 195, 491-499, 1984.
8.Yamamoto, K., Shiroo, M. & Migita, S. Science 232, 227-229, 1986.
9.Benton, W.D. & Davis, R.W. Science 196, 180-182, 1977.
10.Stearman, R.S., Lowell, C.A., Pearson, W.R., et al. Ann. N.Y. Acad. Sci. 389, 106-115, 1982.
11.Beacage, S.L. & Caruthers, M.H. Tetrahedron Lett. 22, 1859-1862, 1981.
12.Maxam, A.M. & Gilbert, W. Meth. Enzym. 65, 499-560, 1980.
13.Miyamoto, H.: personal communication.
14.Yaoita, Y. & Honjo, T. Biomed. Res. 1, 164-175, 1980.
15.Southern, E.M. J. Mol. Biol. 98, 503-517, 1975.
16.Chirgwin, J.M., Przybyla, A.E., MacDonald, R.J., et al. Biochemistry 18, 5294-5299, 1979.
17.Aviv, H. & Leder, P. Proc. Natl. Acad. Sci. USA 69, 1408-1412, 1972.
18.Thomas, P.S. Proc. Natl. Acad. Sci. USA 77, 5201-5205, 1980.
19.Laemmli, V.K. Nature 227, 680-685, 1970.

IV.7 AMYLOIDOGENIC PROTEINS IN HUMAN CENTRAL NERVOUS SYSTEM DISEASES

Colin L. Masters[1] and Konrad Beyreuther[2]

Laboratory of Molecular and Applied Neuropathology
Neuromuscular Research Institute
Department of Pathology
University of Western Australia
Western Australia, 6009.[1]
and
Department of Neuropathology
Royal Perth Hospital
Western Australia, 6001.[1]

Institute of Genetics
University of Cologne
Cologne
Federal Republic of Germany.[2]

1.Introduction

The amyloid proteins which are deposited in the central nervous system fall into two major categories: first, as an involvement incidental to the occurrence of the various forms of systemic amyloidosis; second, amyloid deposits which are restricted to the central nervous system (Table I). This essay is concerned with the latter category, but it is important to consider the implication of this division of nervous system amyloidoses: in the systemic amyloidoses, deposition occurs in the brain in areas where there is an inherently increased permeability of the blood-brain barrier; in contrast, the amyloidoses which are restricted to the brain have a rather distinctive parenchymal and vascular distribution, suggesting that the origin of the amyloid protein (or its precursor) is not hematogenous. It will become apparent later that we favor the concept of a neuronal origin of these brain-restricted amyloidoses, although it is admitted at the start that much of this concept is still hypothetical and speculative.

The protein components in three of the brain-restricted amyloidoses (Alzheimer's disease; the unconventional virus diseases; Icelandic hereditary congophilic angiopathy with cerebral hemorrhage) have now been isolated and characterized in some detail (1-4). In common with the amyloidogenic proteins of the systemic diseases, they are small proteins which appear to have a marked tendency for polymerization into β-sheet fibrillar structures. Their relative insolubilities and resistance to proteolysis forms the basis of their harmful action when deposited in the brain.

TABLE I: CLASSIFICATION OF NERVOUS SYSTEM AMYLOID DEPOSITS

Category	Area involved	Protein component	Protein subunit Kdalton
1. Incidental nervous system involvement in systemic amyloidosis	Dura, leptomeninges, subpial and subependymal areas, choroid plexus, pituitary, infundibulum, area postrema, motor and sensory nerves	Transthyretin Ig light chains Amyloid A protein	14 5-18 8.5
2. Amyloid deposits restricted to the central nervous system			
a. Alzheimer's disease i.neurofibrillary tangles ii.amyloid/neuritic plaques iii.amyloid angiopathy: "angiopathie congophile" (Pantelakis) "drusige Entartung" (Scholz)	Cerebral cortex, subcortical grey matter (cerebellum)	Polymers of A_4 (β protein)	4
b. Down's syndrome, after the age of 30 years	Distribution similar to Alzheimer's	Polymers of A_4 (β protein)	4
c. Pick's disease	Distribution similar to Alzheimer's	?	?
d. Diverse "neurofibrillary tangle-associated diseases": i.progressive supranuclear palsy (PSP; Steele--Richardson-Olszewski) ii.Guamanian amyotrophic lateral sclerosis/ Parkinsonism dementia complex (ALS/PD)	Generally subcortical Generally subcortical	? ?	? ?
e. Unconventional virus-induced subacute spongiform encephalopathies i.scrapie ii.kuru iii.Creutzfeldt-Jacob disease iv.Gerstmann-Straussler syndr.	Cerebral cortex, subcortical grey matter, cerebellum	Polymers of scrapie associated filament protein (PrP)	10-35
f. Icelandic hereditary congophilic angiopathy with cerebral hemorrhage	Cerebral cortex	Cystatin C (gamma-trace)	13.3
g. Other forms of primary cerebrovascular amyloidosis	?	?	?

2. Amyloidogenic proteins in Alzheimer's disease

Alzheimer's disease (AD) is the most frequent cause of intellectual impairment in late adult life. While the incidence and prevalence of AD are difficult to define, it is clear that at least 10% of the population can be expected to show evidence of AD in the eighth and higher decades.

At present, a definitive diagnosis of AD can only be made by neuro-pathological examination of brain tissue. The pathognomonic changes are fibrillar amyloid deposits occurring intracellularly and extracellularly. The intracellular amyloids are the neurofibrillary tangles (NFT) which are composed of paired helical filaments (PHF) and single "straight" filaments. These filaments also accumulate within pre-synaptic axonal terminals which surround the plaque, and terms such as "neuritic degeneration" and "dystrophic neurites" have been used to describe them. Cajal (5) believed that some of the neuritic change around the periphery of a plaque was regenerative, rather than degenerative. We suspect that he may still prove to be correct, for in the center of the plaque lies extracellular deposits of amyloid fibrils. These extracellular deposits of amyloid fibrils are arranged either as amorphous or compact amyloid plaque cores (APC). The extracellular amyloid may also be found around small arterioles in the parenchyma and subarachnoid space, and is termed amyloid congophilic angiopathy (ACA). Sometimes, the amyloid around the arterioles extends well into the parenchyma, and is itself associated with neuritic changes (somewhat analogous to the "drusige Entartung" of Scholz).

For many years neuropathologists have argued over the relationships between the intracellular and extracellular amyloids in AD (see, for example, Schwartz's (6) spirited, but pedantic, defence of Divry's hypothesis). Much discussion has been spent on the histochemical and ultrastructural differences between NFT and APC/ACA. Yet the histochemical techniques (such as Congo red birefringence, thioflavin S fluorescence, PAS reactivity, and argyrophilia) lack specificity, and the ultrastructural appearances of amyloid are now known to be similar between most varieties of extracellular amyloid deposits. The rather striking ultrastructural differences between PHF of NFT and the straight filaments of APC/ACA should be evaluated in the context that NFT are the only known examples of amyloid proteins accumulating in the intracellular space.

For as long as the arguments on the nature of NFT, APC and ACA have been conducted, it has always been recognized that the definitive answers will only come from the physical isolation of the amyloid structures and their biochemical analysis. Fortunately, some progress in this area has been made in the last few years. The first structure to yield information was the ACA: Glenner and Wong (7-9) were able to show a subunit protein of about 4 Kdalton in mass, and presented the N-terminal sequence of the first 24-28 residues. The protein appeared unique and was present in the ACA of both AD and aged individuals with Down's syndrome (DS); there is a well recognized association between AD and DS. At about the same time, Allsop et al (10), our laboratories in Perth and Cologne (1) and several other laboratories in the US (11,12 and H. Wisniewski, personal communications) concentrated on the isolation and characterization of the APC in AD and DS. The protein component of the APC was shown to be virtually identical to the subunit of the ACA (1,2,9).

151

The subunit protein of APC/ACA (termed A_4) has now been fully sequenced, revealing only 42 residues (Beyreuther et al, manuscript in preparation). This small protein readily aggregates into dimers (A_8), tetramers (A_{16}) and higher oligomers (molecular mass greater than 64 Kdalton). The aggregational properties of the monomer are pH and concentration dependent (1). It appears not to be glycosylated (1). The A_4 molecule is highly amyloidogenic, to the extent that synthetic peptides corresponding to residues 1-28, 4-28 and 1-40 spontaneously form amyloid fibrils under physiological conditions (Beyreuther et al, manuscript in preparation). We have identified the key amyloidogenic sequence as residing between residues 10-20, and it is also within this region of the A_4 that a strong epitope for native APC/ACA exists (2). A_4 does not show significant sequence homology to any other known protein. While the ACA-A_4 does not show N-terminal heterogeneity (7,8), the APC-A_4 is considerably degraded in the N-terminal region. We have interpreted this as possibly due to in situ processing (1).

Having established the identity of the APC/ACA protein, our initial studies did not allow comment on the possible site of origin (1), although Glenner (7,9) favoured a hematogenous source. If the A_4 polymer or its precursor is derived from the blood, one must provide explanations for (i) localization to subregional areas of brain, (ii) absence from other organs, (iii) its arteriolar and not venular distribution, and (iv) the spherical nature of the plaque without obvious relationship to the microvasculature. In our opinion, plausible explanations on these four points have yet to be accommodated within the hematogenous origin hypothesis. In contrast, and with hindsight, if the A_4 polymer and its precursors are produced within the brain, then each of these four points are readily explicable: (i) and (ii) are the result of the production of the molecule within the cerebral cortex of brain; (iii) the polymerized A_4 fibril is unable to pass through the wall of arterioles, and accumulates in the Virchow-Robin spaces and overlying subarachnoid space, whereas the locally-produced A_4 polymer does pass through capillaries and venules into the blood; (iv) the spherical nature of the plaque is due to its local origin in a focal area, from which the polymerization of A_4 proceeds in a radial fashion.

But where does the intracellular NFT fit within this story? At the same time that we were struggling with the solubilization of the APC, Selkoe et al (13,14) recognized that the NFT was as equally resistant to the usual denaturants and laboratory solvents. Other laboratories, skilled at purifying NFT, had used these preparations as immunogens (15,16), without being able to precisely define the major protein component of NFT. That NFT share epitopes with normal neurofilaments (NF-H,M) (17-20), microtubule associated proteins (MAP2, tau) (21-24), a phosphorylated determinant (25), vimentin (26) as well as containing their own unique determinants, led to a bewildering array of information, not at all congruous. Agreement seems to be emerging that tau, or a related protein, shares a major epitope with the NFT. Refined ultrastructural studies have tended to emphasize the unique arrays of globular subunits that comprise the NFT (27-31). While most of these studies point to differences between the NFT and APC/ACA, some biochemical data have now emerged that suggests that NFT are built from the same subunit protein (A_4) as APC/ACA.

TABLE II: COMPARISON OF AMYLOID SOLUBILITY PROFILE WITH INACTIVATION OF SCRAPIE

Condition	NFT/APC solubility	Inactivation of scrapie
Detergents		
Triton X-100 (1%)	-	-
CTAB (1%)	-	-
Satkosyl (10%)	-	-
DOC (10%)	-	-
SDS (10%) + heat + sonication	±	+
Acid		
Acetic acid (100%)	-	? (pH <2.1)
Formic acid (70%)	+	? (pH <2.1)
Alkali		
NaOH (0.2-0.5 M)	+	+
Inorganic ions		
Na$^+$, K$^+$, Cl$^-$	-	-
Chaotropic ions		
Guanidine HCl	±/- (6.0 M)	+ (0.2 M)
Guanidinium thiocyanate	+ (6.0 M)	+ (0.2 M)
Potassium thiocyanate	- (6.0 M)	+ (0.2 M)
Trichloroacetate	- (1.0 M)	+ (0.2 M)
Denaturing agent		
Urea (8.0 M)	±/-	±/-
Organic solvents		
Ethanol	-	-
Methanol	-	-
Phenol	+ (≥80%)	+ (5-90%)

First, Kidd et al (32) showed that the amino acid compositions of isolated NFT were the same as APC. Second, Kirschner et al (33) have shown by X-ray diffraction that NFT have the same cross-β conformation as APC. Third, our studies (2) on enriched preparations of NFT show (a) the same solubility profile between NFT and APC (Table II), as predicted from the studies of Selkoe et al (13,14); (b) the same amino acid compositions between NFT and APC/ACA, in agreement with Kidd et al (32); (c) after extraction in formic acid and solubilization in SDS, both NFT and APC have similar HPLC gel permeation chromatography profiles and the same major species of protein (A_4) is identifiable by SDS-urea PAGE; (d) the N-terminal sequence of the NFT protein component shows a highly degraded A_4 sequence, more so than the APC; (e) using synthetic peptides as immunogens, we have been able to show that there is a weak epitope for NFT present in the region of residues 1-11 of the A_4 molecule. From this evidence we concluded that A_4 was the major component common to both NFT, APC and ACA, and by implication, that all three amyloid components had a common origin (2). Moreover, the relative proportions of N-terminal raggedness (NFT>APC>ACA) suggested to us that the NFT was the oldest of the three components, with the ACA being the most recently formed. This conclusion also strongly implied that the A_4 subunit was probably of neuronal origin. The lack of sequence homology between any of the known cytoskeletal elements in the nervous system also indicated that the A_4 or its precursor was unlikely to be derived from any of the known normal neurofilaments, microtubules, or their associated proteins. From the small size of A_4, it is unlikely to represent a primary gene product - it is more likely to derive from a larger precursor molecule. Research is now being directed in the area of identifying the gene for A_4 and its full length precursor.

Our conclusions on the common identity of NFT and APC/ACA have been challenged (12) on the ground that the NFT preparation contained a significant contamination with APC or ACA. It is true that our NFT preparations are not as "clean" as are the APC preparations, and that by electron microscopy fibrillar masses of straight filaments together with PHF can be identified. Nevertheless, by light microscopy, most of the birefringent material is flame-shaped and whorled, typical of the intracellular NFT. Quantitative estimates of the amounts of protein solubilized in the formic acid show that most of the protein ($\geq$90%) is extracted. It is still possible that the buffers used in the gel permeation chromatography or SDS-urea PAGE selectively solubilize the A_4 components, and do not effectively solubilize the postulated NFT protein(s). In view of the strong evidence for a MAP2/tau-like epitope being present on NFT (21-24), we think it possible that the underlying filaments of the NFT are indeed decorated on their surfaces by such microtubule associated proteins. The A_4 polymers which are assembled in the extracellular space escape such decoration. This would be consistent with the known behaviour of these microtubule associated proteins. If this hypothesis is correct, it should be possible to dissociate the MAP2/tau immunoreactivity from the underlying A_4 polymer.

The differences in ultrastructure which have led most authors to conclude that NFT and APC/ACA must be chemically different can also be explained on the basis of different packing densities of the subunits (2,27-31). Other factors such as the interaction of the A_4 with MAP2/tau-like molecules might induce the formation of PHF rather than the straight filaments. It is also worth keeping in mind that NFT may be composed of straight filaments as well as PHF - but the literature is rather ambiguous on this issue.

Finally, we (2) and others (34,35) have shown that aluminium and silicate may be present in the APC, somewhat analogous to the accumulation of aluminium in the NFT (36,37). At this stage we are uncertain whether the presence of these elements is of biological significance.

3. Amyloidogenic proteins in the unconventional virus-induced subacute spongiform encephalopathies

A variable proportion of cases with the virus-induced subacute spongiform encephalopathies develop amyloid plaques during the late stages of the incubation periode (38). It has recently been recognized that amyloid deposition around blood vessels also occurs (39). The deposition of amyloid is strongly influenced by host genetic factors and the strain of infective virus (40).

There is now a considerable body of evidence that the scrapie associated fibril (SAF) represents a form of these amyloid deposits, and that the subunit of the SAF is a host-encoded polymer derived from the PrP 33-35 protein (see references 41-54). We have recently analyzed the amyloid component of the human disease by direct biochemical examination. The subunit protein may be much smaller than the PrP 33-35, with a mass of only 10-12 Kdalton (Beyreuther et al, manuscript in preparation), suggesting that the PrP 33-35 is processed in some manner before extracellular amyloid formation occurs. It is also clear that infectivity co-purifies with the SAF and PrP 33-35. The question which has not yet been settled is whether the infectious agent is an integral part of the SAF/PrP 33-35, or whether these structures represent merely a pathologic by-product of infection. The nucleic acid which is necessary for infectivity has not yet been identified, and indeed there is good evidence that large coding sequences are not required for infectivity. Nevertheless, a small nucleic acid may still be complexed within or adjacent to the polymerized SAF/PrP 33-35.

As these investigations proceed, the similarities in pathogenesis of AD and the unconventional virus diseases become more intriguing than ever. Morphologically, the SAF resemble PHF more closely than the straight filaments of APC/ACA. It is likely that the SAF are assembled intracellulary (55,56) and in this case would be strictly analogous to the assembly mechanism of NFT/APC as discussed in the preceeding section. The chemical inactivation profile or scrapie infectivity bears a resemblance to the solubility profile of NFT/APC (Table II). We suspect that the amyloid filaments in both categories of disease share a common mechanism for this generation of self-aggregating polypeptides of low molecular weight and that these macromolecular assemblies are stabilized by similar forces.

4. Icelandic hereditary congophilic angiopathy with cerebral hemorrhage

There are several reports of unusual forms of primary cerebrovascular amyloidosis, one group constituting an Icelandic disease which occurs as an autosomal dominantly inherited disorder. Recent studies have elucidated the biochemical nature of the amyloid (4,57-58), and have pointed to its possible origin within a subpopulation of neurons within the central nervous system. The protein subunit is cystatin C (gamma trace), of relatively small molecular mass of 13 Kdalton. An amino acid substitution at residue number 58 (glutamine for leucine) appears to underlie the amyloidogenic variant (57). How this protein comes to accumulate around cerebral blood vessels has not been elucidated, although we might predict that the basic mechanism will be similar to that eventually determined for the ACA of AD.

References

1. Masters, C.L., Simms, G., Weinman, N.A. et al. Proc. Natl. Acad. Sci. USA 82, 4245-4249, 1985.
2. Masters, C.L., Multhaup, G., Simms, G. et al. EMBO J. 4, 2757-2763, 1985.
3. Oessch, B., Westaway, D., Wälchli, M. et al. Cell 40, 735-746, 1985.
4. Cohen, D.H., Feiner, H., Jensson, O. & Frangione, B. J. Exp. Med. 158, 623-628, 1983.
5. Cajal, S. & Ramon, Y. In Degeneration and Regeneration of the Nervous System. R.M. May, Ed. Oxford University Press, London, vol. II, 734-760, 1928.
6. Schwartz, P. In Pathology of the Nervous System. Minckler, J. Ed. McGraw-Hill, New York, volume III, 2812-2849, 1972.
7. Glenner, G.G. & Wong, C.W. Biochem. Biophys. Res. Commun. 120, 885-890, 1984.
8. Glenner, G.G. & Wong, C.W. Biochem. Biophys. Res. Commun. 122, 1131-1135, 1984.
9. Wong, C.W., Quaranta, V. & Glenner, G.G. Proc. Natl. Acad. Sci. USA 82, 8729-8732, 1985.
10. Allsop, D., Landon, M. & Kidd, M. Brain Res. 259, 348-352, 1983.
11. Roher, A., Wolfe, D., Palutke, M. & Kukuruga, D. Proc. Natl. Acad. Sci. USA 83, 2662-2666, 1986.
12. Selkoe, D.J., Abraham, C.R., Podlisny, M.B. & Duffy, L.K. J. Neurochem. 46, 1820-1834, 1986.
13. Selkoe, D.J., Ihara, Y. & Salazar, F.J. Science 215, 1243-1245, 1982.
14. Selkoe, D.J., Abraham, C. & Ihara, Y. Proc. Natl. Acad. Sci. USA 79, 6070-6074, 1982.
15. Grundke-Iqbal, I., Johnson, A.B., Wisniewski, H.M. et al. Lancet i, 578-580, 1979.
16. Grundke-Iqbal, I., Iqbal, K., Tung, Y.C. & Wisniewski, H.M. Acta Neuropathol. 6, 52-61, 1985.
17. Anderton, B.H., Breinburg, D., Downes, M.J. et al. Nature 298, 84-86, 1982.
18. Dahl, D., Selkoe, D.J., Pero, R.T. & Bignami, A. J. Neurosci. 2, 113-119, 1982.
19. Gambetti, P., Autilio-Gambetti, L., Perry, G., et al. Lab. Invest. 49, 430-435, 1983.
20. Perry, G., Rizzuto, N., Antilio-Gambetti, L. & Gambetti, P. Proc. Natl. Acad. Sci. USA 82, 3916-3920, 1985.
21. Nukina, N. & Ihara, Y. Proc. Japan Acad. 59, 284-292, 1983.
22. Brion, J.P., van den Bosch de Aguilar, P. & Flament-Durand, J. In Senile Dementia of the Alzheimer Type. Early Diagnosis, Neuropathology and Animal Models. Traber, J., Gispen, W.H., Eds. Springer-Verlag, Berlin, 164-174, 1985.
23. Nukina, N. & Ihara, Y. J. Biochem. 99, 1541-1544, 1986.
24. Grundke-Iqbal, I., Iqbal, K., Quinlan, M. et al. J. Biol. Chem. 261, 6084-6089, 1986.
25. Sternberg, N.H., Sternberger, L.A. & Ulrich, J. Proc. Natl. Acad. Sci. USA 82, 4274-4276, 1985.
26. Yen, S.H.C., Gaskin, F. & Terry, R.D. Am. J. Pathol. 104, 77-89, 1981.
27. Wen, G.Y. & Wisniewski, H.W. Acta Neuropathol. 64, 339-343, 1984.
28. Wisniewski, H.W. & Wen, G.Y. Acta Neuropathol. 66, 173-176, 1985.
29. Wischik, C.M., Crowther, R.A., Stewart, M. & Roth, M. J. Cell. Biol. 100, 1905-1912, 1985.
30. Wischik, C.M. & Crowther, R.A. Br. Med. Bull. 42, 51-56, 1986.
31. Crowther, R.A. & Wischik, C.M. EMBO J. 4, 3361-3365, 1985.
32. Kidd, M., Allsop, D. & Landon, M. Lancet i, 278, 1985.
33. Kirschner, D.A., Abraham, D. & Selkoe, D.J. Proc. Natl. Acad. Sci. USA 83, 503-507, 1986.
34. Nikaido, T., Austin, J., Trueb, L. & Rinehart, R. Arch. Neurol. 27, 549-554, 1972.
35. Candy, J.M., Oakley, A.E., Klinowski, J. et al. Lancet i, 354-357, 1986.
36. Perl, D.P. & Brody, A.R. Science 208, 297-299, 1980.
37. Garruto, R.M., Fukatsu, R., Yanigahara, R.Y. et al. Proc. Natl. Acad. Sci. USA 81, 1875-1879, 1984.
38. Masters, C.L., Gajdusek, D.C. & Gibbs, C.J. Jr. Brain 104, 559-587, 1981.
39. Gilmour, J.S., Bruce, M.E. & MacKellar, A. Neuropathol. Appl. Neurobiol. 12, 173-183, 1986.
40. Bruce, M.E. & Dickinson, A.G. J. Neuropathol. Exp. Neurol. 44, 285-294, 1985.
41. Barry, R.A., McKinley, M.P., Bendheim, P.E. et al. J. Immunol. 135, 603-613, 1985.

42. Bendheim, P.E., Bockman, J.M., McKinley, M.P. et al. Proc. Natl. Acad. Sci. USA 82, 997-1001, 1985.
43. Bockman, J.M., Kingsbury, D.T., McKinley, M.P. et al. N. Engl. J. Med. 312, 73-78, 1985.
44. Bolton, D.C., Meyer, R.K. & Prusiner, S.B. J. Virol. 53, 596-606, 1985.
45. Braig, H.R. & Diringer, H. EMBO J. 4, 2309-2312, 1985.
46. Cho, H.J. J. Gen. Virol. 67, 243-253, 1986.
47. DeArmond, S.J., McKinely, M.P., Barry, R.A. et al. Cell 41, 221-235, 1985.
48. Diringer, H., Gelderblom, H., Hilmert, H. et al. Nature 306, 476-478, 1983.
49. Manuelidis, L., Valley, S. & Manuelidis, E.E. Proc. Natl. Acad. Sci. USA 82, 4263-4267, 1985.
50. McKinley, M.P., Bolton, D.C. & Prusiner, S.B. Cell 35, 57-62, 1983.
51. Merz, P.A., Somerville, R.A., Wisniewski, H.M. et al. Nature 306, 474-476, 1983.
52. Multhaup, G., Diringer, H., Hilmert, H., et al. EMBO J. 4, 1495-1501, 1985.
53. Prusiner, S.B., McKinley, M.P., Bowman, K.A. et al. Cell 35, 349-358, 1983.
54. Chesebro, B., Race, R., Wehrly, K. et al. Nature 315, 331-333, 1985.
55. Kretzschmar, H.A., Prusiner, S.B., Stowring, L.E. & DeArmond, S.J. Am. J. Pathol. 122, 1-5, 1986.
56. Meyer, R.K., McKinley, M.P., Bowman, K.A. et al. Proc. Natl. Acad. Sci. USA 83, 2310-2314, 1986.
57. Ghiso, J., Jensson, O. & Frangione, B. Proc. Natl. Acad. Sci. USA 83, 2974-2978, 1986.
58. Grubb, A., Jensson, O., Gudmundsson, G. et al. N. Eng. J. Med. 311, 1547-1549, 1984.

IV.8   STRUCTURE OF THE ALZHEIMER PAIRED HELICAL FILAMENT

R.A. Crowther[1] and C.M. Wischik[1,2]

Medical Research Council,
Laboratory of Molecular Biology,
Hills Road, Cambridge CB2 2QH, England[1].

Cambridge Brain Bank Laboratory,
Addenbrooke's Hospital,
Hills Road, Cambridge CB2 2QQ, England[2].

1. Introduction

In senile dementia of the Alzheimer type three principal kinds of fibrillary deposit occur in the brains of affected individuals. These comprise neurofibrillary tangles, neuritic plaque cores and cerebrovascular amyloid. All three lesions consist of dense fibrous aggregates and have been called amyloid on the basis of the histopathological test of showing green birefringence when stained with Congo red dye (1). However, the principal fibrous component of the tangle, the paired helical filament (2), is ultrastructurally quite distinct from the fibrils found in cerebrovascular amyloid deposits or in plaque cores (3) or from the fibrils found in other types of amyloidosis (4). This paper will deal with the detailed structure of the paired helical filament and compare it with the amyloid-like fibrils of the plaque core.

Neurofibrillary tangles form in the large pyramidal cells of the cortex and hippocampus, as fibrous bundles that fill the perikarya of affected neurones. These bundles appear histologically as flame-shaped features (Figure 1). When plastic-embedded thin sections are examined in the electronmicroscope, it becomes clear that the tangle is formed from locally aligned groups of a morphologically highly distinctive fibrous element, the paired helical filament or PHF. The PHF appears a twisted structure displaying a characteristic alternation of 20-22 nm wide loops and 8-10 nm wide cross-overs, with an apparent period of about 80 nm. This appearance is quite different from that of any of the normal components of the neuronal cytoskeleton, such as neurofilaments or microtubules.

The neuritic plaque is a complex structure consisting of a region of abnormal swollen and degenerating neuronal processes (neurites), surrounding a more-or-less developed dense core. It has been proposed (5) that the size of the core reflects the history of the plaque, with a young plaque being composed entirely of neurites with little or no extracellular material (such as that shown in Figure 1), while a classical senile plaque consists of a halo of neurites surrounding a well-defined core. Finally in a burned out plaque, in which the neurites have completely degenerated, only an extracellular core is left. Structures apparently identical with the PHFs of the neurofibrillary tangles are found also within the dendritic neurites of the neuritic plaque (5,6).

The number of plaques and tangles found post-mortem correlates with the degree of dementia observed in life (7-9). It also correlates with deficits in major neurotransmitter systems (10) and with the loss of large cortical neurones which accompanies early-onset dementia (11). The occurrence of PHFs both in neurofibrillary tangles and in the dendritic neurites of neuritic plaques, suggests that this morphologically abnormal assembly may play a key role in the degenerative process and provides a rationale for studying its structure and biochemistry.

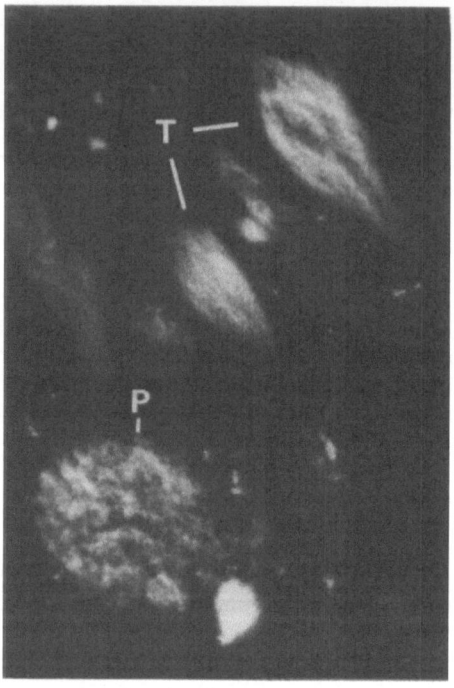

Figure 1: Tissue section from an Alzheimer brain, stained with a fluorescent dye and imaged in the light microscope, showing neurofibrillary tangles (T) and a neuritic plaque (P).

2. Ultrastructure of PHFs

Although PHFs can be clearly recognized from their gross morphology in electron micrographs of thin sections of plastic embedded tissue, the detailed substructure of such filaments is better investigated in negatively stained preparations of extracted tangles (12). We found that negative staining with sodium phosphotungstate gave the clearest pictures of substructure within the filaments, though uranyl acetate gave high contrast images particularly suitable for visualizing fragments of filaments. The characteristic appearance of negatively stained PHFs is seen in Figure 2. The axial spacing between cross-overs is about 80 nm but can be quite variable, ranging from as little as 60 nm to greater than 200 nm in almost completely flattened ribbons (e.g. Figure 4f) (12, 13). Unidirectional shadowing of the filaments shows that the two strands of the PHF wind round one another in a left-handed sense (12).

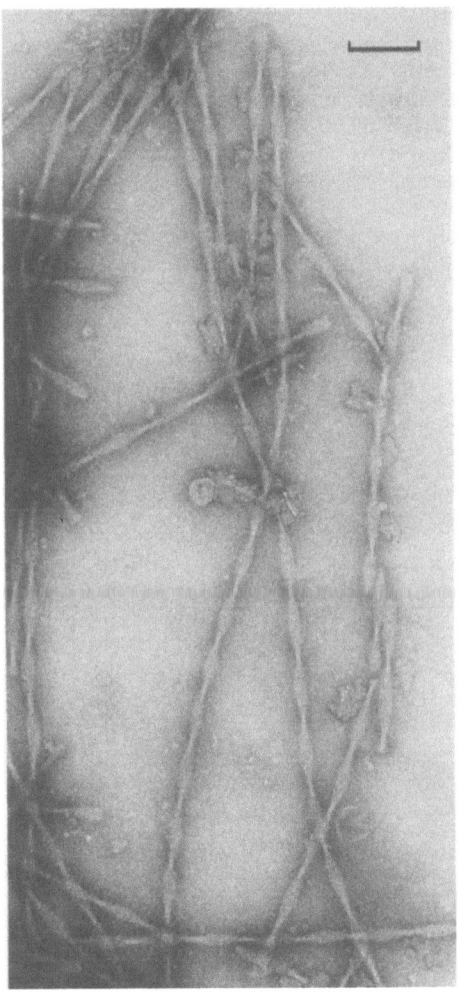

<u>Figure 2</u>: Isolated PHFs negatively stained with Na-phosphotungstate and imaged in the electron microscope. Scale bar = 100 nm.

Some insight into the molecular architecture of the PHF can be derived from a study of the fragmentation patterns observed, since these reveal the likely subunit interfaces. Such an assignment of boundaries for the structural subunit is difficult, if not impossible, on the basis of the features seen in low resolution images of intact filaments. However by studying how the PHF comes apart, some clues can be obtained about the overall shape and dimensions of the subunit which constitutes the assembly.

Two different kinds of fragmentation pattern are observed (12). Firstly PHFs show sharp transverse breaks at apparently random positions along the filament. Sometimes the breakage is extensive and gives rise to an assortment of fragments (Figure 3a), some as short as 20-30 nm. There appears to be no favoured longitudinal unit and a sharp transverse break is almost invariably observed. Much more rarely, a second type of fragmentation is found, in which there is a longitudinal break along the axis of the filament, resulting in a single-stranded region (Figure 3b). The single strand left after such a break continues to have an observable twist, retaining the periodicity and substructure of the complete PHF.

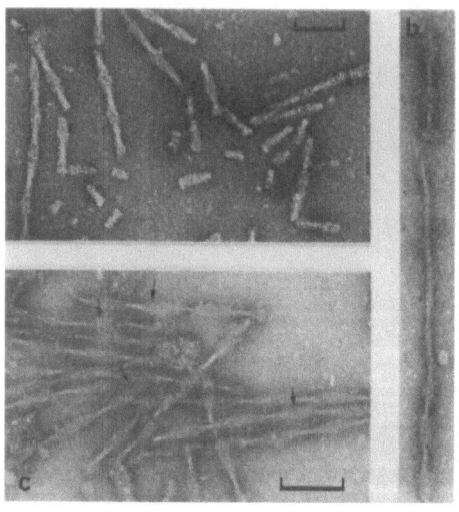

Figure 3: Fragmentation patterns of PHF's. (a) Small fragments showing sharp tranverse breaks, stained with uranyl acetate. (b) Half-PHF, stained with Na-phosphotungstate. Note that the half-PHF retains the characteristic twist and period of the whole PHF. (c) Area of PHF's with some showing transverse striping (arrows). Scale bars 100 nm.

Thus the PHF is indeed a bifilar structure, as first suggested by Kidd (2). The bonds between adjacent subunits along a half PHF are sufficient to confer some degree of structural integrity, though from the comparative rarity of such structures we conclude that the half PHF is less stable than the double stranded PHF. The pattern of sharp transverse fragmentation, with no sign of longitudinal fraying into subfilaments, apart from the single-stranded regions just noted, implies that the subunit is axially compact and not an extended fibrous molecule. The appearance in some regions of PHFs of transverse striping with an axial spacing of about 3 nm (Figure 3c) is consistent with the presence of such a subunit and suggests that its axial extent is about 3 nm. The PHF is therefore a double helical stack of transversely oriented units each of small axial extent, giving the overall shape of a ribbon twisted into a left-handed helix. If one were to draw an analogy with the much better understood filaments in muscle, then the molecular architecture of the PHF resembles the stacking of globular molecules found in the actin filament rather than the extensive overlapping of fibrous coiled-coil molecules seen in the myosin filament. Furthermore the proposed packing structure is quite different from that believed to occur in intermediate filaments in general or neurofilaments in particular.

3. Image of analysis of PHFs

Further information about the nature of the subunit comes from analysis of the detailed substructure seen within PHFs. Several distinctive patterns are observed. These were first interpreted by model building and image simulation by computer (see Figure 5a-c) (12). Subsequently images of PHFs have been analyzed more rigorously and objectively by image reconstruction (13). The results of the two approaches are in good agreement.

The use of image reconstruction techniques is complicated both by the lack of straightness and by the variable loop length observed in PHFs (Figure 4a-e). Computational techniques were therefore used to straighten filaments and to interpolate the images to constant loop length. After such treatment the computed diffraction patterns (Figure 4g-h) reproducibly show the first four orders of the 80 nm cross-over spacing. Combining such data from several images, it is possible to compute an average cross-sectional map through the PHF (Figure 5d-e), thus defining the internal structure of the regularly repeating subunit from which the PHF is constructed. The overall cross-section is elongated and the changing aspect produced by the helical arrangement thus gives rise to the wide to narrow modulation characteristic of PHFs. Each subunit appears to consist of three domains, the arrangement of which gives it an overall C-shape with a large central cleft. From the longitudinal fragmentation patterns it is unlikely that this cleft represents a subunit boundary. Rather when the two halves of a PHF separate, the cleavage occurs in the region of contact between the C-shaped subunits, establishing them as structural subunits. The lining up in an axial direction of these domains gives rise to the characteristic pattern of three and four longitudinal striations within a loop seen in the original micrographs. The pattern arises from the changing superposition of the domains of the subunit as these rotate helically and not from a protofilamentous organization, as has been suggested as an alternative interpretation of the structure (14, 15).

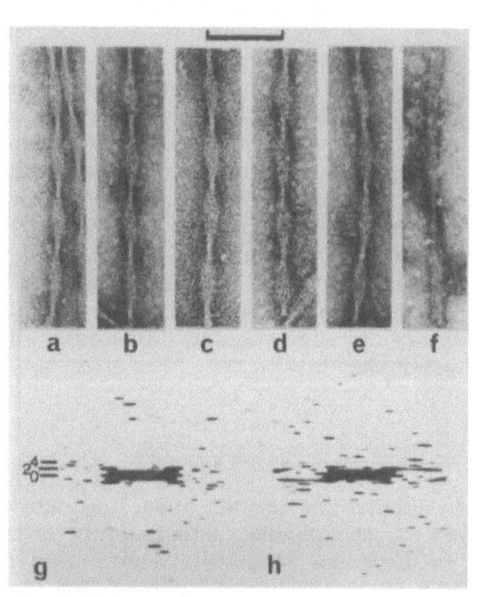

Figure 4: (a)-(f) Electron micrographs of PHF's negatively stained with lithium phosphotungstate. The filaments (a)-(e) are in a native conformation but the untwisted ribbon-like fragment in (f) results from treatment of PHF's on the grid with strong alkali. Scale bar 100 nm. (g)-(h) Computed diffraction patterns (Fourier transforms) of the two particles shown in (a) and (b), with the first four layer lines of the 80 nm cross-over spacing indicated. This figure is taken from Crowther and Wischik (1985).

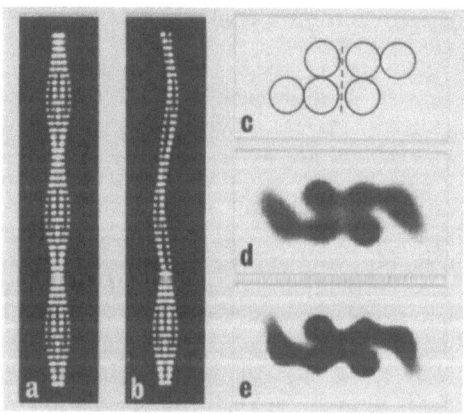

Figure 5: Structure of the PHF. (a) and (b) are simulated images of PHF's showing respectively a whole and a half filament, based on a helical arrangement of the three domain model subunit shown in cross-section in (c) (Wischik et al., 1985). The dotted line in (c) indicates the likely boundary between subunits in the two strands, based on the observed longitudinal splitting into the half PHF. (d) and (e) are two independently computed cross-sections coming from different sets of micrographs. That shown in (d) comes from the PHF's in Figure 4 (Crowther and Wischik, 1985). The computed cross-sections show a subunit consisting, like the crude model in (c), of three domains, though bent more markedly into a C-shape.

4. Comparison of PHFs with amyloid-like fibrils

Our crude preparations of PHFs contain small amounts of a much thinner fibril, which morphologically resembles the amyloid fibrils isolated from Alzheimer plaque cores (3, 16) or from other types of amyloidosis

(4). These thinner fibrils usually occur in clumps, sometimes of large size, which we presume represent the remnants of plaque cores. The small clump shown in Figure 6 was chosen because the fibrils are well stained and because there are PHFs close by for direct comparison. The amyloid-like fibrils are about 10 nm in diameter at their widest, narrowing to about 6 nm in diameter every 30-40 nm and they seem to consist of two sub-fibrils wound round one another. The axes of the fibrils appear to trace a rather irregular path. The morphology of the amyloid--like fibrils is clearly quite different from that of whole PHFs and, more importantly, quite different from that of half PHFs (Figure 3b). It therefore seems unlikely that the PHF consists of a pair or tetrad of these amyloid-like fibrils.

Figure 6: Comparison between PHF's (lower part) and amyloid-like fibrils (upper part), sometimes found in the preparations of PHF's and believed to represent the remnants of plaque cores. The two amyloid-like fibrils arrowed show the twisted structure particularly clearly. Scale bar 100 nm.

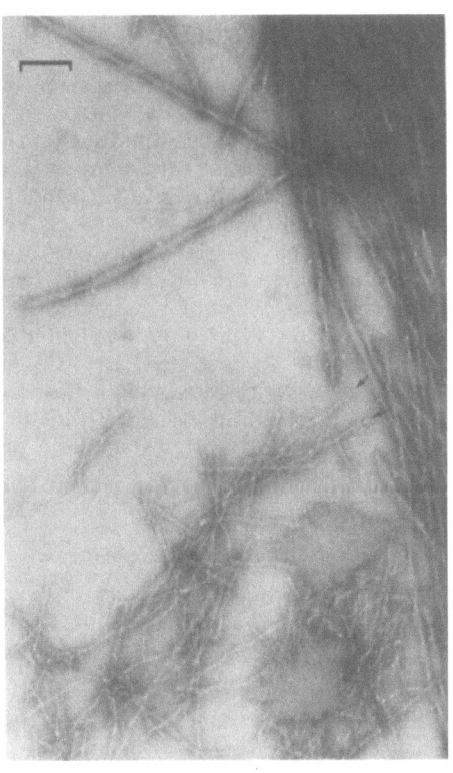

5. Discussion

Our current view of the PHF, summarized in Figure 5, is that it consists of two structural strands of subunits. Each subunit is of small (3nm) axial extent and contains three domains. Estimates of the stain excluding volume of the structural subunit suggest that is has a molecular weight of about 200 Kdalton, but exact positions of boundaries are difficult to locate in negatively stained material. A more precise method of determining the mass distribution is required, such as STEM (scanning transmission electron microscope) measurements of unstained specimens and this we are attempting to do. It is possible that the three-domained structural subunit we have described comprises more than one polypeptide chain.

The biochemical nature of the PHF core subunit is unknown. Recent immunocytochemical results (reviewed by Miller et al (17)) have suggested that PHFs contain epitopes in common with the side arms of both the 210 Kdalton neurofilament protein and the microtubule associated protein 2 (MAP 2), but there is no compelling evidence that these epitopes are intrinsic to the PHF core structure. Cerebrovascular amyloid from Alzheimer brains contains a 4 Kdalton polypeptide (18, 19) and plaque core amyloid contains a similar peptide with almost identical N-terminal sequence (20). However the results of Roher et al (16), with a different amino acid composition, suggest that plaque cores consist of a large protein or a heterogeneous mixture of medium-sized proteins. It has been suggested (21) that the neurofibrillary tangle and hence the PHF itself also consists of an aggregate of the 4 Kdalton polypeptide. However, antibodies raised to a synthetic peptide homologous to the N-terminus of cerebrovascular amyloid, which cross-react with neuritic plaque amyloid, fail to cross-react with neurofibrillary tangles (22).

On the basis of our structural studies presented here it is hard to understand how the PHF subunit could arise entirely from an assembly of a repeating 4 Kdalton polypeptide. Moreover as discussed above, the morphology of PHFs and amyloid-like fibrils is quite different. It is thus difficult to see how the PHF could be formed from a simple assembly of amyloid-like fibrils. Rather the PHF appears to be the sort of structure that might arise by the _de novo_ assembly of a large subunit, possibly arising from an aberrant protein, whose biochemical nature is still to be discovered.

References

1. Cohen, A.S. Int. Rev. Exp. Pathol. 4, 159-243, 1965.
2. Kidd, M. Nature 197, 192-193, 1963.
3. Merz, P.A., Wisniewski, H.M., Somerville, R.A. et al. Acta Neuropathol. 60, 113-124, 1983.
4. Cohen, A.S., Shirahama, T. & Skinner, M. In Electron Microscopy of Proteins Vol. 3. Harris, J.R., Ed. Academic Press, London, 165-205, 1982.
5. Terry, R.D. & Wisniewski, H.M. In Alzheimer's Disease and Related Conditions. Wolstenholme, G.W., O'Connor, M.O., Eds. Churchill, London, 145-168, 1970.
6. Kidd, M. Brain 87, 307-320, 1964.
7. Roth, M., Tomlinson, B.E. & Blessed, G. Proc. Roy. Soc. Med. 60, 254-260, 1967.
8. Blessed, G., Tomlinson, B.E. & Roth, M. Br. J. Psychiatry 114, 797-811, 1968.
9. Wilcock, G.K. & Esiri, M.M. J. Neurol. Sci. 56, 343-356, 1982.
10. Mountjoy, C.Q., Rossor, M.N., Iverson, L.L. & Roth, M. Brain 107, 507-518, 1984.
11. Mountjoy, C.Q., Roth, M., Evans, N.J.R. & Evans, H.M. Neurobiol. Aging 4, 1-11, 1983.
12. Wischik, C.M., Crowther, R.A., Stewart, M. & Roth, M. J. Cell Biol. 100, 1905-1912, 1985.
13. Crowther, R.A. & Wischik, C.M. EMBO J. 4, 3661-3665, 1985.
14. Wisniewski, H.M., Merz, P.A. & Iqbal, K. J. Neuropathol. Exp. Neurol.43, 643-656, 1984.
15. Wisniewski, H.M. & Wen, G.Y. Acta Neuropathol. 66, 173-176, 1985.

16.Roher, A., Wolfe, D., Palutke, M. & KuKuruga, D. Proc. Natl. Acad. Sci. USA 83, 2662-2666, 1986.
17.Miller, C., Haugh, M., Kahn, J. & Anderton, B. Trends in Neurosciences 9, 76-81, 1986.
18.Glenner, G.G. & Wong, C.W. Biochem. Biophys. Res. Commun. 120, 885-890, 1984.
19.Glenner, G.G. & Wong, C.W. Biochem. Biophys. Res. Commun. 122, 1131-1135, 1984.
20.Masters, C.L., Simms, G., Weinman, N.A. et al. Proc. Natl. Acad. Sci. USA 82, 4245-4249, 1985.
21.Masters, C.L., Multhaup, G., Simms, G. et al. EMBO J. 4, 2757-2763, 1985.
22.Wong, C.W., Quaranta, V. & Glenner, G.G. Proc. Natl. Acad. Sci. USA 82, 8729-8732, 1985.

IV.9 THE SIGNIFICANCE OF NON-PROTEIN AA MATERIAL IN
WATER-SOLUBLE BOVINE AA-AMYLOID FIBRILS

Adriaan C.J. van Andel, Theo A. Niewold, Bert T.G. Lutz,
Marcel W.J. Messing and Erik Gruys

Department of Veterinary Pathology, University of Utrecht,
P.O. Box 80.158,
3508 TD Utrecht, The Netherlands.

1. Introduction

The electron microscopically rigid, non-branching amyloid fibrils can
be extracted from amyloid containing tissue with distilled water after
removal of more soluble materials by repeated saline washings (1). A
common feature of all types of amyloid fibrils is their β-pleated sheet
structure (2). They can be solubilized by treatment with chaotropic
agents like urea or guanidine plus a reducing agent. Gel filtration after
solubilization generally gives two major fractions: a high molecular
weight amyloid fibril type-unspecific void-volume fraction and an
amyloid fibril type-specific low molecular weight fraction. Minor fractions of intermediate molecular weight are also frequently observed
(2-5). In reactive and some idiopathic cases of amyloidosis, the low
molecular weight fraction contains a 8-10,000 dalton polypeptide
designated protein AA. The amino acid sequence of protein AA is
homologous to the amino terminal portion of the 12,000 dalton serum
amyloid A protein, SAA. Recently evidence has been presented
supporting that protein SAA can be deposited as amyloid A fibrils in
vivo (6). The minor intermediate weight fractions in AA-amyloid are
described as showing a relation to amyloid P-component (7) which is not
a structural amyloid protein (8), to protein AA (9) and to protein SAA
(10). Moreover, intermediate weight proteins with a molecular weight
larger than 12,000 dalton might be protein AA dimers (11).

Although even very pure amyloid fibril preparations contain considerable amounts of void-volume material, it is still unclear whether it
represents an integral part of the fibril or not (12). The void-volume
fraction has not yet been completely characterized. Immunological
similarities have been found between the V_o-fractions of various amyloid
types and the presence of normal tissue components has been described
(12-14). By extraction and reaggregation studies we have tried to determine whether the V_o-material represents a structural fibril component
or a contaminant.

2.Materials and methods

2.1.Isolation of amyloid fibrils

Amyloid fibrils were isolated from renal papillae (C_1-C_4) of cattle with spontaneous idiopathic AA-amyloidosis (5) using the water extraction method of Pras et al (1). Briefly, $\pm$ 30 gram wet tissue was homogenized in 200 ml 0.15 M NaCl on ice for 5 minutes. The homogenate obtained was subsequently centrifuged at 48,000 g for 30 minutes. This procedure was repeated with the pellet until the supernatant showed an OD_{280} < 0.1. The pellet was then homogenized in 100 ml distilled water and centrifuged at 48,000 g for 30 minutes. This was repeated 7 times. Amyloid fibrils were present in the water extracts 2-7. The renal papillae of non-amyloidotic cattle (C_5-C_7) were subjected to the same procedure, yielding a normal tissue preparation (15). All water extracts were stored at -20 $^{\circ}$C.

2.2.Extraction experiments

In a first experiment water soluble amyloid fibrils (approximately 20 mg) were precipitated with 2 mM $CaCl_2$ and collected by centrifugation. The wet amyloid fibrils were subsequently homogenized in 5 ml 0.55 M Tris-HCl buffer, pH 7.0, containing either 1% Triton or 10 mM EDTA or 0.1 M dithiothreitol or in 5 ml Tris-HCl, 10 mM EDTA, pH 7.0, containing 1 or 2 M guanidine, with and without the addition of 0.1 M dithiothreitol and centrifuged for 30 min. at 50,000 g (Table I). This procedure was repeated three times with the residues. The combined supernatants and residues were dialyzed against distilled water and lyophilized.

In a second experiment wet purified amyloid fibrils (C_1-C_3) and a normal tissue extract (C_5) were extracted as above with 0.55 M Tris-HCl buffer, pH 7.0, containing 5 mM EDTA. This procedure was repeated until the optical density of the supernatants was < 0.1 at 280 nm. The obtained residues and extracts were dialyzed against distilled water and lyophilized. Samples were analyzed by Congo red staining (16), gel filtration, electron microscopy and infrared spectroscopy (4).

2.3.Gel filtration and reaggregation experiments

Samples were solubilized (1-2 mg/ml) in 0.55 M Tris-HCl buffer, pH 8.5, containing 2 mM EDTA, 0.1 M dithiothreitol and 6 M guanidine (Gu-HCl-TED buffer). After filtration through a 0.22 μM Millex GV filter, 100 μl aliquots were gel-filtered on a Superose 12 column (Pharmacia, Uppsala, Sweden) equilibrated with 50 mM Tris-HCl buffer, pH 8.6, containing 6 M guanidine. The composition of the samples was estimated from the peak areas at 280 nm.

Solubilized samples were allowed to reaggregate by dialysis against 1 M acetic acid or 0.55 M Tris-HCl as described (3,4).

3. Results

3.1. Isolation of amyloid fibrils and normal tissue extracts

Application of the water extraction method of Pras et al (1) on amyloid laden renal papillae of C_{1-4} yielded water soluble amyloid fibril preparations of C_{1-3}. Amyloid fibrils, however, were also observed in the saline washings and the residues of C_{1-4}. No water soluble amyloid fibrils could be obtained from the renal papillae of C_4. The gel filtration profiles of the solubilized amyloid preparations were all similar and revealed a major void volume fraction with a shoulder, two minor intermediate fractions, and a major retarded fraction (protein AA). On going from the 2nd to the 7th water extract a gradual increase of the protein AA fraction and a concomitant decrease of the void volume fraction was noted. In the last extracts a high molecular weight non-void volume peak became apparent (Fig. 1).

Figure 1(bottom): Gel filtration on Superose 12 in 6 M guanidine, 50 mM Tris-HCl (pH 8.6) of the solubilized amyloid fibril water extracts 3, 5 and 7 of C_2 and the solubilized normal tissue preparation (N) of C_5.

Figure 2(right): Gel filtration on Superose 12 in 6 M guanidine, 50 mM Tris-HCl (pH 8.6) of varying guanidine solubilized amyloid fibril fractions of C_2:(A) Water soluble amyloid fibrils, (B) the combined first four Tris/EDTA extracts, (C) the residue after four Tris/EDTA extractions, (D) the residue after exhaustive Tris/EDTA extractions.

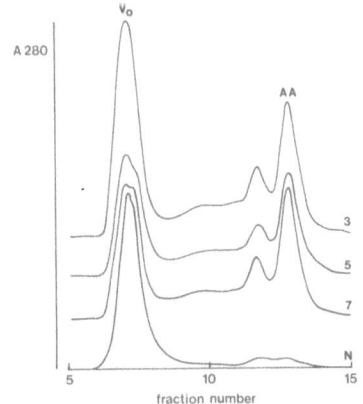

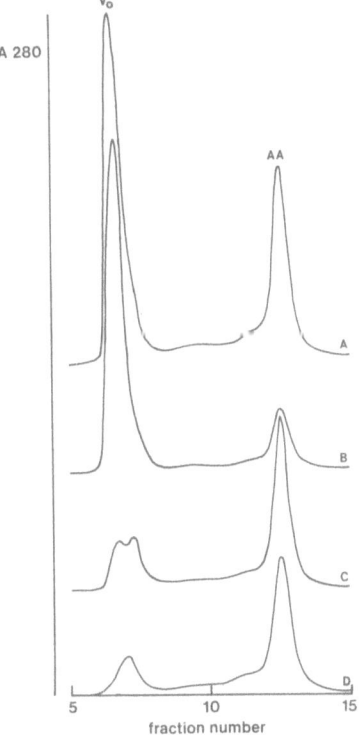

Subjection of normal bovine renal papillae to the water extraction method yielded normal tissue preparations neither showing fibrils on electron microscopy nor any green birefringence after Congo red staining. On gel filtration these preparations revealed large void volume fractions and some retarded material (Fig. 1).

3.2. Extractions

All extracts and residues obtained by further extracting water soluble amyloid fibrils (C_1) with varying buffers for four times (Table I) did stain with Congo red and exhibited apple green birefringence in polarized light. On negative contrast electron microscopy characteristic amyloid fibrils were observed in all extracts and residues.

TABLE I: EXTRACTION OF WATER-SOLUBLE AA-AMYLOID FIBRILS (C_1) FOR FOUR TIMES WITH VARYING BUFFERS

		% extracted[#]	Observed peak area at 280 nm on gel filtration in 6 M guanidine/50 mM Tris-HCl, pH 8.6	
			HMW fraction	retarded fractions
0.55 M Tris-HCl/6 M guanidine/5 mM EDTA/0.1 M DTT, pH 7.0	extract	100 %	55 %	45%
	residue	0 %		
0.55 M Tris-HCl/5 mM EDTA, pH 7.0	extract	60 %	75 %	25 %
	residue	40 %	25 %	75 %
0.55 M Tris-HCl/1 % Tween, pH 7.0	extract	*	67 %	33 %
	residue	*	32 %	68 %
0.55 M Tris-HCl/0.1 M DTT, pH 7.0	extract	61 %	74 %	26 %
	residue	39 %	26 %	74 %
0.55 M Tris-HCl/1 M guanidine/5 mM EDTA, pH 7.0	extract	62 %	75 %	25 %
	residue	38 %	22 %	78 %
0.55 M Tris-HCl/1 M guanidine/5 mM EDTA/0.1 M DTT, pH 7.0	extract	73 %	70 %	30 %
	residue	27 %	14 %	86 %
0.55 M tris-HCl/2 M guanidine/5 mM EDTA, pH 7.0	extract	94 %	56 %	44 %
	residue	6 %	38 %	62 %
0.55 M Tris-HCl/2 M guanidine/5 mM EDTA/0.1 M DTT, pH 7.0	extract	96 %	50 %	50 %
	residue	4 %	54 %	46 %

DTT = dithiothreitol
HMW = high molecular weight fraction. The HMW-fraction is composed of a V_o peak and a slightly retarded fraction.
 * = data were influenced by the presence of Tween.
 # = percentage was calculated from the gelfiltration profile assuming no changes took place in the ratio of the retarded peaks.

Gel filtration of the solubilized fibrils of C_1 revealed that the high molecular weight fraction constituted approximately 55 % of the fibril material. In the extracts obtained using the varying Tris buffers the high molecular weight fraction represented approximately 75 % of the fibril material. In the residues, however, only $\pm$ 25 % eluted in the high molecular weight fraction, composed of a void volume peak and a slightly retarded fraction (Fig. 2).

Gel filtration of the solubilized residues obtained by exhaustive extraction of the water soluble fibrils with a Tris/EDTA buffer, revealed a slightly retarded high molecular weight non-void volume peak, two intermediate weight fractions and a major retarded protein AA fraction. Upon exhaustive extraction of the 2 mM $CaCl_2$ precipitate of normal tissue preparation (C_5) with a Tris/EDTA buffer >95 % of the material was recovered. The residue and extract of the normal tissue preparation of C_4 showed similar gel filtration profiles after solubilization i.e. a void volume fraction accounting for 89 % of the material and a small amount of retarded material (Fig. 1).

3.3. Reaggregation experiments

The reaggregates formed on dialysis of the solubilized extract and residue obtained by exhaustive extraction of water soluble amyloid fibrils with a Tris/EDTA buffer revealed electronmicroscopically fibrillar and at Congo red staining green birefringent material. The reaggregate formed from the solubilized residue, however, showed more numerous areas of green birefringent material (Table II).

TABLE II: CHARACTERISTICS OF THE REAGGREGATES

	dialysis against	Prec.	CR	EM	IR		
Residue	1 M acetic acid	+++	+++	+++	1630	1655	1695 cm^{-1}
	0.55 M Tris pH 7,0	++	++	++	1630	1655	1695 cm^{-1}
Extract	1 M acetic acid	+++	+	++	1628	1650	1695 cm^{-1}
	0.55 M Tris pH 7.0	++	+/-	+++	1630	1653	1695 cm^{-1}

Prec. : formation of precipitates.
CR   : green birefringence in polarized light after staining with Congo red.
EM   : fibrillar appearance on electronmicroscopy.
IR   : main features of the amide 1 band of the infra-red spectra

3.4. Infrared spectroscopy

The infrared spectra of native amyloid fibrils display in the amide 1 band absorptions at 1635 and 1655 cm^{-1} indicating β-pleated sheet and coil/α-helix as the major conformations (4). The residues obtained by exhaustive extraction of the water soluble amyloid fibrils with Tris/EDTA buffer revealed a similar ($C_{1,2}$) or a slightly more intense absorption at 1635 cm^{-1} (C_3) than the water soluble amyloid fibrils. The absorptions at 1635 and 1655 cm^{-1} in the infrared spectra of the native fibrils appeared to be shifted to lower wavenumbers in the reaggregates (Table II) indicating minor differences in conformation between the native amyloid fibrils and the reaggregates.

4. Discussion

During the isolation of the water soluble amyloid fibrils it was noted that in some cases considerable amounts of amyloid fibrils appeared in the saline washings. Large amounts of amyloid fibrils were also found in the residues after completion of the water extraction. This shows that one may find amyloid fibril "subpopulations" within one patient differing considerably in their solubility characteristics. Gel filtration of the solubilized amyloid fibrils from subsequent distilled water extracts revealed that the first extracts contained relatively large V_o-fractions and small protein AA fractions, while the last extracts contained relatively small V_o-fractions and large protein AA peaks. This indicates that the amyloid fibrils in subsequent water extracts differs in composition and/or contains varying amounts of high molecular weight contaminants.

Extraction of pooled water soluble amyloid fibrils with varying Tris--buffers yielded extracts containing large V_o-fractions and residues with small V_o-fractions. In the residues a slightly retarded fraction became apparent, seen only as a shoulder of the V_o-fraction in the gel filtration profile of the solubilized water extracts. The extraction was not significantly influenced by the addition of dithiothreitol, Tween-20, EDTA or 1 M guanidine to the Tris buffers. This suggests that the separation is based on differences in solubility of the amyloid fibril "subpopulations" in the Tris-buffer. Exhaustive extraction of water soluble amyloid with Tris/EDTA buffer yielded a residue virtually devoid of void volume material. This shows that there is at least a "subpopulation" of amyloid fibrils containing no void volume material. Reaggregation of the solubilized residue and extract revealed more green birefringent material after Congo red staining in the reaggregate formed by the residue. It is therefore concluded that the void volume material is not a necessarily integral part of the AA-amyloid fibril. The minor intermediate fractions and the slightly retarded high molecular weight fraction, however, are likely to represent integral amyloid fibril proteins.

Virtually all of the amyloid void volume material and normal tissue preparation are recovered from the Tris/EDTA extract. Immunologically the amyloid void volume fraction shows cross-reactivity with normal tissue components (13). This strongly suggests the void volume fraction to be a contaminant in the amyloid fibril preparation. The extracts, however, also contained amyloid fibrils which could not be sedimented by centrifugation for 30 minutes at 100,000 g. Therefore it is suggested that part of the void volume material is closely associated with an amyloid fibril "subpopulation" soluble in Tris-buffers.

References

1.Pras, M., Schubert, M., Zucker-Franklin, D., et al. J. Clin. Invest. 47, 924-933, 1968.
2.Glenner, G.G. & Page, D.L. Int. Rev. Exp. Pathol. 15, 1-92, 1976.
3.Hol, P.R., Langeveld, J.P.M., Beuningen-Jansen, E.W. van, et al. Scand. J. Immunol. 20, 53-60, 1984.
4.Andel, A.C.J. van, Hol, P.R., Maas, J.H. van der, et al. In Amyloidosis. Glenner, G.G., Osserman, E.F., Benditt, E.P., Calkins, E., Cohen, A.S., Zucker-Franklin, D., Eds. Plenum Press, New York, 39-48, 1986.
5.Gruys, E. & Timmermans, H. Vet. Sci. Commun. 3, 21-37, 1979.
6.Husebekk, A., Skogen, B., Husby, G. & Marhaug, G. Scand. J. Immunol. 21, 283-287, 1985.
7.Holck, M., Husby, G., Sletten, K. & Natvig J.B. Scand. J. Immunol. 10, 55-60, 1979.
8.Pepys, M.B., Dash, A.C., Munn, E.A., et al. Lancet i, 1029-1031, 1977.
9.Lian, J.B., Benson, M.D., Skinner, M. & Cohen, A.S. Arch. Biochem. Biophys. 171, 197-205, 1975.
10.Westermark, P. & Sletten, K. Clin. Exp. Immunol. 49, 725-731, 1982.
11.Eriksen, N. & Benditt, E.P. In Amyloidosis. Glenner, G.G., Osserman, E.F., Benditt, E.P., Calkins, E., Cohen, A.S., Zucker-Franklin, D., Eds. Plenum Press, New York, 3-10, 1986.
12.Husby, G. & Sletten, K. Acta Pathol. Microbiol. Scand. (C) 85, 153-160, 1977.
13.Natvig, J.B., Westermark, P., Sletten, K., et al. Scand. J. Immunol. 14, 89-94, 1981.
14.Scott, D.L., Marhaug, G. & Husby, G. Clin. Exp. Med. 52, 693-701, 1983.
15.Pras, M. & Glynn, L.E. Br. J. Exp. Path. 54, 449-456, 1973.
16.Romhanyi, G. Virchows Arch. [A] 354, 209-222, 1971.

IV.10 FIBRIL DERIVED AMYLOID ENHANCING FACTOR (FAEF) IN HAMSTER: EVIDENCE FOR A CLOSE RELATIONSHIP BETWEEN AEF AND AA-AMYLOID FIBRILS

Theo A. Niewold, Adriaan C.J. van Andel, Paul R. Hol and Erik Gruys

Department of Veterinary Pathology, University of Utrecht
P.O. box 80.158,
3508 TD Utrecht, The Netherlands.

1. Introduction

In AA-amyloidosis, the most frequently occurring type of amyloidosis, the major component of the amyloid fibril is a 8,000 to 10,000 dalton protein, the protein AA (1). The latter is formed in tissues by degradation of its precursor serum amyloid protein A (SAA) which is an acute phase reactant synthetized by hepatocytes(2).

Sustained high levels of SAA in patients with chronic inflammatory diseases, predispose them to AA-amyloidosis but only a small percentage actually develops amyloidosis (3). In laboratory animals AA-amyloidosis can be induced experimentally by repeated injections of inflammation inducing substances. They develop high levels of SAA and, different from the situation in man, all do develop amyloidosis after some weeks or months (4).

The conjunction of circumstances that actually results in the formation of amyloid fibrils is not clear. High levels of the precursor alone are not sufficient. Other possible contributing factors are the existence of amyloidogenic species of SAA (5), and an impaired SAA-catabolism. It was demonstrated that mononuclear phagocytes from amyloidotic animals degrade SAA partially into an AA-like product, whereas the same cells from non-amyloidotic animals completely degraded SAA (6). Miura et al (7) suggest that the organs of preference for amyloid deposition, spleen, liver and kidney, are involved in the normal pathway of SAA-catabolism, showing an abnormal catabolism in amyloidosis.

Neither hypotheses provide an answer to the question of how fibrils are constituted from the produced protein-AA. Purified protein-AA alone does not spontaneously form amyloid fibrils. From in vitro reconstitution experiments it is known that other components of isolated fibrils are essential (8). The nature of these components is unclear, they could be normal tissue (matrix) components (9). Preceding amyloid deposition an increased vascular permeability is demonstrable in the organs of preference (10), enabling SAA to encounter matrix factors (11).

Another factor of importance is the amyloid enhancing factor (AEF). This factor considerably shortens the amyloid induction time in ex-

177

perimental amyloidosis. It can be isolated from organs of (pre)-
amyloidotic animals and from cases of spontaneous amyloidosis, being
able to cross interspecies borders. Furthermore, extracts can be made
of spleens from patients with other types of amyloidosis, enhancing
amyloidosis in mice (Table I). The exact nature of AEF is unknown. As
described (12,13), AEF is neither to be related to amyloid fibrils, nor
to be associated with them. In contradiction to this, in mice AEF-
-activity increased simultaneously with increasing amyloid deposition
(14). Evenmore, AEF can only be isolated from amyloidotic animals or
animals that are amyloidogenically stimulated. In addition to that, in a
transplantation experiment with mice an amyloidotic spleen was placed on
one of the kidneys and amyloid was deposited in the vicinity of the
transplanted amyloid (15). These data suggest an association of AEF
with the amyloid substance.

To investigate whether the AEF is associated with amyloid fibril or
not, we have tried to isolate AEF from purified hamster amyloid fibrils.

TABLE I: LITERATURE DATA ON ENHANCEMENT OF INDUCED AMYLOIDOSIS[#]
Pre-amyloidotic or amyloidotic donor factors were given to recipient animals that received
an SAA-inducing treatment (irradiation, nitrogen mustard, casein, silver nitrate).

Donor	Source	Nature	Acceptor	AEF	Characteristics	Ref
Mouse	spleen	whole cells	mouse	+		15[*]
	spleen	T-cells	"	-		"
	lung	whole cells	"	+		"
	thymus	"	"	-		"
	liver	"	"	+		"
	bone marrow	"	"	-		"
	periton. macrophages	"	"	-		"
	lymph nodes	"	"	-		"
	ly-cytes	"	"	-		"
	spleen	graft	"	+		"
	spleen	nuclear fraction	"	+		"
	spleen	DNA/RNA	"	+		"
	spleen	homogenate	"	+		"
Mouse	spleen	reticular cells	"	+		16
	spleen	homogenate/fr.	"	+	M.W. <15,000 d	17
	spleen/ly-nodes	whole cells	"	+		18
	liver	homogenate	"	+		18
	spleen	homogenate	"	+		19
	spleen	extracts	"	+	glycoprotein	12
	liver	extracts	"	+		12
Hamster	spleen/liver	homogenate/fr.	hamster	+	M.W. >12,000 d	13
Man	spleen	homogenate	mouse	+		20
Man	spleen	fractions	mouse	+	glycoprotein	21
Cattle	kidney	homogenate	mouse	+		22
Dog	blood	serum	mouse	+		23
Man	spleen	homogenate/fr.	mouse	+		24
Man	spleen (AL)	homogenate/fr.	mouse	+		24
Man	spleen (Aprealb.)	homogenate/fr.	mouse	+		24
Hamster	liver	amyloid fibrils	hamster	+	M.W. >50,000 d	**

[#] all donors had AA amyloidosis if not indicated otherwise; all recipients developed AA
  amyloidosis.
[*] data from separate experiments as reviewed in (15)
** this study.
d= dalton.

2. Materials and methods

Fibril AEF (FAEF) was extracted from water purified (25) hamster amyloid fibrils. Briefly, lyophilized hamster amyloid fibrils were extensively sonificated in Tris/HCl buffer (0.5 M, pH 7.6). After centrifugation (30 min, 50,000 g) the supernatant was taken off and the procedure repeated using the residue. In the underlying experiment the supernatants of the 5th, 6th and 7th extraction were pooled. This pool was tested for AEF-activity in hamsters by intraperitoneal injection as described (13). The extract was subjected to Sephadex G-50 gel filtration. Lyophilized samples of the extract, the original fibrils and the residue after centrifugation were analyzed on Superose-12 gel filtration (Pharmacia) in guanidine (to be published elsewhere).

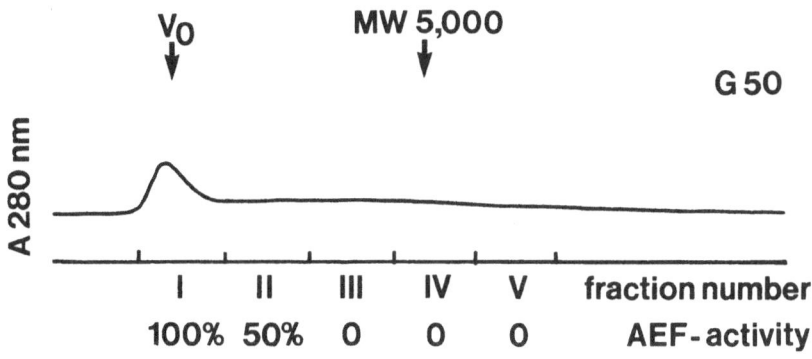

Figure 1: Sephadex G-50 elution profile of the fibril extract. AEF-activity: expressed as percentage of animals (n=6) which developed amyloidosis after 7 days of casein/LPS treatment upon injection of the corresponding fraction in hamsters.

3. Results

From hamster amyloid fibrils an extract was obtained which evidently had AEF-activity. All animals injected with the extract and subsequent casein/LPS treatment developed splenic and hepatic amyloidosis within 7 days, whereas the animals that received only the extract or only casein/LPS did not. Upon Sephadex G-50 gel filtration the extract appeared to contain proteinaceous material of >50,000 dalton only (Fig. 1). Preliminary experiments showed that the AEF-activity was restrained to this peak. Superose-12 gel filtration in guanidine of this material indicated that it was almost identical to the original amyloid fibrils, apart from a higher proportion of high molecular weight proteins in the extract (Fig. 2). The extracted material did not exhibit any green birefringence upon staining with Congo red and no amyloid fibrils were detectable by electron microscopical examination. We therefore conclude that our FAEF-extract very likely consists of small fibril fragments and that the AEF-activity is tightly associated with amyloid fibrils. Preliminary results showed the extract to be immunologically identical to the original fibrils on Western blotting. Furthermore, the extract appeared to contain a β-pleated sheet conformation similar to the original fibrils, as judged by infra-red spectroscopy (to be published).

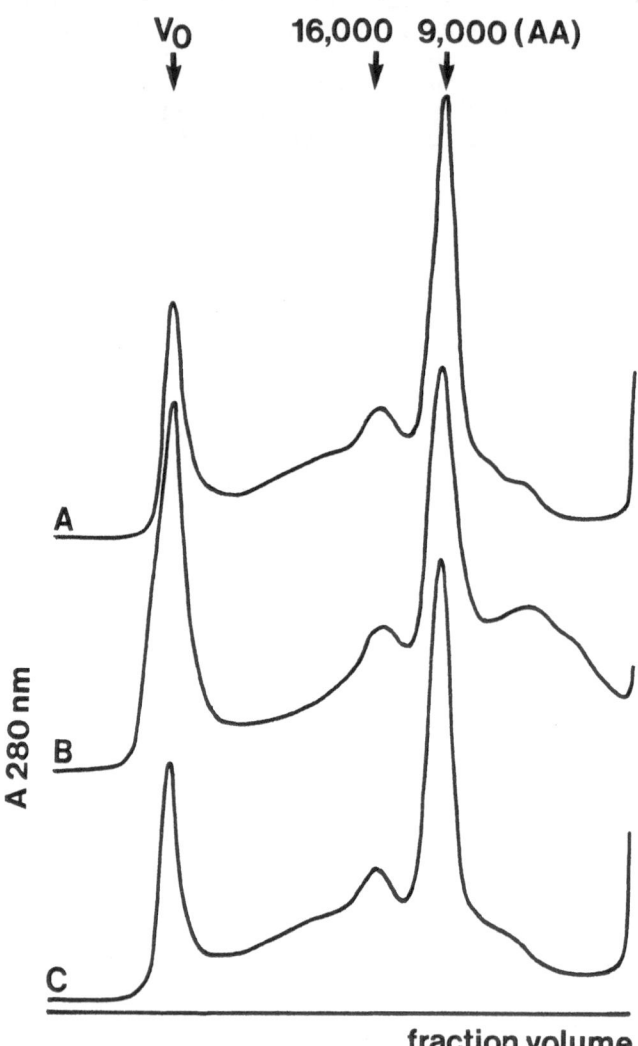

Figure 2: Superose-12 elution profiles of the original fibrils (A), the extract (B) and the residue (C). Note the occurrence of a 16,000 dalton peak, a distinct 9,000 dalton protein AA peak and material of lower molecular weight.

4.Discussion

In mice AEF can be isolated from tissue shortly before amyloid deposits are histologically detectable (14). Very small amounts of amyloid, however, are not encountered by this method, i.e. so called pre-amyloidotic animals could be in fact already amyloidotic. Moreover AEF-activity increased simultaneously with increasing amyloid deposition (14). Tissue derived AEF-preparations from both mice (12) and hamster (13) did not contain any protein AA-cross reactive material. This could be due to the low sensitivity of the techniques used. It remains possible that AEF is indeed not immunologically related to protein AA, being an important non-protein AA component of the fibril. The finding that from spleens of cases of non AA-amyloidosis in man extracts can be made that enhance AA-amyloidosis in mice support this possibility (24). Non-protein AA components have been found in purified amyloid fibril preparations. Some are identified as normal tissue components (9). It was also demonstrated that non protein AA components are essential for fibril formation in in vitro reaggregation experiments (26). The coincidence of occurrence of AEF with amyloid makes it unlikely that AEF is identical to a normal tissue constituent. In this context the role of AEF in fibril formation is rather one of initiation of fibrillogenesis than one of aggregation.

AEF is thought to be of proteinaceous nature (likely a glycoprotein) and capable of forming a complex with itself and other molecules (13), which is possibly an explanation for the conflicting data on the size of the AEF-molecule (Table I). According to us AEF could be an intrinsic part of the amyloid fibril, essential for fibril formation and thereby catalyzing its own production. This hypothesis of a selfgenerating AEF may provide an explanation for the fatal course of amyloid disease once amyloid deposits are formed. Presumably, our FAEF-extract consists of small fibril fragments (being the AEF or containing it), serving as a template for fibrils to grow on. Research is in progress in order to elucidate the nature of the FAEF and that of the classical tissue AEF-preparations.

References

1.Husby, G. Scand. J. Rheumatol. 9, 60-64, 1980.
2.Ramadori, G., Sipe, J.D., Dinarello, C.A., et al. J. Exp. Med. 162, 930-942, 1985.
3.Franklin, E.C. & Gorevic, P.D. In Progress in Immunology IV, vol 3, Fougereau, M. & Dausset, J., Eds. Academic Press, London, 1219-1230, 1980.
4.Sipe, J.D., McAdam, K.P.W.J. & Uchino, F. Lab. Invest. 38, 110-114, 1978.
5.Hoffman, J.S., Ericcson, L.H., Eriksen, N. et al. J. Exp. Med. 159, 641-646, 1984.
6.Fuks, A. & Zucker-Franklin, D. J. Exp. Med. 161, 1013-1028, 1985.
7.Miura, K., Takahashi, Y. & Shirasawa, H. Lab. Invest. 53, 453-463, 1985.
8.Hol, P.R., Langeveld, J.P.M., van Beuningen-Jansen, E.W. et al. Scand. J. Immunol. 20, 53-60, 1984.
9.Scott, D.L., Marhaug, G. & Husby, G. Clin. Exp. Immunol. 52, 693-701, 1983.
10.Schultz, R.T. & Pitha, J. Am. J. Pathol. 119, 127-137, 1985.
11.Gruys, E. Thesis, University of Utrecht, Utrecht, 157-162, 1979.
12.Axelrad, M.A., Kisilevsky, R., Willmer, J.C. et al. Lab. Invest. 47, 139-146, 1982.
13.Hol, P.R., van Andel, A.C.J., van Ederen, A.M. et al. Br. J. Exp. Pathol. 66, 689-697, 1985.

14. Axelrad, M.A. & Kisilevsky, R. In Amyloid and Amyloidosis, Glenner, G.G., Costa, P.P., Freitas, A.F. Eds. Excerpta Medica, Amsterdam, 527-533, 1980.
15. Hardt, F. & Ranløv, P. Int. Rev. Exp. Pathol. 16, 273-334, 1976.
16. Jakob, W., Hilgenfeld, M. & Karasek, E. Exp. Pathol. 6, 141-144, 1972.
17. Kedar, I., Bleiberg, I. & Sohar, E. Br. J. Exp. Pathol. 56, 244-246, 1975.
18. Tanaka, O., Tsubura, E. & Tokushima J. Exp. Med. 25, 67-74, 1985.
19. Wohlgetan, J.R. & Cathcart, E.S. Lab. Invest. 42, 663-667, 1980.
20. Shirahama, T., Lawless, O.J. & Cohen, A.S. Proc. Soc. Biol. Med. 130, 516-519, 1969.
21. Keizman, I., Rimon, A., Sohar, E. & Gafni, J. Acta Pathol. Microbiol. Scand. [A] 80, Suppl. 233, 172-177, 1972.
22. Jakob, W. & Hilgenfeld, M. Zbl. Allg. Pathol. 116, 94-97, 1972.
23. Hilgenfeld, M. & Jakob, W. Z. Gesamte Inn. Med. 27, 60-63, 1972.
24. Varga, J., Flinn, M.S.M., Shirahama, T., et al. Virchows Arch. B. (Cell Pathol.) 51, 177-185, 1986.
25. Pras, M., Schubert, M., Zucker-Franklin, D. et al. J. Clin. Invest. 47, 924-933, 1968.
26. van Andel, A.C.J., Hol, P.R., van der Maas, J.H. et al. In Amyloidosis. Glenner, G.G., Osserman, E.F., Benditt, E.P., Calkins, E., Cohen, A.S., Zucker-Franklin, D., Eds. Plenum Press, New York, 39-48, 1986.

SECTION V

FAMILIAL AMYLOIDOSIS

sub-editor: Mordechai Pras

V.1 THE HEREDITARY AMYLOIDOSES

Mordechai Pras

Department of Internal Medicine
Heller Institute of Medical Research
Sackler School of Medicine, Tel-Aviv University
Sheba Medical Center
52621 Tel-Hashomer, Israel.

1. Introduction

The inherited amyloidoses represent nature's experimental models of amyloidosis in man and provide great promise as a research tool (1). Being genetically determined, their clinical course is highly predictable and investigations can be planned and carried out at various stages of the disease. Genetic disorders, when elucidated, have proven to be simple inborn errors of metabolism. Abnormal products of the metabolic aberrations already characterized biochemically in some of the genetic amyloidoses indicate that they may represent point mutations. Eventually, the aberrant metabolic pathways and the defective genes will be identified. This knowledge will permit detection and treatment of the affected before penetrance, be invaluable in genetic counseling and also provide important insights regarding amyloidosis in general and its pathogenesis.

The clinical syndromes of the inherited amyloidoses show considerable diversity. In some entities, this is due to localized, highly selective deposition of amyloid at very specific sites. Examples are deposition limited to the skin in familial lichen amyloidosis, the tumor and its metastases in familial medullary carcinoma of the thyroid, and meningeal and cerebral arterioles in hereditary cerebral hemorrhage (2-4). Most entities of hereditary amyloidosis are marked by systemic deposition. Even when amyloid deposition is widespread, it is not random. Factors apparently related to the nature of the amyloid or the ground substance in which it accumulates or both are responsible for a preferential affinity for certain vital organs, resulting in characteristic, entity-specific patterns of deposition and resultant clinical presentation (Table I) (5).

The inherited systemic amyloidoses can be divided accordingly into three groups:
1. In the nephropathic group, amyloidosis is manifest by proteinuria that progresses through the nephrotic syndrome to renal insufficiency. This group includes several diseases whose genetic heterogeneity is established by differences in the mode of inheritance, the absence or presence of pleiotropic effects of the mutant gene and differences in the pleiotropic manifestations when these occur. In studies of two entities that are genetically and clinically distinct, amyloid was of the AA type but biochemical heterogeneity remains to be established.

TABLE I: HEREDITARY AMYLOIDOSES

Clinical	Ethnic origin	Chemical characterization	
		Serum precursor protein	Amyloid variant* protein
SYSTEMIC			
Polyneuropathy Lower limb	Portuguese, Japanese, Swedish	Prealbumin	30 (met/val)
	Jewish	Prealbumin Prealbumin	33 (ile/phe) 49 (gly/thr)
Upper limb	German, Swiss	Prealbumin	84 (ser/ile)
Face	Finnish		
Cardiopathy	Danish	Prealbumin	
	German-English-Irish (Appalachian)	Prealbumin	60 (ala/thr)
Nephropathy			
FMF	Sephardic Jews, Turks, Armenians	SAA	
Urticaria, deafness	English, French	SAA	
LOCALIZED			
Cerebral hemorrhage	Icelandic, Dutch	gamma-trace	68 (glu/leu)

* position and type of substitution [e.g. methionine substituting valine at position 30]

2. In the neuropathic group the picture is dominated by a progressive symmetrical polyneuropathy. Three prototypic forms have emerged. One affects initially and predominately the lower extremities; a second, the upper extremities; and a third, the face. Autonomic dysfunction is severe in the first, moderate in the second and minimal in the last. The ethnic segregation of these clinical patterns and their constancy are indicative of genetic heterogeneity. Within the lower limb form, further genetic heterogeneity has been proven biochemically by the characterization of different variant prealbumins as the protein subunit of amyloid fibrils. Still another prealbumin is apparently the substrate of the upper limb form.

3. In the cardiopathic group, intractable heart failure leads to progressive incapacitation and death. There are suggestions that the protein component of their amyloid is also prealbumin.

In the following we shall emphasize those disorders whose amyloid protein has been fully characterized and for the sake of completeness, briefly review the remainder. It is noteworthy that no familial entity of immunoglobulin-related (AL-) amyloidosis has been reported to date.

2.Familial systemic amyloidosis dominated by nephropathy

2.1.Familial Mediterranean fever

The immigration of Sephardic Jewry from North African and Middle Eastern countries to Israel made possible the delineation of the clinical, genetic and pathologic features of familial Mediterranean fever (FMF) (6). Notable sequels of the interest stimulated by clinical research were water solubilization for the isolation and purification of amyloid (7), the first complete amino acid sequence analysis of an amyloid protein, amyloid A (or AA) protein obtained from a patient with FMF (8), and identification of the previously unknown acute phase reactant from which it derives, serum amyloid A protein (SAA) (9). AA-protein is a 9100 dalton polypeptide made up of 76 amino acids, completely homologous with the amino terminal portion of SAA. This highly characteristic amino terminal is laden with phenylalanine residues at positions 3,4,6 and 11:

Arg-Ser-Phe-Phe-Ser-Phe-Leu-Gly-Glu-Ala-Phe-

In contrast to immunoglobulin (AL)-related and prealbumin-related amyloidoses that have been found only in man, AA-protein is the major constituent of the amyloidosis that is ubiquitous in the animal kingdom (10). In man, AA-protein is the structural subunit of the more prevalent forms of amyloidosis, those that are acquired in association with a variety of predisposing diseases (e.g. tuberculosis, osteo-myelitis, rheumatoid arthritis, Hodgkin's disease) (8), inherited as in FMF (8), or idiopathic (11) in etiology.

FMF is the most common form of hereditary amyloidosis. Over 1500 patients with FMF are being treated by our group at the Heller Institute at Sheba Medical Center, Tel-Hashomer. Several hundreds have been reported from other countries, bringing the total to well over 2000 patients. The disease is transmitted as an autosomal recessive trait; it is the only known hereditary amyloidosis that is not transmitted by a dominant gene. The disorder is most common in Jews of Sephardi ancestry (6), Anatolian Turks (12), Armenians (13) and Arabs of the Middle East. The disease has two phenotypic manifestations which are independent of one another - amyloidosis and febrile attacks. In most patients febrile attacks precede clinical evidence of amyloidosis (phenotype I) but in some, amyloid nephrosis has been the first indication of disease (phenotype II) (14,15). Phenotype II can be diagnosed only if another member of the patient's family is of phenotype I or the patient himself eventually develops attacks.

The diagnosis of FMF is based on the characteristic febrile attacks. In two-thirds of the afflicted these appear during the first decade of life, and in 90% by the end of the second. Only rarely is the onset delayed beyond the age of thirty. Thereafter, attacks recur at irregular, unpredictable intervals and are accompanied by signs of peritonitis, pleuritis, synovitis or an erysipelas-like erythema. Except for an occasional joint attack that may assume a protracted course (16), the attacks are brief and self-limited, usually subsiding completely within 24-48 hours. Acute phase reactants, SAA-protein among them, are often elevated during attack-free intervals and rise strikingly during attacks (17).

Amyloidosis occurs frequently in FMF but its prevalance varies in different ethnic groups (12,13,18). Among afflicted Sephardic Jews and Anatolian Turks the development of systemic amyloidosis and early death in renal failure is their genetically determined fate. Our youngest patient died at the age of five after amyloidosis had been manifest for three years. The paucity of survivors beyond the age of 40 in our patient population is striking.

The major manifestation of FMF-amyloidosis is nephropathy. Its course progresses from a preclinical stage that is diagnosable only by a fortuitous biopsy through clinically overt proteinuric, nephrotic and uremic stages. The lives of patients in terminal renal failure have been prolonged by dialysis and kidney transplantation. Transplantation was performed in 26 amyloidotic patients between 1970 and 1982, at the Sheba Medical Center (19). Fourteen are alive with grafts normally functioning, several more than six and one more than 12 years after transplantation. Six patients rejected their grafts and returned to dialysis. Six others died, four early in our experience due to septicemia abetted by over-intensive immunosuppressive measures. Live-threatening complications and deaths in the transplantation setting have been gratifyingly reduced by the application of a less aggressive immunosuppressive regime, a greater willingness to sacrifice a trouble-making graft and, lately, the introduction of cyclosporin.

A new era in FMF followed Goldfinger's suggestion in 1972 that colchicine may prevent its attacks (20). The drug quickly became the mainstay of therapy after its efficacy was proven in controlled clinical trials (21,22). More than 90% of our patients enjoy a complete remission or a marked amelioration of attacks as long as they take 1-2 mg colchicine daily, children requiring full adult dosage. In the remainder, the attacks recur even on larger dosage.

Evaluation of the effect of the drug on amyloidosis required a longer trial. A recent analysis of 1070 patients followed-up 4-11 years after being advised to begin colchicine revealed a prevalence of amyloidosis that was one-third of that observed in our patient population before the use of colchicine (23). Among 960 patients who initially had no evidence of amyloidosis, proteinuria appeared in only 4 of 906 (0.44%) who adhered to the prophylactic schedule. This compliant group included 34, none of whom developed proteinuria, whose attacks failed to respond. This is a striking contrast to the development of proteinuria in 16 of 54 (29.6%) patients who admitted non-complaince and served as an unplanned and unanticipated concurrent control group. Among 110 patients with overt amyloid nephropathy, 86 were in the proteinuric stage when colchicine was started. The drug has apparently prevented progression in 68 and permitted resolution in 5. Thirteen patients in the proteinuric stage and all 24 in the nephrotic and uremic stage deteriorated. With the objective of preventing amyloidosis in the non-amyloidotic patient and blocking continuing deposition of amyloid in the amyloidotic patient, we recommend daily lifelong administration of colchicine for all our patients with FMF - including those whose attacks do not respond and those with irreversible renal lesions.

2.2.Familial nephropathic amyloidosis with febrile urticaria and deafness

An unusual syndrome was described in 1962 by Muckle and Wells in an English family where an autosomal dominant trait was transmitted over four generations, affecting nine of 18 members-at-risk (24).

The constant feature of the disease, appearing at adolescence and recurring thereafter, was the "aguey bout". These bouts lasted as long as 36 hours and were characterized by the appearance of an urticarial rash during episodes of fever with rigors, malaise and pain in the limbs. The rash consisted of large, geographic, flattened red papules which were irritating or painful.

Progressive perceptive deafness was a second manifestation. It began as early as the first decade of life, sometimes preceding the febrile urticarial episodes.

Three siblings died in renal failure between the ages of 39 and 57. Laboratory findings were those classical in the nephrotic syndrome. Autopsies revealed systemic amyloidosis and contracted kidneys as the only findings of note. There was massive replacement of renal glomeruli, severe adrenal cortical involvement, a "lardaceous" spleen and small quantities of amyloid in the pulmonary capillaries; hepatic sinusoids were spared. Amyloid was not found in the inner ear or cochlear nerve. By 1979, Muckle was able to collect 63 additional cases that had been reported in more than one generation of one Danish, two English and six French families (25). These families confirm autosomal dominant inheritance. It is not surprising, therefore, that the disease has been recorded as occurring apparently sporadically in patients of Danish, English, Spanish and German stock. A protein extracted from formalin-fixed tissue obtained from the German patient at autopsy was shown by sequence analysis to be homologous with AA-protein for amino terminal residues 2-30 (26).

2.3.Additional families with nephropathic systemic amyloidosis

Nephropathic amyloidosis has been recorded in at least eight additional families of varying ethnic stock. All their pedigrees are compatible with transmission of a dominant trait. In none has the amyloid been chemically characterized. How many different genetic mutations these families represent is unknown. Pleiotropic effects of the mutant gene were clearly present in two families. In a Swedish family, all four affected had experienced, from childhood, recurrent bouts of fever and abdominal pain that often lasted for two weeks or more. The father, who died in renal failure at the age of 58, transmitted his disease to three sons, progeny of two marriages, who died between 19 and 33 years of age (27,28). In an American family of undesignated ethnic stock, the six affected in three generations suffered brief bouts of fever and chills in childhood. Two children in the third generation experienced severe transient joint pains and slight maculopapular rashes during these episodes but had no evidence of renal disease when reported. Their father, paternal grandfather and two paternal grand-uncles died at ages 39-45 of renal amyloidosis (29,30). The differences in the pleiotropic effects of the mutant gene in these two families indicate that each is a distinct entity, different from FMF and the Muckle-Wells syndrome and the families to be summarized below. Not available for review is the report of a Russian family, whose afflicted had "allergic" features before the appearance of amyloid nephropathy (31).

In five additional families, no pleiotropic effects of the mutant gene were evident. The German family of Ostertag was the first familial amyloidosis recorded (32). Amyloid nephropathy in the five affected in three generations was accompanied by hypertension and hepato-splenomegaly. Since then, families of Polish, Irish, English and "American" stock have been recorded (33-36). All patients presented with nephrotic syndrome. Hypertension was absent in patients seen relatively early in their nephropathy. Amyloidotic hepatosplenomegaly was not common to all these families. Sicca syndrome due to amyloid deposition in lacrimal and salivary glands, present in one of the English afflicted, was not noted in any other family. It seems, therefore, that the mutant gene is not a pleiotropic one. Whether or not the ethnic variation of these families indicates genetic heterogeneity cannot be established on the basis of available data.

3. Familial systemic amyloidosis dominated by cardiopathy

The cardiopathic froms are the least common of the hereditary system-ic amyloidoses, having been described in but a few families. The first was a Danish family recorded in 1962 by Frederiksen et al in which three males and four females of a sibship of 12 were affected (37). The disease became manifest in the fourth and fifth decade of life when fa-tigue and dyspnea appeared on exertion. Signs of right heart failure developed and ran a relentness course until death after two to five years. Post-mortem examinations of two cases revealed massive amyloid deposition in the myocardium and endocardium and infiltrations in the tongue, peripheral veins, gastrointestinal tract and lungs. Although the

190

ratio of affected to unaffected in this sibship suggested inheritance of an autosomal dominant trait, proof was delayed until the son of one of the siblings developed the disease (38). His death at the age of 43 provided the opportunity for characterization of his amyloid. Partial amino acid sequence analysis of polypeptide fragments obtained from proteolytic digestion of amyloid fibrils established homology with prealbumin but was inadequate to identify this as a variant prealbumin.

In a kindred of German-English-Irish stock recently uncovered in the Appalachian region of the United States (39), all affected members suffered and succumbed to congestive heart failure in their 60's. Sequence analysis of the subunit protein of isolated cardiac amyloid fibrils revealed that it was a variant prealbumin having a heterogeneous amino terminal region (residues starting from positions one to six of the parent molecule) and containing an alanine for threonine substitution at position 60. This variant was also present in the plasma of affected individuals and some asymptomatic members of the kindred. Although detailed clinical descriptions are lacking, some of the affected had experienced carpal tunnel syndrome and peripheral neuropathy and the eponym familial amyloidotic polyneuropathy (FAP), Appalachian type, has been proposed. While these have features simulating upper limb FAP in which cardiac involvement is often prominent, the progression of their disease is apparently not the same. Their variant prealbumin differs from that of upper limb FAP, the latter being marked by a serine for isoleucine substitution at position 84 (40).

In an additional American family of undesignated ethnic stock, four members, a father and three of his offspring, suffered from congestive heart failure that developed between the ages of 53 and 60 (41). Amyloidosis was proven in one by endomyocardial biopsy and to be systemic in another at autopsy. The amyloid in this family has not been studied.

Clinically unique is a Latin-American family in which four siblings, all alive at reporting, presented between the ages of 33 and 43 with slow heart rates due to persistent atrial standstill (42,43). This was accompanied by cardiomegaly and mild decompensation. Two experienced systemic embolization. A fifth sibling with an enlarged heart and the mother died suddenly of strokes at an early age and may have had the disease. In only one of the sibship was amyloidosis established histologically, by biopsy of the right atrial appendage. A variety of other biopsies from three affected - liver, bone marrow, skin, rectum, skeletal muscle - were negative. Whether this curious familial amyloidosis is localized to the heart or systemic will be known after a case has come to autopsy.

4. Familial localized amyloidosis: hereditary cerebral hemorrhage with amyloidosis

This disorder, described originally in Iceland where 75 cases have been documented (4), has also been recorded in 11 patients in The Netherlands (44). It is transmitted as an autosomal dominant trait. Previously healthy, non-hypertensive young individuals, ranging in age from 15 to 58 years, suffered sudden catastrophic, often multifocal hemorrhages from small cerebral and meningeal arteries and arterioles extensively infiltrated with amyloid. Post-mortem examinations have shown the amyloid to be localized to these vessels alone; there is no evidence of extra-cranial deposition of amyloid.

Complete amino acid sequence analysis has been performed on amyloid fibrils isolated from pooled leptomeningeal tissues and meningeal vessels of six Icelandic patients. The major protein component is identical with residues 11-120 of gamma-trace basic protein (Cystatin C) except for a single amino acid substitution, glutamine for leucine, at position 68 (position 58 of the amyloid variant) (45,46). This is the only biochemical characterization to date of a localized form of hereditary amyloidosis (presumably the amyloid of familial medullary carcinoma of the thyroid will prove to be related to calcitonin, as has been shown in sporadic cases of this disease).

References

1. Gafni, J., Sohar, E. & Heller, H. Lancet i, 71-74, 1964.
2. Sagher, F. & Shanon, J. Arch. Dermat. 87, 171-175, 1963.
3. Schimke, R.N. & Hartman, W.H. Ann. Intern. Med. 63, 1027-1039, 1965.
4. Gudmundsson, G., Hallgrimsson, J., Jonasson, T.A. et al. Brain 95, 387-404, 1972.
5. Heller, H. Gafni, J. & Sohar, E. In The Metabolic Basis of Inherited Disease, 2nd Ed. Stanbury, J.B., Wyngaarden, J.B., Fredrickson, D.S., Eds. McGraw Hill, New York, 995-1014, 1965.
6. Sohar, E., Gafni, J., Pras, M. & Heller, H. Am. J. Med. 43, 227-253, 1967.
7. Pras, M., Schubert, M., Zucker-Franklin, D. et al. J. Clin. Invest. 47, 924-933, 1968.
8. Levin, M., Franklin, E.C., Frangione, B. & Pras, M. J. Clin. Invest. 51, 2773-2776, 1972.
9. Levin, M., Pras, M., Franklin, E.C. J. Exp. Med. 138, 373-380, 1973.
10. Pras, M. & Gafni, J. Immunochemistry, Glynn, E.L., Steward, M., Eds. John Wiley and Sons, Publ. Co. Ltd. 509-533, 1977.
11. Pras, M., Zaretzky, J., Frangione, B., Franklin, E.C. Am. J. Med. 68, 291-294, 1980.
12. Ozdemir, A.L. & Sokmen, C. Am. J. Gastroenterol. 51, 311-316, 1969.
13. Schwabe, A.D. & Peters, R.S. Medicine 53, 453-462, 1974.
14. Heller, H., Sohar, E., Gafni, J. & Heller, J. Arch. Intern. Med. 107, 539-550, 1961.
15. Blum, A., Gafni, J., Sohar, E. et al. Ann. Intern. Med. 57, 795-799, 1962.
16. Sneh, E., Pras, M., Michaeli, D. et al. Rheumatol. Rehab. 16, 102-106, 1977.
17. Knecht, A., de Beer, F.C. & Pras, M. Ann. Intern. Med. 102, 71, 1985.
18. Pras, M., Bronshpigel, N., Zemer, D. & Gafni, J. Johns Hopkins Med. J. 150, 22-26, 1982.
19. Jacob, E.T., Siegal, B., Bar-Nathan, N. & Gafni, J. Transplant. Proc. 14, 41-45, 1982.
20. Goldfinger, S.E. N. Engl. J. Med. 287, 1302, 1972.
21. Zemer, D., Revach, M., Pras, M. et al. N. Engl. J. Med. 291, 932-934, 1974.
22. Dinarello, C.A., Wolf, S.M., Goldfinger, S.E. et al. N. Engl. J. Med. 291, 934-937, 1974.
23. Zemer, D., Pras, M., Sohar, E. et al. N. Engl. J. Med. 314, 1001-1005, 1986.
24. Muckle, T.J. & Wells, M. Q. J. Med. 31, 235-248, 1962.
25. Muckle, T.J. Br. J. Dermatol. 100, 87-92, 1979.
26. Linke, R.P., Heilmann, K.L., Nathrath, W.B.J. & Eulitz, M. Lab. Invest. 46, 698-704, 1983.
27. Nilsson, S.E. & Floderus, S. Acta Med. Scand. 175, 341, 1964.
28. Bergman, F. & Warmenius, S. Am. J. Med. 45, 601-608, 1968.
29. Maxwell, E.S. & Kimball, I. Med. Bull. VA. 12, 365-369, 1936.
30. Mahloudji, M., Teasdall, R.D., Adamkiewicz, J.J. et al. Medicine 48, 1-37, 1969.
31. Vinogradova, O.M., Tareeva, I.E., & Serov, V.V. Therap. Arch. 41, 105-109, 1969.
32. Ostertag, B. Z. Menschl. Vererbungs Konstit. Lehre 30, 105-115, 1950.
33. Alexander, F. & Atkins, E.L. Am. J. Med. 59, 121-128, 1975.
34. Mornaghi, R., Rubinstein, P. & Franklin, E.C. Am. J. Med. 73, 609-614, 1982.

35.Lanham, J.G., Meltzer, M.L., de Beer, F.C. et al. Q. J. Med. 201, 25-32, 1982.
36.Weiss, S.W. & Page, D.L. Am. J. Med. 72, 447-460, 1973.
37.Fredriksen, T., Gøtzsche, H., Harboe, N. et al. Am. J. Med. 33, 328-348, 1962.
38.Husby, G., Ranløv, P.J., Sletten, K. & Marhaug, G. In Amyloidosis. Glenner, G.G., Osserman, E.F., Benditt, E.P., Calkins, E., Cohen, A.S., Zucker-Franklin, D., Eds. Plenum Press, New York, 391-399, 1986.
39.Benson, M.D. Personal Communication, 1986.
40.Benson, M.D. & Dwulet, F.E. Clin. Res. 33, 590A, 1985.
41.Ruder, M.A., Alpert, M.A., Sanfelippo, J.F. et al. South. Med. J. 77, 831-833, 1984.
42.Allensworth, D.C., Rice, G.J. & Lowe, G.W. Am. J. Med. 47, 775-784, 1969.
43.Harrison, W.H., Derrick, J.R. & Adamkiewicz, J.J. Angiology 20, 610-617, 1969.
44.Wattendorff, A.R., Bots, G.T., Went, L.N. & Endtz, L.J. J. Neurol. Sci. 55, 121-135, 1982.
45.Cohen, D.H., Feiner, H., Jensson, O. & Frangione, B. J. Exp. Med. 158, 623-628, 1983.
46.Ghiso, J., Jensson, O. & Frangione, B. Proc. Natl. Acad. Sci. USA 83, 2974-2978, 1986.

V.2 FAMILIAL AMYLOIDOTIC POLYNEUROPATHIES
Portugese, Japanese, Swedish, British, Jewish, German-Swiss and Finnish forms

Shukuro Araki

Department of Internal Medicine
Kumamoto University Medical School
1-1-1, Honjo, Kumamoto, 860 Japan.

1. Introduction

The hereditary amyloidotic polyneuropathies are a heterogeneous collection of familial diseases with the systemic accumulation of amyloid fibrils in the peripheral nerves and other organs. At the present time, our knowledge concerning the biochemical nature of the amyloid fibril proteins in the hereditary syndromes is still limited. Consequently, the only current classification is based on the 3 prototypic clinical forms as follows: Type I with onset in the lower limbs (Portuguese, Japanese, Swedish and Jewish families), Type II with onset in the upper limbs (Swiss-German families), and Type III with cranial neuropathy plus lattice corneal dystrophy (Finnish families) (1) (Table I).

TABLE I: CLINICAL PROTOTYPES OF FAMILIAL AMYLOIDOTIC POLYNEUROPATHY [Gafni, J. 1985 (1)]

EPONYM	ANDRADE		RUKAVINA	MERETOJA	
Ethnic origin	Portuguese		Swiss	Finnish	
- first report	- Andrade	(2)	- Rukavina (3)	- Meretoja	(7)
- later reports	Japanese		German	Danish	
	- Araki	(6)	- Mahloudji (8)	- Boysen	(14)
	- Kito	(13)		Dutch	
	Swedish			- Winkelman	(12)
	- Andersson	(11)		Scottish-Irish	
	British			- Sack	(15)
	- Van Allen	(9)			
	Polish				
	- Kulisiewicz	(4)			
	German				
	- Delank	(5)			
	Greek				
	- Dyck	(10)			
	Jewish				
	- Pras	(16)			
	- Gafni	(1)			
Major Involvement	Lower limbs		Upper Limbs	Face	
Autonomic symptoms	Early, severe		Moderate	Rare, mild	
Ocular feature	Vitreous opacities		Vitreous opacities	Corneal lattice dystrophy	
Age of onset (yrs)	20-30		>40	>40	
Progression	Rapid		Insidious	Insidious	
Age at death (yrs)	30-40		Old age	Old age	

This paper reviews the recent studies of the familial amyloidotic polyneuropathies (FAP) from various laboratories in different countries and this review might offer insight in the pathogenesis of amyloidosis and provide new approach to therapeutic trials in a disease of increasing significance.

2. Characteristics of the hereditary syndromes

2.1. Lower limb neuropathy (Portuguese, Andrade)

Type I neuropathy is characterized by sensorimotor polyneuropathies affecting the lower extremities more severely than the upper. Autonomic dysfunction occurs early in the illness. The initial description of this disease was in Portuguese subjects (2) and subsequently, a similar polyneuropathy appeared in Portuguese immigrants in Brazil, Africa and France (17-19). Reports of this type I neuropathy in subjects of non-Portuguese descent have emanated from the United States (10,20), Germany (5), Poland (4), Japan (6,13), Sweden (11), Great Britain (21) and Israel (16).

Though these syndromes reported from several countries have no apparent genetic link to the Portuguese disease, their clinical and pathological similarity to it is striking.

2.1.1. Portuguese families

2.1.1.1. History and clinical features

The first case of familial amyloidotic polyneuropathy was observed in the Department of Neurology of the Hospital of Santo Antonio in Oporto in 1939 by Andrade. In 1952, he reported a peculiar peripheral neuropathy, endemic, known by the inhabitants as "foot disease", in Povoa de Varzim, a small town on the coast 30 km from Oporto (2). Until up to 1969, 173 affected families have been detected with 696 patients of which 284 have been examined by Andrade. The disease is inherited in an autosomal dominant mode with equal sex ratio of affected patients and a high penetrance rate (17,22).

The age of onset is between 25 and 35, but may occur as early as the second or as late as the sixth decade. Progression of the disease is relentless, with death usually from cachexia, intercurrent infection, or cardiovascular failure within 10 to 12 years after the first symptoms.

Neurological symptoms begin in the lower extremities, with paresthesia and hypesthesia advancing in a distal to proximal fashion to produce a stocking-type disturbance (2). Distal upper extremities become involved later, and sensory loss may occur at the trunk. Objectively, thermal and painful sensations are lost before vibration and proprioception. Motor impairments occur relatively late in the illness and are more pronounced in the lower extremities. Foot drop was prominent in more severely affected patients. Absence of deep reflexes, trophic cutaneous changes and muscle wasting are common features.

Symptoms and signs of autonomic dysfunction are frequent. Sexual impotence is a very early symptom among affected men and presumed secondary to hypogastric autonomic plexus infiltration (23). Orthostatic hypotension is common in the advanced stages of illness. Hypohydrosis, gastrointestinal motility disturbances and urinary and fecal incontinence are other manifestations of autonomic neuropathy.

Gastrointestinal motility disturbances are prominent and may precede symptoms of neurologic involvement. Constipation is the most frequent initial complaint, but alternating bouts of constipation and diarrhea are characteristic as the disease progresses. Anorexia, vomiting and abdominal fullness are common and these symptoms are due to gastrointestinal malfunction.

Andrade described anisocoria, irregular pupillary margins and delayed reaction to light in several patients. Vitreous opacities are occasionally seen in the affected individuals. Electrocardiographic abnormalities are frequent. Renal failure, carpal tunnel syndrome and macroglossia are uncommon.

2.1.1.2.Pathology

The pathology was investigated by Silva Horta et al (23). The deposits of amyloid were distributed in the vessels of all viscera. The liver and spleen were not extensively involved. The heart, kidney, pancreas, tongue, stomach and skin were invariably affected by amyloid infiltration.

In the peripheral as well as the sympathic nervous system, an extensive gross involvement of nerves was observed. Central nervous system involvement was limited to the choroid plexus, with extensive involvement of the meninges of the cerebral hemispheres and spinal cord.

Electron microscopic studies of the peripheral nerve changes revealed abnormalities in the Schwann cells, which contained multivesicular bodies and myelin globules with breakdown of the myelin lamellas and collaps of the myelin sheath. Coimbra and Andrade suggested that neuronal changes preceeded amyloid deposition in the blood vessels of the endo- and perineurium and in the endoneurium itself (24).

2.1.2.Japanese families

2.1.2.1.History and clinical features

In 1968, Araki et al reported a kindred with amyloid neuropathy from the Arao city region, Kumamoto prefecture of Japan (6). Of 70 members in four generations, 25 are believed affected, and 10 have been examined by Araki et al. The disease was inherited in an autosomal manner, with equal sex predilection. The clinical features were remarkably similar to the Portuguese disease.

In 1973, Kito reported a large focus of familial amyloidotic polyneuropathy in the Ogawa village region, Nagano prefecture, central area of main land of Japan (13). Later thirty-four families with 242 affected individuals were found by epidemiological studies from 1972 to 1978 (25). Twenty-one had amyloid deposits documented by tissue examination. The disease was inherited in an autosomal dominant manner. Age of onset ranged from 15 to 77 years with a mean of 33 years. The sex ratio of the 242 affected patients was 3:2 and there was a tendency that female patients showed later onset and slower progression than males. The clinical features of the familial amyloidotic polyneuropathy in Ogawa village were virtually identical to the Portuguese disease and the disease in Arao city region of Japan.

In 1980, Araki et al summarized the clinical and genetic manifestations of familial amyloidotic polyneuropathy in 69 individuals from 7 pedigrees in Kumamoto (26). The symptoms started between 20 and 45 years of age with a mean of 32.1 years. The symptoms of sensory dominant mixed type peripheral neuropathy started in the lower limbs. Dissociation of sensory impairment was common, with pain and temperature sensation most severely affected. The upper limbs were also frequently involved, starting a few years after the lower limbs.

Features of autonomic nervous system involvement, such as dishydrosis, sexual impotence, disturbance of gastrointestinal motility (alternating type of diarrhea and constipation), orthostatic hypotension and urinary incontinence, were frequent. The disease is always progressive and fatal in about 10-20 years (27).

2.1.2.2.Laboratory studies

Laboratory investigations revealed that routine blood counts, urinanalysis, ESR, serum Wasserman reactions and serum electrolytes were within normal limits in all familial cases. Anemia was found in some cases. Serum proteins and liver function tests were unremarkable. Cerebrospinal fluid showed that the protein concentration was moderately increased, ranging from 100 to 200 mg/dl.

The sensory nerve conduction velocity (SCV) revealed a prominent decrease in FAP with illness over 4 years. The MCV showed electrical silence in 50% of FAP patients with illness over 4 years. A marked decrease in MCV parallelled the severity of the illness. The decrease in the M-wave amplitude was more prominent than the slowing of MCV.

The cardiovascular system was examined in 19 cases of FAP (28). In a group of patients with neurological involvement, various cardiac abnormalities were common, including orthostatic hypotension, prominent apex cardiographic A waves, abnormal apical systolic waves (bulges), systolic murmur, mid-systolic clicks, QS waves, atrioventricular blocks, left bundle branch blocks, and abnormalities of the ejection time and pre-ejection period. Though there was one case with pronounced cardiac abnormality despite a normal neurological state, and though cardiovascular symptoms appeared later than neurological symptoms, the degree of cardiac involvement generally parallelled the severity of the neurologic disorder.

On vectorcardiography, the QRS loop in the horizontal plane showed counterclockwise rotation in all patients in the early stage of neurological involvement. The His-Purkinje conduction time (AV interval) of FAP was prolonged.

Some of the FAP patients were in a state of latent hypothyroidism. Other common clinical symptoms including impotence and menstrual irregularities were considered to be due to autonomic dysfunction since the result of gonadal function studies were normal.

The concentrations of all free amino acids in serum and urine in FAP were less than in the control.

2.1.2.3. Pathology

The pathology was investigated by Shirabe et al, and Kimura et al (29,30). In the central nervous system, they found that amyloid was mainly seen in the subarachnoid membrane and choreoid plexus. Amyloid in slight amounts was seen in the subependyma. Amyloid deposition was not found in the parenchyma of the brain or the spinal cord. The peripheral nerves, autonomic ganglia and spinal nerve roots consistently showed the greatest degree of involvement with amyloid deposition.

TABLE II: THE PATHOGENESIS OF AMYLOID NEUROPATHY

	Theoretical Backgrounds	Discrepancy
Local compression	Amyloid deposits are found around nerve fibres. Wallerian degeneration is a prominent finding.	Small calibre nerve fibres are affected more severely than large calibre fibres.
Ischemia	Stenosis and occlusion of vasa nervorum due to amyloid deposition has been reported.	Some cases do not show occlusion of vasa nervorum. Unmyelinated fibres are affected more severely.
Metabolic disorder	Some cases show changes of nerve fibres preceeding the deposition of amyloid.	Changes apparently based on local compression or ischemia are sometimes observed.
Schwann-cell disorder	Changes of Schwann-cells are prominent. Some cases mainly show segmental demyelination.	Numerous reports of axonal degeneration.

It is observed in amyloid neuropathy that there is a widespread endoneural deposition of amyloid and also amyloid deposition within the walls of the vasa nervorum of both the epineurium and the endoneurium. The latter two patterns of amyloid deposition are accompanied by severe depletion of unmyelinated and small-diameter myelinated fibers.

In other general organs, amyloid deposition was chiefly seen in intestinal vessel walls and muscle fibers. The organs predominantly involved were kidney, thyroid, spleen, liver, adrenal glands, testis, ovarium, heart and urinary bladder.

It is unknown as yet why amyloid is deposited predominantly in the peripheral and autonomic nervous system in FAP. Metabolic, mechanical and ischemic factors are thought to participate in the pathogenesis of amyloid neuropathy (Table II).

2.1.2.4.Histochemical reaction with the potassium permanganate method

The potassium permanganate (PP) method, described by Wright et al, in 1977, is now considered as a simple and useful histochemical method for distinguishing AA protein from non-AA protein of amyloid fibrils. However, the mechanism of the action of PP is unknown. Specimens were obtained from the rectum or thyroid of 13 FAP patients in Kumamoto prefecture, 5 cases of secondary amyloidosis and 8 cases of FAP. The tissue sections were pretreated with PP. After this treatment, the specimens were stained with Congo red and examined under a polarizing microscope. When most of the amyloid deposits lost their affinity for Congo red after PP treatment, the specimen was considered to be sensitive to the agent, and when the affinity for Congo red was remained, the specimen was considered to be resistant. Without any relation to the pretreatment time intervals with PP, the amyloid deposits of secondary amyloidosis appeared to be sensitive, and those of FAP were resistant. The amyloid protein of FAP is non-AA protein (31).

2.1.3.Swedish families and Swedish ancestry in USA

2.1.3ᵃ.Swedish families

2.1.3ᵃ.1.History and clinical features

Since 1965, Andersson and colleagues have reported about 30 patients with Type I neuropathy from northern Sweden (11). The onset was at a mean age of 45 years in men and a decade later in women. The clinical features of the affected patients were similar to those in the Portuguese cases. According to Andersson's preliminary report, 9 of 12 patients had electrocardiographic abnormalities, and 3 had evidence of cardiomegaly and congestive failure early in their illness. Of 18 cases, 3 had pronounced vitreous opacities. Anisocoria, irregular pupils, and sluggish pupillary reactions were also observed. Steatorrhea was documented in 7 of 18 cases.

2.1.3[a].2.Laboratory studies

Electromyographic changes of denervation were most severe in the lower extremities and motor nerve conduction velocities were also abnormal. Genitourinary abnormalities were studied (32). Of the 24 men evaluated, 16 had total impotence. Urinary retention as well as overflow incontinence were frequently observed and considered to be secondary to amyloid infiltration of the bladder nerves and muscles.

2.1.3[b].Swedish ancestry in USA

In 1977, Benson and Cohen have described a new FAP kinship (LIN), with hereditary dominant FAP of Swedish origin living in Western USA (33). This family immigrated into the United States from Sweden in about 1880. A progressive polyneuropathy beginning in the third decade and a clinical picture similar to FAP are characteristic of this family.

In 1980, Cohen et al described a new family of Swedish origin with FAP (34). This family originated from the town of Ljusdal in Sweden about 200 miles northwest of Stockholm. The oldest traceable ancestor emigrated to the United States in 1905 and settled in South Dakota. She later moved to Seattle, Washington. She died in 1933 at an age of 50 years and autopsy was not performed. She had 3 children, all of whom developed FAP between the ages of 35 and 45 years and died 5-10 years thereafter.

2.1.4.British families (Iowa, Van Allen)

2.1.4.1.History and clinical features

In 1969, Van Allen et al have described a syndrome of amyloidosis in 0 individuals from 2 generations of an Iowa kindred of Scottish, English and Irish descent (9). Three instances of father-to-son transmission suggested an autosomal dominant mode of inheritance. Major symptoms were neuropathy, nephropathy and peptic ulceration. The onset of symptoms is usually in the third of fourth decade (range from 26 to 44 years) and the average survival is about 12 years (range 6 months to 26 years) from the onset of symptoms (35).

Early symptoms of neuropathy are restricted to the lower extremities. Shooting pain, dysesthesia and then loss of pain sensation are the earliest findings. Lower extremities are regularly involved. Evidence of weakness, muscle atrophy and the absence of deep-tendon reflexes occur late in the illness. Autonomic symptoms develop in many patients. Renal insufficiency is the most common cause of death. In 1974, Gimeno et al have described a family with Iowa type of neuropathy. The propositus, a 68-year-old man of Irish descent developed polyneuropathy, clouded vision after a previous history of infantile nephritis with spontaneous resolution (36).

2.1.4.2.Laboratory studies

Cerebrospinal fluid protein values are elevated from 84 to 204 mg/ml. Nephropathy may progress slowly or rapidly to renal failure. Duodenal ulcers are common (9). Constipation and diarrhea do occur but are less common than in Type I neuropathy. Electrocardiographic changes consistent with amyloid cardiac involvement are common, but progressive congestive heart failure is not observed. Hearing deficit and cataracts without vitreous opacities have been found in some cases.

2.1.4.3.Pathology

Van Allen et al have described the pathologic findings in 5 autopsy cases. Two patients had severly contracted kidneys with renal arterial amyloid deposits (9). Three patients had marked glomerular involvement. Amyloid deposits were found in the adrenals, testis, liver, spleen, nerve roots and peripheral nerves. Amyloid infiltration was also observed in symptomatic nerves and ganglions as well as in the dorsal root ganglions.

2.1.5.Jewish families

In 1981, Pras et al described the occurrence of hereditary amyloidotic polyneuropathy in a family of Jewish origin (37). The patient (S.K.O.), a 28-year-old Ashkenazi Jew, suffered from progressive neuropathy as well as blindness because of vitreous amyloid deposits. His father had died at the age of 29 from an identical disease. Tissues were obtained from the patient (S.K.O.) at autopsy. Amyloid fibrils were isolated from spleen and thyroid. Amino acid analysis and amino acid sequence studies were performed (see section 3 of this chapter).

In 1985, Gafni et al reported the first instance of FAP in 2 generations of an Ashkenazi Jewish family (1). The father, J.S. was born in Poland in 1923. He was well until the age of 30 when he began to complain of spots before his eyes. On examination vitreous opacities were noted. Shortly thereafter, impotence, difficulties at micturition, diarrhea and paresthesias in the lower limbs occurred in rapid succession. All modalities of sensation were diminished or absent in the legs but deep tendon reflexes were preserved. Two years later weakness and atrophy of the muscles of the lower extremities became prominent and paresthesias in the hands and arms were noted. The patient's course was marked by progressive neurological incapacitation, recurrent urinary tract infections and weight loss. In 1959, during his final hospitalization, the diagnosis of systemic amyloidosis was confirmed by rectal biopsy. Virtually blind, bedridden, cachectic and incontinent of urine and faeces, the patient died of bleeding gastric erosions at the age of 36 after 7 years of illness. At autopsy amyloid was present in the blood vessels of every organ examined. Most massively infiltrated were spinal nerves, including their anterior and posterior roots and autonomic nerves.

The son, H.S., the only child of J.S., was born in Israel in 1952. At the age of 25, his vision began to deteriorate. Numerous vitreous opacities were found. Impotence appeared at the age of 26. Diarrhea, incontinence of urine and faeces and sensory impairment in the lower extremities were noted at the age of 27. Neurological examinations were almost similar to that of his father. After 4 years of illness, he committed suicide.

At autopsy amyloid was present in the blood vessels of all organs of the body. Amyloid deposits were massive between the fibres of spinal nerve roots and peripheral nerves and in autonomic ganglia surrounding ganglia cells.

The amyloid fibril protein appeared to consist of a complete variant monomer of prealbumin, glycine replacing threonine at residue 49. In addition smaller polypeptides resulting from cleavage at the point of substitution were demonstrated.

2.1.6. German-English ancestry in Texas

In 1984, Libbey et al have described a family with autosomal dominant transmitted familial amyloidotic polyneuropathy residing in Texas, USA (38). This family has a German-English ancestry. Clinically, the prominent sensory and severe autonomic nervous system involvement resembles the Andrade (Portuguese) Type I familial amyloidotic polyneuropathy but is unique in the age of onset being the seventh decade in all family members affected to date. Using an immunoperoxidase technique, prealbumin was demonstrated in the amyloid deposits. This finding suggests that this family shares biochemical as well as clinical characteristics consistent with similar kinships with Type I familial amyloidotic polyneuropathy of diverse geographic origin.

2.2. Upper limb neuropathy (Indiana, Rukavina)

Type II amyloid neuropathy is characterized by the carpal tunnel syndrome and diffuse upper extremity neuropathy preceeding significant lower extremity symptoms. Large kindreds with this neuropathy have been reported in Swiss descent from Indiana (3) and German descent from Maryland, USA (7).

2.2.1. Swiss families

2.2.1.1. History and clinical features

Two cousins of Swiss descent from Indiana were seen in 1953 for progressive loss of vision. In 1955, Falls et al have observed sheet-like vitreous opacities in two cousins afflicted with disabling peripheral neuropathy mostly in the hands (39). Gingival biopsy established the diagnosis in each. One cousin died suddenly in 1954 at age of 51 and was found to have widespread amyloid deposition in heart, tongue and in the wall of blood vessels throughout many organs. The other cousin died at age of 55 and was found to have extensive perivascular and cardiac amyloid depositions. Systematic evaluation of this family by Rukavina and his colleagues disclosed a hereditary amyloidotic polyneuropathy which differed from the Portuguese neuropathy in several respects (40,35). The prominent features were carpal tunnel syndrome, generalized sensorimotor neuropathy with salient upper extremity involvement, vitreous opacities and frequent electrocardiographic abnormalities.

This family of Swiss origin emigrated to the United States in 1883. The genealogy was traced to the 16th century and association with other amyloidotic kindred was not apparent. Of 66 family members evaluated, 13 had clinical evidence of amyloidosis. The inheritance was autosomal dominant (35).

Symptoms start generally in the fourth to fifth decade. Early symptoms of neuropathy are restricted to the hands. Pain, paresthesia and numbness in the hands and thenar atrophy characteristic of carpal tunnel syndrome dominate the early picture. Diffuse sensory and motor changes eventually develop in the arms and later in the legs.

Autonomic disturbances with impotence and impairment of gastrointestinal motility occur later in the disease. Hepatosplenomegaly and macroglossia have not been observed. Visual impairment associated with the vitreous opacities was prominent, generally with onset in the sixth decade. Chronic congestive heart failure tends to occur later in the course of the disease.

2.2.1.2. Pathology

Autopsies have been performed in two cases. In the propositus, deceased at age 51, extensive generalized amyloid deposits were found in the myocardium, vessels, tongue, liver, spleen, kidneys and pancreas. Nerve tissue has not been examined. A cousin of the propositus, deceased at age 55, also had extensive perivascular and cardiac amyloid involvement (41).

2.2.2. German families

2.2.2.1. History and clinical features

In 1969, Mahloudji et al have studied 11 families from Washington County, Maryland, with a clinical picture virtually identical to that of the Indiana neuropathy (42). All eleven families were traced back to a couple who emigrated from Germany in 1746. In all, 146 affected individuals have been detected in 7 generations. Of 59 living subjects, 53 were evaluated and the typical presentation patterns were well confirmed. The 18 patients with peripheral neuropathy in familial primary amyloidosis described by Schlesinger belong to this kindred (43).

The disease is inherited in an autosomal dominant mode. The ratio of afflicted men and women is about 1:1, but men are more severely affected than women. Age of onset ranges from 15 to 66 years, with a mean of 43 years.

Upper extremity symptoms dominate the early clinical picture, which may ultimately progress to a generalized sensorimotor polyneuropathy. Autonomic dysfunction, gastrointestinal complaints and cardiac dysfunction are rare. Renal failure and macroglossia have not been observed. Survival is from 14 to 40 years from the onset of symptoms.

Pain, paresthesia and numbness in the median nerve distribution area are the initial complaints. These symptoms progress until the pain is gradually replaced by numbness. Weakness in the thenar and lateral lumbrical muscles develops later. The carpal tunnel syndrome is occasionally the only neurological manifestation for more than 20 years, but in many patients progression to a generalized distal upper and lower extremity polyneuropathy ensues within 8 to 10 years. Objectively, light touch, pain and temperature sensations are lost before vibration and proprioception. Foot drop and diminished deep-tendon reflexes occur late in the illness. Some patients require mechanical support for ambulation 3 to 5 years after the onset of pedal symptoms. Vitreous opacities have been demonstrated in one patient by Mahloudji (42) and in his sib by Schlesinger (43). Electrocardiograms and cerebrospinal fluid examinations were normal (42).

2.2.2.2.Pathology

Mahloudji described the results of necropsies in two cases (42). In one 66-year-old man, amyloid deposition was found in small and medium-sized arteries in most organs. The heart, peripheral nerves and ganglions were extensively involved. No amyloid depositis were found in the spleen. A limited amount of amyloid was found in the medium and small arteries of the liver and kidneys.

In the second case, a 75 year-old man, extensive amyloid deposits were found in the heart, peripheral nerves, large vessels and kidneys.

Amyloid deposits in the flexor retinaculum of Maryland neuropathy patients differed morphologically from deposits in idiopathic carpal tunnel syndrome with amyloidosis and multiple myeloma with amyloidosis (44,45). In the familial neuropathy, amyloid deposits in the flexor retinaculum appeared to replace collagen in a unit-for-unit fashion. In the acquired disease, amyloid deposits occupied the periphery of collagen bundles and were not demonstrable in the vessels of the flexor retinaculum.

2.2.2.3. Treatment

Surgery of the flexor retinaculum has resulted in complete symptomatic improvement in 12 of 13 patients (35).

2.3. Face neuropathy (Finland, Meretoja)

2.3.1. History and clinical features

This type of neuropathy is characterized by lattice dystrophy of the cornea, cranial neuropathy and pendulous skin. The vast majority of patients have been described primarily in the Finnish population.

In 1969, Meretoja reported on 10 cases of a newly identified form of inherited systemic amyloidosis in Finland (7,46) and until 1974 the number of patients diagnosed in Finland with this illness has reached 218, distributed among 60 families (47).

In 1981, Sack et al reported this type of neuropathy from the United States (15) and 7 reports have been described outside of Finland or Denmark. In 1986, Darras et al described the second US case (48).

The onset of this disease occurs at about 20 years of age. The clinical diagnosis can be made either during an ophthalmological slit-lamp examination, which reveals the corneal lattice dystrophy, or later, after a patient reaches the age of 40, from the mask-like and hanging face with bilateral upper, and later lower, facial paresis that typify such patients.

Characteristic of this disease is a very slow progression with rather mild symptoms until the age of about 40 to 50. The eventual corneal dystrophy leads to considerable loss of vision at about the age of 65. Glaucoma and pseudo-exfoliation syndrome are also often present (49).

Cutaneous signs may include cutis laxa, bruises, pruritus and small cheloids. Peripheral neuropathy is mild. Cardiac abnormalities play a pronounced role in the syndrome. Transient proteinuria is observed in about one-half of the patients but uremic signs are rare.

This form of inherited, systemic amyloidosis appears to occur in geographical isolation: in 2 neighbouring southern Finnish districts, South Hame and Kymenlaakso, cases are known to have existed since at least the seventeenth century. It is transmitted by a dominant autosomal mode of inheritance; a rare homozygosity has been documented in 2 patients (50).

2.3.2. Pathology

In 1972, Meretoja et al reported renal biopsy findings observed in 4 patients with this type of amyloidosis. Interstitial accumulation of amyloid was sparse in all patients and was concentrated in the glomeruli (50).

In the postmortem studies reported by Meretoja, amyloid was deposited in the intima and media of arteries throughout the body (51). Myocardial amyloid deposits were variable. Minor branches of the facial nerve were totally replaced by amyloid infiltrates. Moderate deposits were noted in the perineurium and endoneurium of peripheral nerves. Central nervous system involvement was restricted to the leptomeninges and their vessels. Renal deposits were prominent in the glomeruli and their capillaries.

Lattice dystrophy of the cornea may occur as a localized form of amyloid infiltration restricted to the cornea without systemic involvement.

3. Biochemical studies on amyloid fibril protein

The chemical nature of the deposits of human systemic amyloidosis has been clarified in recent years by the discovery of two different types of proteins constituting the β-pleated sheet amyloid fibrils in the acquired amyloidosis syndromes. In the acquired "primary" disease the major fibrillar protein is, in the majority of cases, an intact immunoglobulin light polypeptide chain (AL) and/or its amino-terminal variable region fragment, while in the acquired "secondary" process and in familial Mediterranean fever, the major fibrillar protein constituent is most often a nonimmunoglobulin protein, designated protein AA (52).

In 1978, Costa et al have reported a new finding on the nature of proteins isolated from amyloid fibrils in familial amyloidotic polyneuropathy (FAP) of Portuguese origin (53).

Amyloid fibrils were concentrated from the kidney, thyroid and peripheral nerve of six patients with FAP. The fibril concentrates were solubilized in 6M guanidine-HCL and fractionated on Sephadex G-100 columns. The elution profile of all FAP amyloid fibril concentrates revealed a protein of 14,000 dalton, designated the FAP protein, that was absent from normal human tissues treated by the same procedure and from fibrils of a primary amyloidosis liver. Antisera against whole denatured fibril concentrates prepared in rabbits reacted with FAP protein and a component in normal human serum corresponding to prealbumin. It was further established that the FAP protein shared common antigenic determinants with human prealbumin by its reaction of identity with normal prealbumin using commercial antisera against human prealbumin. Amyloid AL or AA proteins could not be identified in FAP fibrils by sensitive immunochemical assay methods. Costa et al concluded that the FAP protein is a unique and significant component of the FAP amyloid fibrils and that it is closely related to the 13,745 dalton prealbumin subunit (53).

In 1981, Taware et al have reported the study on the nature of the amyloid fibril proteins from patients with FAP in Arao, Japan (54). Amyloid fibrils were isolated from the kidneys of two Japanese patients and fractionated on a Sephadex G-100 gel column. The elution pattern showed three peaks. The molecular weight of the third peak protein was about 14,000 dalton. Using the same procedures no such protein could be demonstrated in the tissues of non-amyloidotic patients. Antisera raised against a denatured amyloid fibril preparation did react with this protein, showing a precipitin arc on immunoelectrophoretic analysis with a slightly cathodal drift compared to prealbumin. The amino acid composition of this protein was different from those of AA protein, AL protein, or the normal human prealbumin subunit. Tawara et al concluded that the major subunit GAM III of amyloid fibril protein appears immunologically related to prealbumin.

In 1981, Skinner and Cohen have reported a study on the prealbumin nature of the amyloid protein in a FAP family (Swedish variety) living in Western USA (55). They have isolated a 15,000 dalton protein from the amyloid laden tissue of a patient. It appeared to be homologous to normal plasma prealbumin as judged by N-terminal sequence analysis. They concluded that the normal plasma protein prealbumin is linked to the disease syndrome.

In 1981, Benson has reported partial amino acid sequence homology between a heredofamilial amyloid protein and human plasma prealbumin (56).

In 1983, Pras et al reported the primary structure of an amyloid prealbumin variant in FAP of Jewish origin (57). The complete amino acid sequence of three related amyloid proteins (14,000, 10,000 and 5,000 dalton) derived from tissues of a Jewish patient with FAP, were elucidated. The protein, which contains 127 amino acid residues, is identical to a human serum prealbumin subunit. Only one amino acid substitution, glycine for threonine, was detected at position 49. At this position enzymatic cleavage occurred, yielding 5,000 and 10,000 dalton fragments which represent the amino terminus (residues 1-48) and carboxyl terminus (residues 49-127) of the molecule, respectively. They concluded that a prealbumin variant and its fragments constitute the amyloid fibrils in FAP of Jewish origin.

In 1983, Taware et al have described the structural identification of an amyloid fibril protein of 14 Kdalton (designated AFj-INO), isolated from the kidney of a Japanese patient with FAP, named Ino (58). In the study, AFj-INO protein, repurified after conversion to the reduced and S-carboxymethylated form RCM-AFj-INO was subjected to sequence analyses. Peptide maps prepared from cyanogen bromide fragments and tryptic digests of RCM-AFj-INO were compared with those of normal RCM-prealbumin to precisely identify structural differences between AFj-INO and normal plasma prealbumin. Sequence analyses indicated that only a valine residue at position 30 in prealbumin is replaced by a methionine residue. Furthermore, it was also proven that AFj-INO consists of four components: the prealbumin variant and its three related proteins, which are derived by successively accumulated deletion of the N-terminal three amino acid residues (Gly^1, Pro^2, and Thr^3) from the prealbumin variant (Table III).

TABLE III: AMINO ACID SEQUENCE OF THE PREALBUMIN VARIANT IN A JAPANESE FAP PATIENT SERUM

1	5	10	15	20

Gly-Pro-Thr-Gly-Thr-Gly-Glu-Ser-Lys-Cys-Pro-Leu-Met-Val-Lys-Val-Leu-Asp-Ala-Val-

　　　　　　　　　　　　　　　　　*

Arg-Gly-Ser-Pro-Ala-Ile-Asn-Val-Ala-<u>Met</u>-His-Val-Phe-Arg-Lys-Ala-Ala-Asp-Asp-Thr-

Trp-Glu-Pro-Phe-Ala-Ser-Gly-Lys-Thr-Ser-Glu-Ser-Gly-Glu-Leu-His-Gly-Leu-Thr-Thr-

Glu-Glu-Glu-Phe-Val-Glu-Gly-Ile-Tyr-Lys-Val-Glu-Ile-Asp-Thr-Lys-Ser-Tyr-Trp-Lys-

Ala-Leu-Gly-Ile-Ser-Pro-Phe-His-Glu-His-Ala-Glu-Val-Val-Phe-Thr-Ala-Asn-Asp-Ser-

Gly-Pro-Arg-Arg-Tyr-Thr-Ile-Ala-Ala-Leu-Leu-Ser-Pro-Tyr-Ser-Tyr-Ser-Thr-Thr-Ala-

　　　　　　　　　　　　　　　127

Val-Val-Thr-Asn-Pro-Lys-Glu

* Valine at position 30 in normal prealbumin is replaced by methionine.

In 1984, Kametani et al have reported that a variant prealbumin-related low molecular weight amyloid fibril protein was found in FAP patients in the Nagano region of Japan (59).

In 1984, Dwulet and Benson have determined the entire primary structure of an amyloid prealbumin from a patient with FAP of Swedish origin and have found an amino acid substitution that is also present in the circulating plasma prealbumin (60). Prealbumin from an individual with FAP was isolated from plasma by using a three-step procedure involving ion exchange, Affi-gel Blue affinity chromatography and gel filtration. This prealbumin and its associated amyloid fibril subunit protein were digested with trypsin and the resulting peptides were separated by high performance liquid chromatography. Comparison with normal prealbumin peptides showed that an amino acid substitution of a methionine for a valine had occurred at position 30. In the plasma prealbumin the abnormal residue accounted for 1/3rd of the material while in the amyloid fibrils it accounted for 2/3rd (Table IV).

TABLE IV: AMINO ACID SEQUENCE ANALYSES OF AMYLOIDS & PLASMA PREALBUMIN OF PATIENTS WITH LOWER LIMB FAMILIAL AMYLOIDOTIC POLYNEUROPATHY

	1	15	23	30	49	127	
Normal	┊----------┊----------┊----------┊----------┊----- / /------┊		lys	ser	val	thr		Kanda, 1974
Jewish	┊---┊----- / /------┊					49 gly		Pras, 1983
Japanese	┊--┊--------------- / /------┊				30 met			Tawara, 1983
Swedish	┊--┊--------------- / /------┊				30 met			Dwulet, 1983
Portuguese	┊--┊--------------- / /------┊				30 met			Saraiva, 1984

209

In 1984, Nakazato et al have investigated whether the prealbumin variant could also be demonstrated in the serum of a Japanese FAP patient and, if present, whether or not it was identical to the amyloid prealbumin variant in organs with amyloid deposition. They have found that serum prealbumin consists of a mixture of normal prealbumin and a prealbumin variant which contains a methionine for valine substitution at position 30. The prealbumin variant in the serum was identical to the prealbumin variant derived from amyloid fibrils of a Japanese patient. They suggested that FAP likely results from the deposition of abnormal serum prealbumin in various organs as amyloid fibrils (61). Recently, Koeppen et al have described that amyloid fibrils were isolated from the myocardium of 2 patients with FAP living in upstate New York.

From the studies by immunochemical and immunocytochemical methods, they suggested that FAP with cardiomyopathy is due to infiltration of susceptible tissues by an anomalous transthyretin (prealbumin) (85).

From these limited data in 1985, Gafni et al have suggested that a) derivation of amyloid from prealbumin is the biochemical common denominator of lower limb familial amyloidotic neuropathies regardless of the ethnic derivation of the afflicted; b) to the extent that ethnic diversity reflects genetic heterogeneity, this will be demonstrable in the amyloid of the afflicted as entity-specific variant prealbumin monomers distinguished by different single amino acid substitutions; c) on clinical and biochemical grounds, lower limb familial amyloidotic neuropathies include at least three genetic entities (1).

In the upper limb and facial forms of familial amyloidotic polyneuropathy first recorded in Swiss and Finns respectively, the differences in their patterns of neurological disease and ocular lesions could be the result of their amyloid deposits being derived from proteins other than prealbumin (1).

4.Recent advances of diagnostic procedures

4.1.Biopsy

A number of methods for the diagnosis of systemic amyloidosis have been used during the last 50 years. In 1960, Gafni and Sohar introduced the method of rectal biopsy (63). They reported abnormal results in 26 biopsies performed on 30 patients with amyloidosis. No false-positive results were recorded. The rectal biopsy is rated as very valuable because of its high reliability, but it has the limitation of causing discomfort to the patient and of technical difficulty to perform.

4.1.1.Fine-needle biopsy of subcutaneous fat

In 1973, Westermark and Stenkvist introduced a method for the diagnosis of systemic amyloidosis (64). Subcutaneous biopsies were performed in five different places between the symphysis and the xiphoid process on all patients. By employing disposable syringes, multiple aspirations can be performed. The needle had a diameter of 0.7 mm and length of 50 mm. The aspirated material was spread on a glass slide and allowed to air-dry. The sample was covered with a clean glass slide before it was stained. The material was stained with alkaline Congo red. After this, the slide was dipped into concentrated (99.6%) alcohol and xylene, mounted with canada balsam, and examined for green birefringence in an ordinary microscope with polarization equipment. The described method was used in the examination of 28 patients who were clinically suspected of systemic amyloidosis. Eight patients had abnormal results from fine-needle biopsy of subcutaneous abdominal fat. The abnormal results were later confirmed by rectal biopsy or autopsy. In addition, seven of the 19 patients with normal results also had normal results from rectal biopsies. They proved that a fine-needle biopsy of subcutaneous fat is a simple and reliable method for diagnosing secondary systemic amyloidosis. This method is expected to be applicable to the diagnosis of FAP.

4.1.2. Gastric biopsy

In 1982, Ikeda et al performed gastric and rectal biopsy in familial amyloidotic polyneuropathy and reported that amyloid deposition was found in 6 cases by gastric biopsy and in all 7 cases by rectal biopsy (65) In the stomach, amyloid was mainly deposited in the muscularis mucosae and less frequently in the lamina propria or submucosa. In the rectum, amyloid was frequently found in the muscularis mucosae and submucosa, especially in the vessel wall. Gastroendoscopy requires no premedication and is readily accepted by patients. Complications of gastric biopsy were rare. Although gastroendoscopy itself is uncomfortable, gastric biopsy should be considered preferable for the diagnosis of familial amyloidotic polyneuropathy.

In 1985, Yamada et al reported the results of gastric biopsy in AL (primary or myeloma-associated) amyloidosis and concluded that gastric biopsy was more valuable than rectal biopsy in the diagnosis of AL amyloidosis (66).

4.2. Radioimmunoassay for detecting abnormal prealbumin in the serum

In 1984, Nakazato et al have developed a highly sensitive and specific method for quantitative analysis of the prealbumin variant in the sera of FAP patients by using a radioimmunoassay for a nonapeptide corresponding to subsequence 22-30 of the prealbumin variant (67).

This peptide was produced from the prealbumin variant by cyanogen bromide cleavage followed by tryptic digestion. The serum concentration of the prealbumin variant in five Japanese FAP patients ranges from 40 µg/ml to 78 µg/ml, which is 100 times or even higher than normal controls. This should be helpful for an early diagnosis of this hereditary disease.

In 1985, Skinner et al have developed a radioimmunoassay technique for measurement of serum prealbumin in patients with amyloidosis (68). The prealbumin levels in 24 patients with FAP were 149.2 $\pm$ 38.2 µg/ml (mean $\pm$ S.D.). The 56 unaffected, but at-risk relatives had levels of 169.0 $\pm$ 57.9 µg/ml. In the 22 normal individuals, prealbumin levels were 232.9 $\pm$ 64.3 µg/ml. These differences in prealbumin levels of FAP patients and their at risk relatives when compared to normals showed a statistically significant difference by analysis of variance (p <0.01). The mean prealbumin level in 29 patients with the secondary (AA) form of amyloidosis was 211.7 $\pm$ 93.7 µg/ml, and in 30 patients with the primary (AL) form of amyloidosis was 221.9 $\pm$ 110.8 µg/ml.

The significantly lowered levels of prealbumin in FAP patients and in unaffected, but at-risk relatives suggest that a serum precursor variant or a metabolic or catabolic abnormality may be present in this form of disease.

4.3. DNA method for diagnosis

In recent years, restriction endonuclease analysis has been increasingly used as a tool for diagnosing genetic disorders such as several types of hemoglobinopathies (69), phenylketonuria (70) and Huntington's disease (71).

To apply restriction endonuclease analysis for the diagnosis of FAP, Mita et al cloned a human prealbumin cDNA and determined the entire nucleotide sequence (72). The cDNA sequence suggested the possibility that a carrier of the mutant prealbumin gene is directly detectable by digesting genomic DNA's with either NsiI or BalI, followed by Southern blot analysis (73), using the ^{32}P-labelled prealbumin cDNA as a probe.

The DNA's were extracted from white blood cells and 5 to 10 µg of genomic DNA's was digested to completion with NsiI. Fourteen individuals from 5 families with the Japanese type of FAP and 10 disease-free individuals showed 2 bands (6.6 Kb and 3.2 Kb) complementary to a human prealbumin cDNA, whereas digests from 11 individuals with FAP and 3 asymptomatic ones exhibited 2 additional bands (5.1 Kb and 1.5 Kb) (Fig. 1).

Mita et al (6) interpreted these changes in pattern to be the result of a restriction site for NsiI located in the altered codon and associated with the mutant prealbumin gene. All these individuals with FAP were hereterozygous for the prealbumin gene, carrying one normal and one mutant gene (74). One of the asymptomatic individuals of a FAP family was heterozygous for the prealbumin gene. This individual was a 32 year-old sister of a FAP individual. Because clinical symptoms of the FAP usually appear when the individual is between 20 and 45 years of age, the possibility of unique clinical symptoms occurring in this individual in the near future is predicted to be extremely high. Such an early diagnosis and close follow-up should aid in clarifying the pathogenesis of FAP (74). Sasaki et al have reported the diagnosis of FAP by cDNA techniques (75,76).

Araki

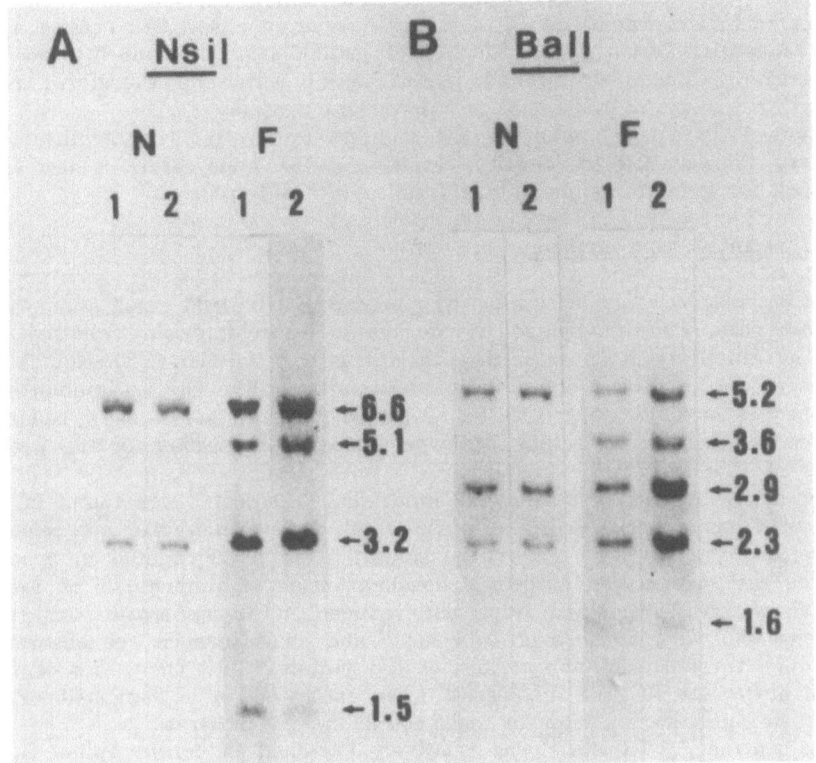

<u>Figure 1</u>: Southern blot analysis of human genomic DNA's. NsiI(A) or BalI(B) digests of DNA's from two normal individuals (N) (lanes 1 and 2), and that from two individuals with FAP (F) (lanes 1 and 2), were subjected to electrophoresis on agarose gels and transferred onto nitrocellulose filters. The filters were hybridized with the ^{32}P-labeled prealbumin cDNA. Sizes of the hybridizable fragments are indicated in Kb on the right.

Restriction endonuclease assay for the mutant gene is expected to be immediately applicable to the prenatal diagnosis of FAP.

4.4. CNBr cleavage and High Performance Liquid Chromatography

In 1985, Benson and Dwulet have described a new method for detecting carriers of a variant plasma prealbumin that is associated with FAP of Swedish origin (77). This method was based on the finding of an extra methionine in the variant prealbumin, at position 30 from the amino terminus. Since normal prealbumin has only one methionine (position 13), treatment with cyanogen bromide (CNBr), which cleaves only at methionine residues, results in 2 peptides. CNBr treatment of the

213

variant prealbumin gives 3 peptides. The extra peptide can then be detected in two ways: by HPLC using a reverse-phase C18 column and by sequential Edman degradation. Each method can detect as little as 1% variant prealbumin in isolated plasma prealbumin, and therefore, can identify carriers of the gene for the variant protein.

Since FAP type I usually is not manifest until after the childbearing years, this method to identify carriers of the gene offers a new approach for genetic counselling of families with this disease.

4.5. Immunoblotting method

Effective and rapid immunoblotting procedures both at small and semi--micro scale were developed by Saraiva et al to determine whether or not a transthyretin (prealbumin) variant with ^{30}Val-Met (TTR-Met^{30}) is present in the plasma of an individual subject (78). The immunoblotting procedure employs only 0.01 ml of serum and can serve as a reliable procedure for the screening of large numbers of persons for the presence of TTR-Met^{30}.

In family studies of seven FAP kindreds, TTR-Met^{30} was found in 21 out of 41 asymptomatic FAP offspring and its presence was not related to either age or sex. Thus, the mutant TTR is segregated in accordance with the known autosomal dominant mode of inheritance of FAP. Total plasma TTR levels were not reduced in asymptomatic FAP offspring who were carriers of TTR-Met^{30} and no difference was observed between carriers and noncarriers of the mutant TTR. The ratios of the variant to normal TTR in plasma were estimated in asymptomatic FAP offspring and were similar to those found in FAP patients.

In contrast, TTR-Met^{30} was relatively enriched in cerebrospinal fluid samples from 2 FAP patients. The significance of this finding is not known, but might relate to the preferential deposition of amyloid in the nervous system in FAP. The study strongly suggested that the presence of TTR-Met^{30} in plasma constitutes a predictive biochemical marker of FAP in the preclinical phase of the disease.

5. Prealbumin and nervous system

Prealbumin, one of the most completely characterized human proteins, plays an important role in plasma transport of vitamin A and is also involved in the transport of thyroid hormones. The term "prealbumin" refers to its electrophoretic mobility at pH 8.6, which exceeds that of albumin. Prealbumin has been found to be the fibril constituent in two localized forms of amyloid that are associated with aging. In localized senile cardiac amyloid, isolated fibrils have been identified as prealbumin (83). In senile cerebral amyloid of Alzheimer's disease, immunocytochemical studies have suggested that prealbumin is a common constituent in the neuritic plaque, the neurofibrillary tangle and the microangiopathic lesion (84). This latter finding suggests that the prealbumin molecule may play a role in the central nervous system. It is of interest that FAP amyloid begins as a peripheral nervous system disease. Skinner has concluded that prealbumin is important in the nervous system and serves another, undefined physiologic function in nerve tissue in addition to its role in vitamin and hormone transport (68)(Table V).

TABLE V: BIOCHEMICAL TYPE OF AMYLOID PROTEINS AFFECTING THE NERVOUS SYSTEM

1. AL amyloid
      - carpal tunnel syndrome

2. Prealbumin
      - familial amyloidotic polyneuropathy
      - senile cerebral amyloid of Alzheimer's disease
         a. neuritic plaque
         b. neurofibrillary tangle
         c. micro-angiopathic lesion

3. Gamma-trace protein
      - hereditary cerebral amyloid with hemorrhage
        (Iceland)
4. Beta$_2$-microglobulin
      - chronic hemodialysis entrapment syndromes
        (carpal tunnel syndrome)

6. Treatment

The ultimate aim of all our studies is to make it relevant to patient care and to improve the welfare of our patients.

Dimethylsulfoxide (DMSO), a remarkable solvent, was reported to increase the solubility of amyloid fibrils by Osserman et al in 1976 (79). Although there is no specific therapy for amyloidosis, DMSO and other symptomatic treatments have been tried to decrease the symptoms in several countries. Araki et al and Ikegawa et al have reported the results of various therapeutic trials to 18 patients with FAP of Japanese origin.

By DMSO therapy, subjective improvements of diarrhea, sensory and gait disturbances were observed in 8 cases. However, the disease was progressive under the treatment with DMSO. They tried other symptomatic treatments such as MAO-I and tyramine or L-threo-Dops for orthostatic hypotension, isoproterenol for bradyarrhythmias, pacemaker for Adams-Stokes syndrome, loperamide hydrochloride for diarrhea, domperidone or chlorpromazine for severe nausea, and obstructive operation of lacrimal punctum for impairment of visual disturbance (80,81).

Experiences of plasma exchange in a few cases with amyloidosis proved some useful effects. Although the plasma exchange therapy is expensive, further studies are necessary to prove the usefulness of this type of treatment (82).

7. Conclusions

1. Three prototypic clinical forms are distinguishable, with the large foci of patients in Portugal (Lower limb type), Swiss (Upper limb type) and Finland (Face type). Since these original reports, each clinical prototype has been recorded in families of other ethnic origins.

2. Lower limb FAP has been described in many families in Portugal, Sweden and Japan. Clinical, pathological and biochemical data of FAP in the Japanese are strikingly similar to that in the Portuguese. The spread of dominant genetic trait beyond its original ethnic is unclear.

3. For an early diagnosis of FAP, a radio immunoassay system was developed. A diagnosis of FAP can be made by use of restriction endonuclease, a cloned human prealbumin cDNA and Southern blot procedures. High performance liquid chromatography and immunoblotting methods to detect the presence of variant prealbumin in plasma of FAP patients are also newly established. The above described methods are expected to be valuable to the prenatal diagnosis of FAP.

4. Although there is no specific treatment for amyloidosis, DMSO and other symptomatic therapy have been effective to decrease the symptoms in some cases. The results of DMSO treatment were inconclusive.

References

1. Gafni, J., Fischel, B., Reif, R. et al. Q. J. Med. 55, 216, 33-43, 1985.
2. Andrade, C. Brain 75, 408-428, 1952.
3. Rukavina, J.G., Block, W.D., Jackson, C.E. et al. Medicine 35, 239-334, 1956.
4. Kulisiewicz, T., Zielinski, J. & Kozlowska-Kowarska, A. Neurol. Neurochir. Psychiat. Pol. 14, 241-245, 1964.
5. Delank, H.W., Koch, G., Konn, G. & Missmahl, H.P. Arzneimittel-Forsch. 19, 401-406, 1965.
6. Araki, S., Mawatari, S., Ohta, M. et al. Arch. Neurol. 18, 593-602, 1968.
7. Meretoja, J. Ann. Clin. Res. 1, 314-324, 1969.
8. Mahloudji, M., Teasdall, R.D., Adamkiewicz, J.J. et al. Medicine 48, 1-37, 1969.
9. Van Allen, M.W., Frohlich, J.A. & Davis, J.R. Neurology 19, 10-25, 1969.
10. Dyck, P.J. & Lambert, E.H. Arch Neurol 20, 490-507, 1969.
11. Andersson, R. Acta Med. Scand. 188, 85-94, 1970.
12. Winkelman, J.E., Delleman, J.W. & Ansink, B.J.J. Klin. Mbl. Augenheilk. 159, 618-623, 1971.
13. Kito, S., Fujimori, N., Yamamoto, M. et al. Nippon Rinsho 31, 170-182, 1973.
14. Boysen, G., Galassi, G., Kamieniecka, Z. et al. J. Neurol. Neurosurg. Psychiat. 42: 1020-1030, 1979.
15. Sack, G.H., Dumars, K.W., Gummerson, K.S. et al. Johns Hopkins Med. J. 149, 239-247, 1981.
16. Pras, M., Franklin, E.C., Gafni, J. et al. In Amyloidosis E.A.R.S. Tribe, C.R., Bacon, P.A., Eds. John Wright & Sons Ltd, Bristol, 35-38, 1983.
17. Andrade, C. In Amyloidosis. Mandema, E., Ruinen, L., Scholten, H.J., Cohen, A.S. Eds. Excerpta Medica, Amsterdam, 377-389, 1968.
18. Mello, A.R. J. Bras. Med. 1, 161-218, 1959.
19. Juliao, O.F., Queriroz, L.S. & Lopes de Faria, J. Eur. Neurol. 11, 180-195, 1974.
20. Kantarjian, A.D. & De Jong R.N. Neurology 3, 399-409, 1953.
21. Zalin, A., Darby, A., Vaughan, S. et al. Br. Med. J. 1, 65-66, 1974.
22. Klein, D. Acta Neuropath., Suppl. 2, 49-53, 1964.
23. Silva Horta, J. da, Filipe, I. & Duarte, S. Pathol. Microbiol. (Basel) 27, 809-825, 1964.
24. Coimbra, A. & Andrade, C. I. Brain 94, 199-206, 1971, II. Brain 94, 207-212, 1971.

25.Kito,S., Itoga, E., Kamiya, K. et al. Eur. Neurol. 19, 141-151, 1980.
26.Araki, S., Kurihara, T., Tawara, S. & Kuribayashi, T. In Amyloid and Amyloidosis. Glenner, G.G., Costa, P.P., Freitas, A.F. Eds. Excerpta Medica, Amsterdam, 67-77, 1980.
27.Araki, S. Brain Development 6, 128-133, 1984.
28.Sawayama, T., Kurihara, T. & Araki, S. Br. Heart J. 40, 1288-1292, 1978.
29.Shirabe, T., Hashimoto, M., Araki, S. et al. In Progress in Neuropathology Vol 2. Zimmerman, H.M., Ed. Grune & Stratton, New York, 409-420, 1973.
30.Kimura, Y., Araki, S. & Takahashi, K. In Annual Report of the Special Project Research of Selected Intractable Neurological Disorders. Toyokura, Y., Ed. (Tokyo) 338-343, 1985.
31.Nagamine, M., Tawara, S. & Araki, S. J. Jpn. Soc. Intern. Med. 71, 795-801, 1982.
32.Andersson, R. & Hofer, P.A. Acta Med. Scand. 195, 49-58, 1974.
33.Benson, M.D. & Cohen, A.S. Ann. Intern. Med. 86, 419-424, 1977.
34.Cohen, A.S., Rubinow, A., Ginter, D. & Wilson, F. In Amyloid and Amyloidosis. Glenner, G.G., Costa, P.P., Freitas, A.F., Eds. Excerpta Medica, Amsterdam, 78-85, 1980.
35.Andrade, C., Araki, S., Block, W.D. et al. Arthritis Rheum. 13, 902-915, 1970.
36.Gimeno, A., Garcia-Alix, D., Segovia de Arana, J.M. et al. Eur. Neurol. 11, 46-57, 1974.
37.Pras, M., Franklin, E.C., Prelli, F. & Frangione. B. J. Exp. Med. 154, 989-993, 1981.
38.Libbey,C.A., Rubinow, A., Shirahama, T. et al. Am. J. Med. 76, 18-24, 1984.
39.Falls, H.F., Jackson, C.E., Carey, J.H. et al. Arch. Ophthalmol. 54, 660-664, 1955.
40.Rukavina, J.G., Block, W.D., Jackson, C.E. et al. Medicine 35, 239-334, 1956.
41.Jackson, C.E., Falls, H.F., Block, W.D. et al. Am. J. Hum. Genet. 12, 434-439, 1960.
42.Mahloudji, M., Teasdall, R.D., Adamkiewicz, J.J. et al. Medicine 48, 1-37, 1969.
43.Schlesinger, A.S., Duggins, V.A. & Masucci, E.F. Brain 85, 357-370, 1962.
44.Bastian, F.O. Am. J. Clin. Pathol. 61, 711-717, 1974.
45.Lambird, P.A. & Hartmann, W.H. Am. J. Clin. Pathol. 52, 714-719, 1969.
46.Meretoja, J. Clin. Genet. 4, 173-185, 1973.
47.Meretoja, J. In Amyloidosis. Wegelius, O., Pasternack, A., Eds. Academic Press, London, 195-209, 1976.
48.Darras, B.T., Adelman, L.S., Mora, J.S. et al. Neurology 36, 432-435, 1986.
49.Meretoja, J. & Tarkkanen, A. Ophthalmologica (Basel) 170, 337-344, 1975.
50.Meretoja, J., Jokinen, E.J., Collan, Y. et al. Acta Pathol. Microbiol. Scand. [A] 80, Suppl. 223, 228-238, 1972.
51.Meretoja, J. & Teppo, L. Acta Pathol. Microbiol. Scand. (A) 79, 432-440, 1971.
52.Glenner, G.G. & Page, D.L. Int. Rev. Exp. Pathol. 15, 1-92, 1976.
53.Costa, P.P., Figueira, A.S. & Bravo, F.R. Proc. Natl. Acad Sci. USA 75, 4499-4503, 1978.
54.Tawara, S., Araki, S., Toshimori, K. et al. J. Lab. Clin. Med. 98, 811-822, 1981.
55.Skinner, M. & Cohen, A.S. Biochem. Biophys. Res. Commun. 99, 1326-1332, 1981.
56.Benson, M.D. J. Clin. Invest. 67, 1035-1041, 1981.
57.Pras, M., Prelli, F., Franklin, E.C. & Frangione, B. Proc. Natl. Acad. Sci. USA 80, 539-542, 1983.
58.Tawara,S., Nakazato, M., Kangawa, K. et al. Biochem. Biophys. Res. Commun. 116, 880-888, 1983.
59.Kametani, F., Tonoike, H., Hoshi, A. et al. Biochem. Biophys. Res. Commun. 125, 622-628, 1984.
60.Dwulet, F.E. & Benson, M.D. Proc. Natl. Acad. Sci. USA 81, 694-698, 1984.
61.Nakazato, M., Kangawa, K., Minamino, N. et al. Biochem. Biophys. Res. Commun. 122, 712-718, 1984.
62.Gafni, J., Fischel, B., Reif, R. et al. Q. J. Med. 55, 216, 33-43, 1985.
63.Gafni, J. & Sohar, E. Am. J. Med. Sci. 240, 332-336, 1960.
64.Westermark, P. & Stenkvist, B. Arch. Intern. Med. 132, 522-523, 1973.
65.Ikeda, S., Makishita, H., Oguchi, K. et al. Neurology 32, 1364-1368, 1982.
66.Yamada, M., Hatakeyama, S. & Tsukagoshi, H. Hum. Pathol. 16, 1206-1211, 1985.
67.Nakazato, M., Kangawa, K., Minamino, N. et al. Biochem. Biophys. Res. Commun. 122, 719-725, 1984.
68.Skinner, M., Connors, L.H., Rubinow, A. et al. Am. J. Med. Sci. 289, 17-21, 1985.
69.Geever, R.F., Wilson, L.B., Nallaseth, F.S. et al. Proc. Natl. Acad. Sci. USA 78, 5081-5085, 1981.
70.Woo, S.L.C., Lidsky, A.S., Guttler, F., et al. Nature 306, 151-155, 1983.
71.Gusella, J.F., Wexler, N.S., Conneally, P.M. et al., Nature 306, 234-238, 1983.
72.Mita, S., Maeda, S., Shimada, K. & Araki, S. Biochem. Biophys. Res. Commun. 124, 558-564, 1984.
73.Southern, E.M. J. Mol. Biol. 98, 503-517, 1975.
74.Mita, S., Maeda, S., Ide, M. et al. Neurology 36, 298-301, 1986.
75.Sasaki, H., Sakaki, Y., Matsuo, H. et al. Biochem. Biophys. Res. Commun. 125, 636-642, 1984.
76.Sasaki, H., Sakaki, Y., Sahashi, K. et al. Lancet i, 100, 1985.
77.Benson, M.D. & Dwulet, F.E. J. Clin. Invest. 75, 71-75, 1985.
78.Saraiva, M.J.M. Costa, P.P. & Goodman, D. J. Clin. Invest. 76, 2171-2177, 1985.

217

79.Osserman, E.F., Isobe, T. & Farkangi, M. In Amyloidosis. Wegelius, O., Pasternack, A., Eds. Academic Press, London, 533-564, 1976.
80.Araki, S., Kurihara, T., Tawara, S. & Kuribayashi, T. In Amyloid and Amyloidosis. Glenner, G.G., Costa, P.P., Freitas, A.F., Eds. Excerpta Medica, Amsterdam, 67-77, 1980.
81.Araki, S., Ikegawa, W., Nagata, J. et al. Neurological Therapeutics (Japanese) 299-304, 1985.
82.Ikegawa, S., Araki, S., Nagata, J. et al. Clin. Neurol. 26, 175-179, 1986.
83.Westermark, P., Johansson, B. & Natvig, J.B. Scand. J. Immunol. 10: 303-308, 1979.
84.Shirahama, T., Skinner, M., Westermark, P. et al. Am. J. Pathol. 107, 41-50, 1982.
85.Koeppen, A.H., Mitzen, E.J., Hans, M.B. et al. Muscle Nerve 8, 733-749, 1985.

V.3 BIOCHEMICAL AND GENETIC CHARACTERIZATION OF A VARIANT TRANSTHYRETIN CAUSING FAMILIAL AMYLOIDOTIC POLYNEUROPATHY

Masamitsu Nakazato[1], Teruyuki Kurihara[1], Shigeru Matsukura[1], Kenji Kangawa[2], Hiroyuki Sasaki[3], Hirokazu Furuya[3], Yoshiyuki Sakaki[3] and Hisayuki Matsuo[2]

The Third Department of Medicine[1] and Department of Biochemistry[2], Miyazaki Medical College, Kiyotake, Miyazaki 889-16, and Research Laboratory for Genetic Information[3], Kyushu University, Fukuoka, 812, Japan.

1. Introduction

Familial amyloidotic polyneuropathy (FAP) has a worldwide distribution and type I FAP is the most common disorder characterized by progressive polyneuropathy. Very little has been known about the biochemical and genetic nature of this intractable disorder. In addition there has been no diagnostic method for this progressive disorder before symptoms appear around the age of 20 to 40 years. Since this disorder is transmitted by autosomal dominant inheritance and the clinical onset is postmarital, it has long been desired to develop an early diagnostic method to predict possible transmission of the disease.

We have purified amyloid fibril protein from type I FAP of Japanese origin. Sequencing analyses on cyanogen bromide and tryptic peptides of amyloid protein have turned out to be helpful for determining the primary structure of amyloid related to transthyretin (TTR), which was formerly called prealbumin (1). Amyloid protein contains a variant form of TTR with an amino acid substitution of a methionine-for-valine at position 30 (2). This variant TTR is present in the serum of patients along with normal TTR (3).

The diagnosis of FAP has been suggested by clinical manifestations together with biopsy studies. To develop a definitely and noninvasively diagnostic test for the disease, we have established a radioimmunoassay (RIA) specific for the variant TTR (4,5). The amino acid replacement in the variant TTR has led us to study the genetic abnormality in the patients. Guanine to adenine change in the first letter of the Val[30] codon is responsible for the substitution of methionine for valine (6). Since the base change produces new restriction sites for restriction endonucleases: NsiI and BalI, the aberrant TTR gene can be detected by Southern blot hybridization analysis (7).

The purpose of this study is to clarify the biochemical and genetic characterization of FAP and to confirm the applicability as prenatally and presymptomatically diagnostic methods of the RIA and DNA techniques. Here we report the results in Japanese FAP patients, their non-inheriting members and symptom-free children by these methods.

2.Materials and methods

2.1.Subjects

Forty five Japanese FAP patients (23 females, 22 males; mean age 41.6 ± 11.8 (SD) years); 50 non-inheriting members of families with FAP (29 females, 21 males; mean age 47.8 ± 11.7 years); 24 children of 15 FAP patients (13 females, 11 males; mean age 15.3 ± 3.4 years) were examined. All the children did not have any symptoms and signs of FAP when the studies were performed.

2.2.Radioimmunoassay for the variant TTR

The amount of the variant TTR was measured by the RIA based on a nonapeptide (positions 22-30) of the variant (4,5). Five µl of the serum of subjects were lyophilized. The samples were treated with 3 mg of cyanogen bromide in 70% formic acid at room temperature for 36 hr and then re-lyophilized. The resulting fragments were incubated in 100 µl of 0.1 M Tris-HCl to convert COOH-terminal homoserine lactone into homoserine. The fragments were then digested with 8 µg of TPCK-treated trypsin at 37°C for 2 hr. Thereafter, soybean trypsin inhibitor was added to the buffer to stop the reaction. Samples were measured according to the RIA procedure described previously (4).

2.3.DNA analysis

DNA was isolated from leucocytes of 10 ml of blood samples. DNA (5-10 µg) was digested with restriction endonucleases NsiI and/or BalI, and then subjected to Southern blot hybridization analysis with the ^{32}P- -labelled TTR cDNA as a probe (6).

3.Results

Restriction sites for NsiI and BalI in the TTR locus are shown in Fig. 1 and Fig. 2. Normal TTR gene gave only a single hybridization band of 6.35 kilobase (Kb) in digestion with NsiI. Guanine to adenine change in the aberrant TTR gene leads to formation of a new restriction site for NsiI (GTGCATATGCAT). Therefore, the aberrant gene gave two extra bands of 4.90 and 1.45 Kb. In the case of BalI digestion (Fig. 2), normal TTR gene gave two bands of 5.2 and 2.2 Kb, whereas the aberrant gene gave two extra bands of 3.65 and 1.55 Kb due to the new restriction site (TGGCCGTGGCCA) in the 5.2 Kb fragment.

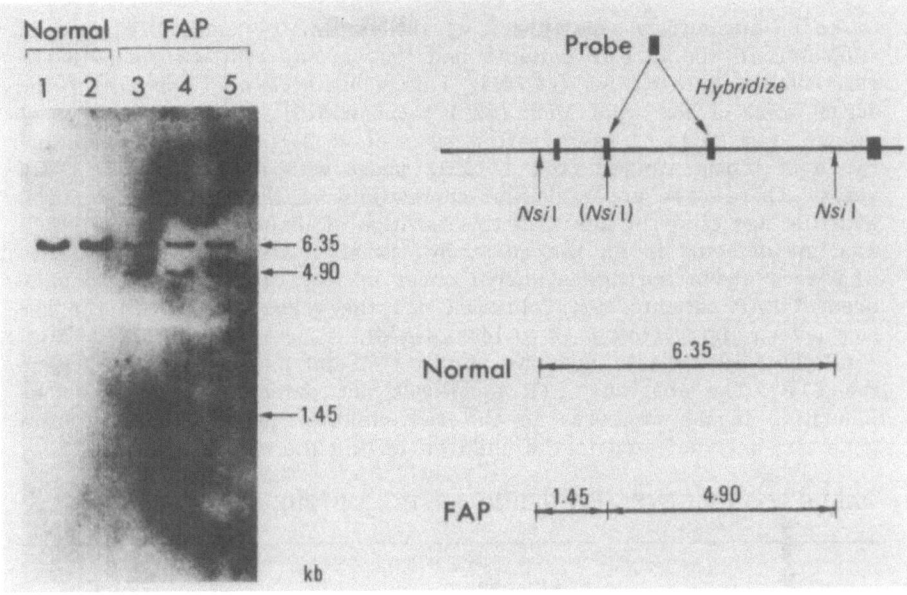

Figure 1: Detection of a new restriction site for NsiI in the mutated TTR gene. The new restriction site is indicated in parentheses. Lane 1 and 2 represent DNA samples from two normal individuals, and 3-5 those from three FAP patients.

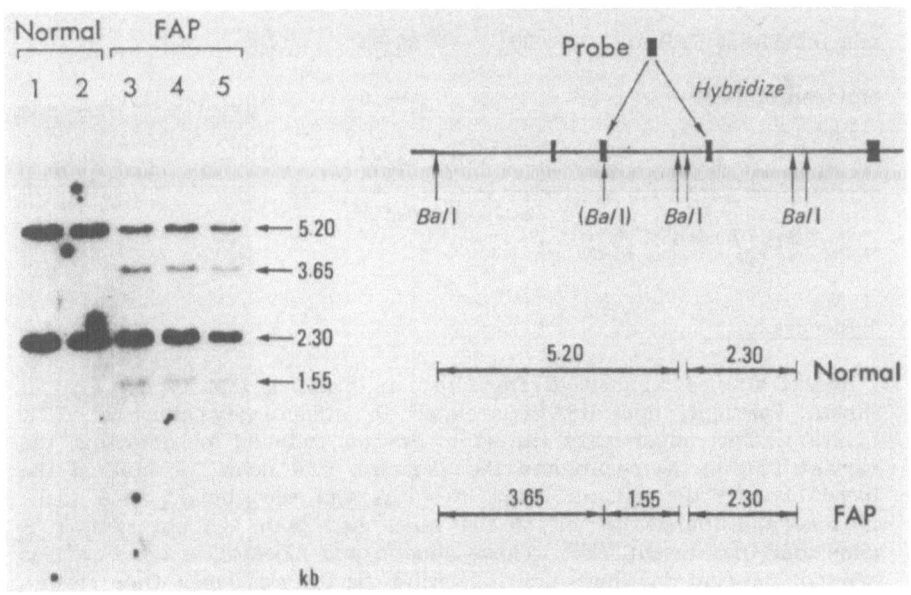

Figure 2: Detection of a new restriction site for BalI in the mutated TTR gene. Samples are the same as in Fig. 1.

221

Table I summarizes serum levels of the variant TTR and TTR gene in subjects. All the 45 FAP patients had the variant TTR with a mean serum level of 9.18 $\pm$ 2.69 (mg/dl). This value accounted for 2/5 of the serum level of the total TTR (22.4 $\pm$ 6.6 mg/dl). Their ages of onset ranged from 23 to 67 years with a mean of 36.3 $\pm$ 11.4 years, and duration of illness ranged from 1 to 17 years with a mean of 5.5 $\pm$ 3.6 years. There were no significant correlations of the variant TTR level with the age of onset nor with the duration of illness. The variant TTR was not detected in all the 50 family members lacking FAP symptoms, who were above the age of usual onset of FAP. In asymptomatic children of FAP patients, 9/24 children had the variant TTR with the serum level ranging from 8.32 to 14.71 mg/dl.

All the FAP patients had one normal (N) and one aberrant (A) gene for TTR. The aberrant TTR gene was not detected in all the non-inheriting family members. In the two children groups, the aberrant gene was only detected in the children having the variant TTR.

TABLE I: TTR GENE AND SERUM LEVELS OF THE VARIANT TTR

Subjects	Number of cases	Age (yrs)	TTR[*] gene	Variant[**] TTR (mg/dl)
FAP patients	45	25-68	NA	9.18 $\pm$ 2.69
non-inheriting FAP	50	33-62	NN	0
children of FAP	9	9-19	NA	11.90 $\pm$ 2.33
	15	7-22	NN	0

[*] N= normal TTR gene; A= aberrant TTR gene.
[**] The data are expressed as the mean $\pm$ SD.

4. Discussion

Recent studies on amyloid fibril protein clarified that type I FAP in Japan, Portugal, and USA is related to structurally abnormal TTR (2,8,9,). This abnormality led us to develop methods for detecting the variant TTR in the serum and the aberrant TTR gene. We studied the blood of 45 FAP patients using the RIA and recombinant DNA techniques, and found that all of the cases had both the aberrant TTR gene and the variant TTR. These genetic and biochemical abnormalities are not present in their non-inheriting family members. Our results indicate that the base change in TTR-DNA, structurally abnormal TTR, and clinical expression of FAP perfectly link together. Quite recently amyloid of type II FAP (Indiana/Swiss type) has been determined as another variant TTR with a serine-for-isoleucine substitution at position 84 (10). Most of, but not all of FAP can be considered as a molecular disorder to TTR. The different clinical manifestations of various types of FAP, at least in part, may be caused by a certain amino acid substitution at various positions.

The RIA showed that the variant TTR already exists in the serum of children inheriting the mutant gene. The close follow-up of inheriting children could give us a valuable clue to clarify the pathogenesis of this disorder in relation to abnormal TTR deposition. Such a study would be helpful for developing a therapy to prevent or to retard amyloid fibril formation. It is well known that there is a wide variety in onset ages and progression of the disease in the world. These variations suggest that factors other than structurally abnormal TTR may influence the onset and progression of the disease.

FAP patients have one normal and one aberrant gene for TTR, indicating that they are heterozygous for the mutant gene. The amount of the serum variant TTR is approximately half of the total TTR in these patients. This ratio shows that the two TTR's are the products of a co-dominant expression of two allelic genes in the heterogeneous state.

The RIA and TTR gene analysis can serve as two independent and consistent diagnostic methods for directly detecting biochemical and genetic abnormalities in type I FAP. We can also predict before usual onset age whether a member of a FAP family is likely to develop the disease in the future. Therefore, members of families with FAP can do better family planning, being assured whether or not they can have children without worrying about transmission of the disorder. These diagnostic methods can be widely applied to type I FAP throughout the world for early diagnosis and genetic counselling before the child-bearing age.

References

1. Nomenclature Committee of IUB (NC-IUB) IUB-IUPAC Joint Commission on Biochemical Nomenclature (JCBN). J. Biol. Chem. 256, 12-14, 1981.
2. Tawara, S., Nakazato, M., Kangawa, K., et al. Biochem. Biophys. Res. Commun. 116, 880-888, 1983.
3. Nakazato, M., Kangawa, K., Minamino, N., et al. Biochem. Biophys. Res. Commun. 122, 712-718, 1984.
4. Nakazato, M., Kangawa, K., Minamino, N., et al. Biochem. Biophys. Res. Commun. 122, 719-725, 1984.
5. Nakazato, M., Kurihara, T., Matsukura, S., et al. J. Clin. Invest. 77, 1699-1703, 1986.
6. Sasaki, H., Sakaki, Y., Matsuo, H., et al. Biochem. Biophys. Res. Commun. 125, 636-642, 1984.
7. Yoshioka, K., Sasaki, H., Yoshioka, N., et al. Mol. Biol. Med. (In Press).
8. Saraiva, M.J.M., Birken, S., Costa, P.P., et al. J. Clin. Invest. 74, 104-119, 1984.
9. Dwulet, F.E. & Benson, M.D. Proc. Natl. Acad. Sci. USA. 81, 694-698, 1984.
10. Benson, M.D. & Dwulet, F.E. Clin. Res. 33, 590A, 1985.

SECTION VI

SENILE AMYLOIDOSIS

sub-editor: George G. Glenner

VI.1 THE NATURE AND PATHOGENESIS OF THE AMYLOID DEPOSITS IN ALZHEIMER'S DISEASE

George G. Glenner and Caine W. Wong

University of California,
San Diego, School of Medicine Department of Pathology (M-012)
La Jolla, CA 92093, U.S.A.

1. Introduction

Up until 15 years ago the twisted filaments of the neurofibrillary tangles and the amyloid fibrils in neuritic plaques and cerebral vessels seen in Alzheimer's disease (AD) were primarily of descriptive interest and their interrelationship unknown. Indeed it was only 10 years ago that necropsy studies of demented and nondemented individuals indicated that the diagnostic presence of plaques and tangles could be found in significant quantities in demented old individuals of an age too advanced to be classified as typical "Alzheimer's disease". Since the diagnostic cerebral lesions in both groups were found to be identical, the definitions of "presenile" and "senile" dementia merged (1). In addition the same lesions (2,3) and similar symptoms (4) were found in Downs's syndrome adults over the age of 40 (5). Did this signify that all Down's syndrome individuals acquired Alzheimer's disease or that an invariable genetic component of Down's syndrome was Alzheimer's disease? What was the significance of these lesions? Slowly, but inexorably, answers to these questions have been forthcoming.

1.2. The Fibrillar Pathology

1.2.1. Neurofibrillary Tangles

Upon the introduction of silver impregnation methods, Alzheimer (6) first described the rigid fibrillar argyrophilic deposits in certain cortical neurons in patients having what we now call Alzheimer's disease. Divry (7), based on the Congo red polarization properties (birefringence and green polarization color) of the tangles, assumed that these represented amyloid (8). This was an iconoclastic view since intracellular amyloid had never been previously described. Electron microscopic examination of the tangles presented two interpretations, one of "twisted tubules" by Terry et al (9) and the other of "paired helical filaments" (PHF) by Kidd et al (10,11). The latter configuration has been validated (12) and its significance (13) in our interpretation of these lesions. Antibodies to neurofilament proteins (150 Kd and 215 Kd) react with the PHF (14,15). X-ray diffraction studies have thus far been inconclusive in defining the nature of the PHF due to the lack of purity of the preparations (16).

1.2.2. Neuritic Plaques

These lesions were first described by Blocq and Marinesco (17) and vary in shape from diffuse to compact. Divry (6) also ascribed the presence in the plaque to amyloid based on their Congophilic polarization properties. Electron microscopy revealed the diffuse (premature) plaques to be composed of a periphery of degenerating neurites containing PHF, with associated microglia and astrocytes and none or a few wisps of amyloid fibers (18). Compact plaques were invariably composed primarily of amyloid "cores" (18). Antibodies to a wide variety of serum proteins (19,21) have been localized to the plaques, but not all these results have been confirmed (22). Neurofilament protein has not been localized to the amyloid of the plaques (15). Considerable lysosomal enzyme activity has been associated with the plaques by several authors (23,24).

1.2.3. Cerebrovascular Amyloidosis (CVA)

First described in the leptomeninges and intracortices by Fischer in 1910 (25) this lesion was also designated as amyloid by Divry (7). Although early writers noted its association with dementia and/or plaques (26,27) it was more often related to normal aging than to Alzheimer's disease until an extensive study of over 400 Alzheimer's disease autopsies revealed its presence in 92% of Alzheimer's disease cases and absence in non-Alzheimer's disease individuals (5,22). It has also been associated with intracortical and leptomeningial hemorrhage (28) usually with Alzheimer's disease. A condition known as hereditary Congophilic angiopathy with hemorrhage (HCHWA) has been reported from Iceland (29) in which the victims die of cerebral hemorrhage, usually at age 20-30 years. The amyloid protein from these cases has been found to be homologous with a serum protein, gamma trace (30).

In this study our objective was to define the chemical nature of the amyloid of plaques and cerebral vessels in Alzheimer's disease in order to decipher the nature of these lesions and their role in the pathogenesis of Alzheimer's disease. We here describe the characteristics and localization of the cerebrovascular β protein, a marker protein for Alzheimer's disease.

2. Materials and Methods

2.1. Amyloid Fibril Concentration

Human brains of Alzheimer's disease victims obtained at autopsy were frozen at -70°C. Histological sections were taken, stained for amyloid and only those with extensive cerebrovascular amyloidosis were selected for amyloid fibril isolation. The brains of a 61 and 62 year old individual diagnosed as having Down's syndrome were similarly processed. Age matched normal brains were used for controls. The meninges were stripped, and gross cortex contaminants removed. The tissue was homogenized in 0.9% sodium chloride-0.1% sodium azide and the homogenate centrifuged in a Sorvall RC-5B (DuPont Instruments) at 12,500 x g for 60 min. at 4°C. The supernatant was discarded. The resultant pellet was made up of two visually distinct layers. The thin brownish top layer was enriched in amyloid fibrils as monitored by polarization microscopy after Congo red staining. The layers were separated by dissection of the frozen pellet. A second homogenization of the lower layer yielded a significant second crop of amyloid fibrils. The amyloid-enriched top layer was homogenized in 0.05 M TRIS-HCl, 3mM NaN_3, 0.01 mM $CaCl_2$, pH 7.5 buffer to make an approximate 4% solution (w/v). Solid collagenase (EC 3.4.24.3 Sigma Chemical type 1) was added in a 1:100 ratio (weight enzyme: weight pellet) and the resultant mixture was incubated in a Dubnoff shaker bath at 37°C for 8 hrs. The digestion by collagenase was monitored by Congo red staining with polarization microscopy. After the digestion was completed, the mixture was centrifuged in a Beckman L5-50B ultracentrifuge at 105,000 x g for 60 min. at 4° C. The supernatant was discarded and the pellet frozen at -20°C (31,32).

2.2.X-ray Crystallography of the Amyloid Fibrils

Samples of the amyloid fibril concentrate were prepared for X-ray diffraction by suspending small pieces of the fresh amyloid in distilled water and concentrating the suspension into the tip of a 0.7 mm diameter thin walled quartz capillary by centrifugation (1000 x g). To prevent moisture-loss during the recording of the diffraction diagram, the capillaries were sealed with wax before mounting in the X-ray camera. The X-ray diffraction diagrams were recorded on film with nickel-filtered copper radiation (1.54 Å) obtained from a fine focus tube operated at 30 kV and 38 mA. Patterns of fresh unlyophilized amyloid depositis were obtained with a 57.3 mm diameter Debye-Scherrer powder camera. Accurate recordings of the amyloid diffraction maxima in purified preparations were made using a 114.5 mm diameter Debye-Scherrer powder camera. The diffraction lines from small amounts of palladium metal mixed with the amyloid deposits were used as internal calibration standards in these latter recordings. The patterns from oriented material were obtained using a Chesley-Philips microcamera having a specimen to film distance of 14.7 mm and equipped with a 100 μ-bore glass capillary collimator. The mechanically oriented specimens were examined with the X-ray beam path either parallel or perpendicular to the direction of applied pressure. The lamellar samples were photographed with the lamellar surface either parallel or perpendicular to the beam. Both the microcamera and the 57.3 mm diameter camera were used in comparing tissue preparations (29) by Dr. E.D. Eanes, National Institute of Dental Research, Bethesda, Maryland.

2.3. Protein Extraction

The collagenase-treated pellet was solubilized in 6 M guanidine-HCl, 0.1 M TRIS-HCl, 24 mM dithiothreitol, 0.34 mM EDTA, pH 8.0 (22% w/v) and stirred at room temperature for 48 hrs. After 48 hrs. the solution was centrifuged in a Beckman L-5-50B ultracentrifuge at 105,000 x g for 60 min. at 4°C. The pellet was separated from the supernatant. The supernatant was placed into 1000 dalton cut off dialysis tubing (Spectra/Por 6, Fisher Scientific) and dialyzed, lyophilized and the resulting powder stored dessicated at -70°C.

2.4. SDS-urea Polyacrylamide Gel Electrophoresis (SDS-urea PAGE)

SDS-urea PAGE was done by the Laemmli system (34) modified only by the addition of 8 M urea in the stacking and resolving gel. Slab gels (15%) were made 0.75 mm thick and run at 10 mA constant current. After electrophoresis, gels were stained with Coomassie Brilliant Blue.

2.5. G-100 Sephadex Column Chromatography

The procedure was identical to that employed previously (32), using a 2.5 x 100 cm G-100 calibrated Sephadex column (Pharmacia) equilibrated with 5 M guanidine-HCl, 1 N acetic acid. The column was calibrated with cytochrome C (horse heart), 12,384 dalton and glucagon, 3,485 dalton. The protein elution profile was monitored at 280 nm with a Beckman 35 spectrophotometer. The protein peak centered at 4,200 dalton was pooled and dialyzed against deionized water, lyophilized and stored dessicated at -70°C.

2.6. High Performance Liquid Chromatography (HPLC)

One hundred µg of the lyophilized protein from peak fractions of the Sephadex column was solubilized into 25 µl of 5 M guanidine-HCl, 1 N acetic acid. This was injected into a Waters HPLC system. The mobile phase was: solvent A: 0.1% trifluoroacetic acid/H_2O, solvent B: 100% acetonitrile. The gradient was linear from 10% to 50% solvent B over 60 min. Flow rate was 0.8 ml/min. and the protein peaks were detected at 229 nm with 2.0 AUFS. The stationary phase was a Vydac 214TP54 C_4 peptide column. Three major protein peaks were found that had no correspondence with control samples. These protein peaks were pooled separately, lyophilized and stored at -70°C.

2.7. Amino Acid Sequencing

HPLC purified samples were dissolved in heptofluorobutyric acid and loaded in a Beckman 890 C spinning cup sequencer. The collected antilothiazolone amino acids were converted to phenylthiohydantoin amino acids (PTH-amino acids) with 1 N HCl/MeOH at 50° C for 10 min. The PTH-amino acids were dried and redissolved in MeOH. The PTH-amino acids were analyzed on a Beckman 322 system fitted with a ETH-Permaphase guard column and a IBM 6μ CN column in line. The eluent was monitored at 254 nm.

2.8. Immunization

A synthetic peptide (OP1) with the sequence consisting of the first 10 residues of the β protein (Asp-Ala-Glu-Phe-Arg-His-Asp-Ser-Gly-Tyr) was synthesized according to Marglin and Merrifield (35). A cysteine residue was added to the carboxyl terminus for coupling the peptide to a carrier protein. OP1 was coupled to keyhole limpet hemocyanin (KLH) through the cysteine with m-maleimidobenzoyl-N-hydroxysuccinimide ester (Sigma) as described by Green (36). Five 10 week old female BALB/c mice were injected intraperitoneally with 4 μg OP1 coupled to KLH (OP1-KLH) in Freund's complete adjuvant (Sigma). The mice were boosted 14 days later with 4 μg OP1-KLH in Freund's incomplete adjuvant (Sigma). Three weeks after initial immunization, the mice were boosted once more with 1.0 μg OP1-KLH in 10 mM Tris, 150 mM NaCl, pH 8.0. Serum was obtained 7 days after the final boost. The mice immune sera were assayed for anti-OP1 and anti-β protein activity by solid phase ELISA (33). Each mouse serum was diluted 1:10,000-1:32,000 in 0.1% ovalbumin, 20 mM Tris, 150 mM NaCl, 0.2% Tween-20, 0.01% Thimerosal, pH 8.0. Assays were performed on polyvinyl chloride microtiter plates (Dynatech) in which 0.05 μg F82B, or 0.1 μg KLH had been dried in the wells. Bound antibodies were detected with peroxidase conjugated goat antimouse IgG at 1:1000 dilution (Cappel). O-phenylenediamine was used as the substrate and quantitation was done with a Multiskan Microplate Reader (Flow Laboratories) at 492 nm. All five immunized mice sera were found immunoreactive to β protein, OP1 and KLH and unreactive to F82B. Normal mouse serum was unreactive to all antigens tested. The mouse serum with the highest titer (A_{492}=1.94 at 1:2000) against β protein was designated OP1MS1 and used for all further work in this manuscript. The specificity of antiserum OP1MS1 for β protein and OP1 was tested. A limiting dilution of OP1MS1 (1:6000) was preincubated with varying concentrations of inhibitors OP1 and F82B (an unrelated 17 amino acid peptide) at 4°C for 12 hrs. and then reacted in a solid phase ELISA.

2.9. Immunohistochemistry

Localization of amyloid deposits was demonstrated with mouse anti-OP1 serum (OP1MS1) by the PAP method of Sternberger (34). Formalin fixed sections of autopsied brain tissues were obtained from Alzheimer's disease, adult Down's syndrome, HCHWA and age-matched control cases. Tissue sections were cut 6.0 microns thick and fixed to glass slides. The sections were then challenged with the following series of antibod-

ies with wash steps in between each: 1) OP1MS1 (experimental) or normal mouse serum (control) at 1:2500 dilution or 1.0% ovalbumin-PBS
(blank), 2) rabbit antimouse IgG at 1:1000, 3) swine anti-rabbit IgG at
1:100, 4) rabbit peroxidase-anti-peroxidase at 1:1000 (Dakopatts). Positive immunoreaction was detected with 3,3'-diaminobenzidine (Sigma).
Congo red (Kodak) staining followed and Mayer's hematoxylin (MCB
Chemicals) was used as counterstain (39). For inhibition experiments, a
1:500 dilution of OP1MS1 was preincubated with 1.0% OP1 or KLH in 20
mM Tris, 150 mM NaCl, 0.2% Tween-20, 0.01% Thimerosal, pH 8.0 for 12
hrs. at 4°C prior to use in the procedure just outlined. A Leitz Ortho-
plan polarizing microscope was employed for visualization and photo-
microscopy.

3. Results

The amyloid fibril concentrates of cerebrovascular amyloid gave un-
oriented X-ray crystallographic patterns having a 4.75 Å outer and 10
Å inner d-spacing (Fig.1).

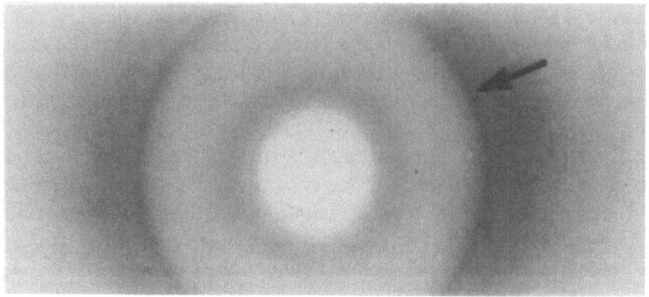

Figure 1: X-ray crystallography of isolated cerebrovascular amyloid fibrils. Diffraction
pattern reveals an outer 4.75 Å band and a 10 Å inner band (d-spacing) indicative of a
β-pleated sheet protein conformation (arrow).

This pattern is indicative of the β-pleated sheet conformation characteristic of all amyloid fibrils. Six Alzheimer's disease cases and three
age-matched control cases were examined by SDS-urea PAGE. The lyophilized material revealed a unique band of protein, β protein, that was
not seen in control samples prepared in identical fashion (Fig. 2). This
protein could be consistently fractionated on a calibrated G-100
Sephadex column with its peak fraction centered at 4,200 dalton.
Because of its uniqueness to amyloid fibril preparations, it was assumed, as shown in numerous, previous studies (31), to be a major
protein constituent of amyloid fibrils. High performance liquid chromato-

graphy fractionated three peaks from the G-100 preparation of both the Alzheimer's disease and adult Down's syndrome β protein (Fig. 3) and these were found to have almost identical amino acid compositions. Two other cases of Alzheimer's disease and an adult Down's syndrome gave identical HPLC profiles.

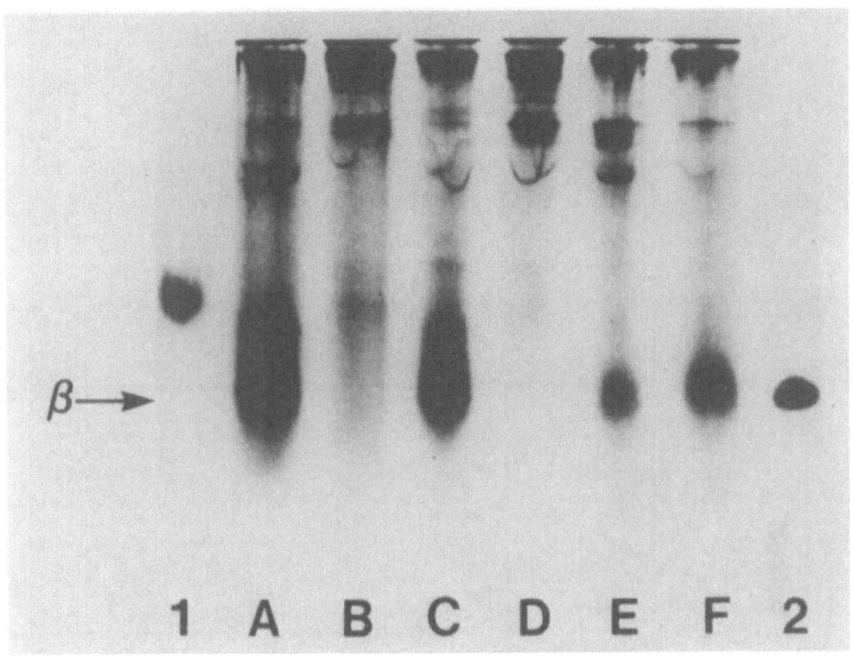

Figure 2: SDS slab gel electrophoresis identification of cerebrovascular amyloid fibril protein β of patients A, C, E and F compared to normal cerebral vessel preparations B and D indentically treated. Molecular weight markers are: 1. cytochrome C (12,300 dalton) and 2. glucagon (3,485 dalton).

Our studies reveal the HPLC elution profiles of the β protein from the cerebrovascular amyloid fibrils of Alzheimer's disease and adult Down's syndrome are almost identical (Fig. 3). The Down's profile revealed a lesser quantity of the β_1 peak. No corresponding peaks were noted in three control preparations. In addition these chromatographs resolved from both protein preparations a β_3 peak, previously obscured within that of β_2 (40). It has been shown that the β_1 and β_2 proteins were homologous by amino acid sequence analysis (41). Since β_3 was initially included in β_2, it is assumed to be homologous to β_2. Why β protein appears as a doublet or triplet on HPLC is presently unknown. The amino acid sequence analysis of the Down's and Alzheimer's disease β_2 protein fraction to residue 28 is presented in Table I.

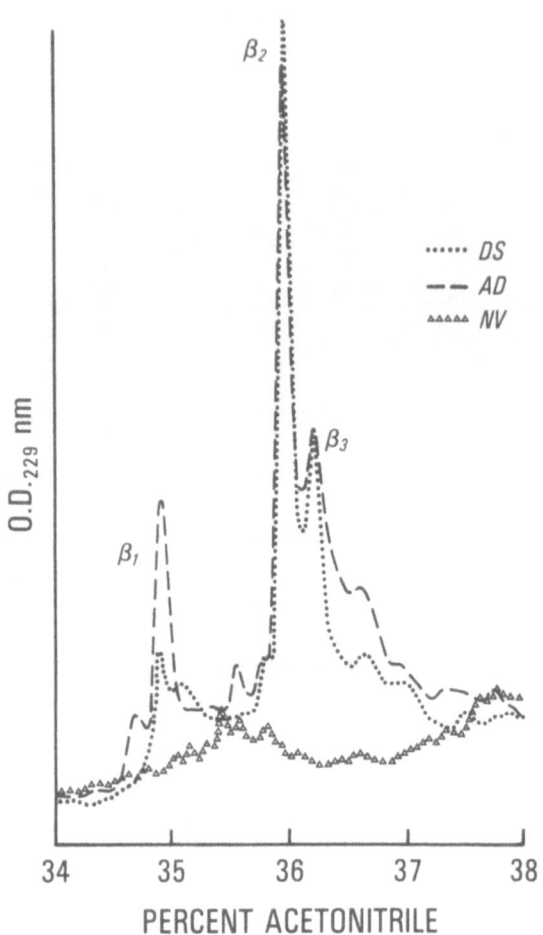

<u>Figure 3</u>: HPLC of the cerebrovascular amyloid fibril β protein from an Alzheimer's disease patient (AD) previously isolated on Sephadex G-100 as compared to the β protein of an adult Down's syndrome individual (DS) demonstrating three major protein peaks (β_1, β_2, and β_3). The β_1 and β_2 proteins have identical amino-terminal amino acid sequences, while the characteristics of β_3 are presently unknown (see text).

This protein was found to have an amino acid sequence identical to that of the Alzheimer's disease β_2 protein (40) through position 28 with the exception of a substitution of Glu for Gln residue at position 11 (Table I). The retention of Gln[15] strongly suggests that Glu[11] is a true substitution and is not due to an artifactual deamidation. The β_2 protein is not homologous to the serum protein gamma trace (30) found to compose the cerebrovascular amyloid protein of the Icelandic HCHWA (30), nor

Glenner & Wong

to any other known sequenced protein. The preparation from the second Down's case gave an HPLC profile with an identical major peak at 35% acetonitrile, but inadequate material was available for sequencing.

TABLE I: AUTOMATED AMINO ACID SEQUENCE ANALYSES OF β_2 PROTEIN TO POSITION 28 FROM CEREBRO-VASCULAR AMYLOID FIBRILS OBTAINED FROM ALZHEIMER'S DISEASE (AD) AND ADULT DOWN's SYNDROME (DS) (Variant residue is underlined)

	1	2	3	4	5	6	7	8	9	10	11	12	13	14
AD	Asp	Ala	Glu	Phe	Arg	His	Asp	Ser	Gly	Tyr	Gln	Val	His	His
DS	Asp	Ala	Glu	Phe	Arg	His	Asp	Ser	Gly	Tyr	<u>Glu</u>	Val	His	His

	15	16	17	18	19	20	21	22	23	24	25	26	27	28
AD	Gln	Lys	Leu	Val	Phe	Phe	Ala	Glu	Asp	Val	Gly	Ser	Asn	Lys
DS	Gln	Lys	Leu	Val	Phe	Phe	Ala	Glu	Asp	Val	Gly	Ser	Asn	Lys

These findings indicate that of the three disease processes most often characterized by cerebrovascular amyloidosis, i.e., Alzheimer's disease (2,5), adult Down's syndrome (5) and Icelandic HCHWA (29), only Alzheimer's disease and adult Down's syndrome share a homologous amyloid protein. This is the first chemical evidence of a relationship between Alzheimer's disease and Down's syndrome.

There is presently no known spontaneous or experimental animal model for Alzheimer's disease. There are mouse models for Down's syndrome (42), but since the trisomic fetuses do not survive beyond term, their value for the study of Alzheimer's disease is limited. The human familial cases of Alzheimer's disease tend to follow an autosomal dominant pattern of inheritance (43) with the usual statistical prediction of affected progeny. However, the great similarity in the cerebral lesions between adult Down's syndrome and Alzheimer's disease (2,5) and the demonstration of chemical homology in the pathologic amyloid fibril β protein strongly suggests that Down's syndrome may represent the first truly predictable model for Alzheimer's disease.

Tissue from six cases of Alzheimer's disease, two cases of adult Down's syndrome, one case of Icelandic HCHWA and three age-matched normal brains were immunohistochemically studied by the Sternberger peroxidase-antiperoxidase (PAP) method (38) using OP1MS1. Amyloid--laden vascular sites in the leptomeningial and intracortical areas in Alzheimer's disease and adult Down's syndrome cases immunostained intensely and corresponded precisely to the areas of Congo red polarization birefringence (Figs. 4a and 4b). This birefringence resulting from Congo red staining is an accepted histochemical marker for the β-pleated sheet structure of amyloid (13). In addition, both diffuse (primitive and compact (mature) neuritic plaques reacted with OP1MS1 in the PAP procedure in Alzheimer's disease and adult Down's syndrome tissue sections (Figs. 4c and 4d).

235

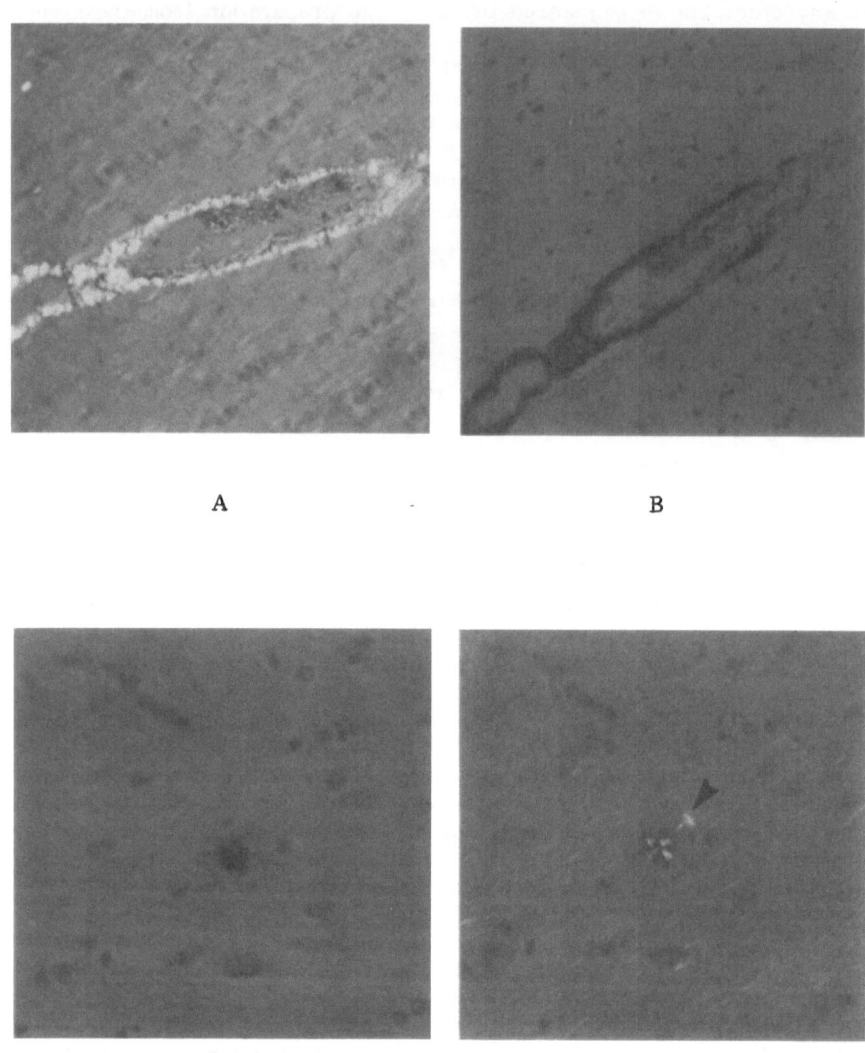

A

B

C

D

Figure 4: Sections of formalin-fixed cerebral tissue from adult Down's syndrome stained by the alkaline Congo red method with hematoxylin counterstain and visualized by polarization microscopy (A & C). The same sections were immunoreacted with the PAP method using anti-bodies to β protein homologue OP1MS1 and visualized by bright field (B & D). Amyloid deposits (A) in vessels - partially obscured by PAP staining - are reactive to β protein homologue OP1MS1 antibody with PAP method (B). Compact neuritic plaque (C) is reactive (C-arrow) to OP1MS1 antibody (D). Note neurofibrillary tangles are unreactive to OP1MS1 antibody (From Proc. Natl. Acad. Sci USA Ref. 49).

There were rare instances in Alzheimer's disease and adult Down's syndrome tissue in which localized PAP staining of sites resembling small diffuse plaques did not have corresponding Congo red birefringence. This could be due to the ability of the PAP procedure to detect localized deposits of β protein that were not in the β-pleated sheet conformation and were, therefore, non-birefringent.

PAP staining of CVA and neuritic plaques could be completely inhibited if OP1MS1 was preincubated with OP1. Preincubation of OP1MS1 with a concentration of KLH that eliminated all anti-KLH activity as detected by ELISA had no effect on the PAP staining of CVA and neuritic plaques. The specific inhibition with OP1 strongly indicates that the specific PAP staining by OP1MS1 was entirely due to antibodies to OP1.

The normal brain tissues examined showed no significant PAP staining beyond the very slight background also obtained when normal mouse serum was used in place of OP1MS1. This confirms the observation by SDS-polyacrylamide gel electrophoresis and high performance liquid chromatography of the uniqueness of the β protein in cerebral tissues to Alzheimer's disease and adult Down's syndrome (40,41). The HCHWA case, though heavily laden with cerebrovascular amyloid as detected by Congo red birefringence, was also unreactive to PAP staining. This is consistent with the fact that HCHWA cerebrovascular amyloid is composed of gamma trace (30) which has no sequence homology with β protein. The lack of reactivity with the HCHWA case further supports the specificity of OP1MS1 for β protein.

No PAP staining was seen associated with neurofibrillary tangles (Fig. 4d). This suggests that the etiology and source of neurofibrillary tangles is either distinct from that of CVA and neuritic plaques or that the anti-OP1 determinants of neurofibrillary tangles are sterically obscured. Kidd et al (44) and Allsop et al (45) have noted that the amino acid compositions of neuritic plaques, neurofibrillary tangles and CVA are similar and suggests that they are all composed of the same protein. Our findings support their suggestion that neuritic plaques are composed of β protein but does not confirm their suggestion that neurofibrillary tangles are also composed of β protein. It should be noted that Anderson et al (14), reported that the monoclonal antibodies used by them to identify the immunochemical relationship between the 155 and 210 Kdalton neurofilament proteins and neurofibrillary tangles did not react with the amyloid in neuritic plaques. Earlier reports have implicated IgG (19) and prealbumin (46) as the CVA and neuritic plaque amyloid protein. We have been unable to duplicate the reported PAP staining of CVA and neuritic plaques with anti-human IgG and anti-human prealbumin antibodies. Furthermore, the amino acid composition of plaque cores and CVA are not consistent with the compositions of either IgG or prealbumin.

4. Discussion

The present studies confirm in part our initial hypothesis (46) as to the pathogenesis of Alzheimer's disease. It is evident from the electron microscopic and X-ray diffraction data that the amyloid of the cerebral vessels (CVA) is a fibril composed of proteins in a twisted β-pleated sheet conformation (5,47). Although suspected of being a β-pleated sheet fibril of different protein composition (5,47) than plaques or vessels, the physico-chemical nature of the PHF is still unknown. In this study antibodies to β protein fail to react with tangles, although those of the 155 and 210 Kdalton neurofilament proteins have been reported to do so (14).

The absence of the cerebrovascular amyloid protein, β protein, in vessels of normal individuals and HCHWA indicates that β protein is a unique marker protein for Alzheimer's disease. While having common cerebral lesions, the almost identical amino acid sequence of β protein of the cerebrovascular fibrils in both Alzheimer's disease and adult Down's syndrome is the first chemical evidence that Down's syndrome is a pathologic model for Alzheimer's disease. Immunohistochemical studies further substantiate the uniqueness of β protein for Alzheimer's disease.

The HCHWA case, though heavily laden with cerebrovascular amyloid as detected by Congo red staining, was unreactive by PAP staining. This was expected since HCHWA cerebrovascular amyloid fibrils are composed of gamma trace protein (30) which has no homology with the β protein. The experiment with the HCHWA case was included as an additional control to demonstrate the specificity of OP1MS1 for β amyloid protein. HCHWA is the only other neuropathologic process that is known to have cerebrovascular amyloidosis as a significant lesion (5,40). Since our isolation and purification scheme for β protein eliminated contamination by intracerebral tissue, it, therefore, eliminated contamination of our original preparations of CVA by plaques and tangles. The localization of β protein antibodies to amyloid deposits in cerebral vessels of both Alzheimer's disease and Down's syndrome (49) was expected (5) in view of the similarity in amino acid sequence of their β protein. Not only was the intended target, CVA, stained by OP1MS1, but also the neuritic plaques in both Alzheimer's disease and adult Down's syndrome (Figs. 4c and 4d). The localization of the β protein antibodies to neuritic plaques in both Alzheimer's disease and Down's syndrome indicates the source of amyloid in both plaques and vessels is the same. It further supports the concept that Down's syndrome is a chemical model for Alzheimer's disease.

What distinguishes our immunohistochemical work from earlier reports (19,21) is that we used antibodies raised to a well-defined, pure synthetic peptide whose sequence was derived from the first 10 residues of a purified protein that appears by three different criteria to be unique specifically to Alzheimer's disease and adult Down's syndrome. We do not know if the PAP reaction with OP1MS1 detects the amyloid fibril protein or a non-fibrillar associated component of the plaque. A definitive statement can only be made following amino acid sequence analysis of the amyloid fibril protein of the plaque.

The amino acid compositions of plaque amyloid "cores" and CVA are similar (44,45). Therefore, it is likely that plaque amyloid fibrils also consist of β protein. This suggests that the amyloid in plaques and CVA have a common plasma source. Recently, Masters et al (50) attempted the amino acid sequencing of the amyloid core plaques obtained from cases of Alzheimer's disease and Down's syndrome. They obtained an inseparable series of at least four polypeptides by HPLC fractionation which had progressive deletions of their N-terminal amino acids. They ordered these according to the amino acid sequence of β protein and obtained homology with it except for discrepancies (49) in positions 11 (Glu for Gln), 27 (Ser for Asn) and 28 (Ala for Lys). It is doubtful that without the known sequence of β protein these polypeptides could have been ordered into sequence since at each cycle at least four amino acids would have been detected. Using antibodies to peptide 1-11 and 11-23 of β protein, Masters et al (51) claimed that not only did antibodies to peptides 11-23 react with cerebrovascular amyloid and amyloid plaque core in Alzheimer's disease but contrary to the findings of Wong et al (49), that antibodies to peptide 1-11 reacted with neurofibrillary tangles. The findings of cerebrovascular wall and plaque amyloid reacting to antibodies to β protein (49) have been confirmed by several authors (52) and in agreement with us no reactivity of neurofibrillary tangles with anti-β protein antibodies was found.

The pathologic implications of our findings strongly support a close association of neuritic plaques with cerebral vessels and/or serum (53). There are six clinical conditions (AL, AA, AF as well as Alzheimer's disease, HCHWA and adult Down's syndrome) that are associated with vascular amyloid fibril deposits. Of the three that have been investigated, all have been shown to be derived from an abnormal serum protein precursor (54). Based on this precedent, we suggest that the three remaining processes Alzheimer's disease, adult Down's syndrome and HCHWA will have an abnormal serum precursor as well.

The present report fills in an important gap in unveiling the pathogenesis of Alzheimer's disease that suggests that the formation of neuritic plaques is the result of breaks in the blood-brain barrier (55). Miyakawa et al (56) found that all neuritic plaques were associated with at least one degenerating amyloidotic capillary. We present here evidence that the β protein found in cerebral vessel amyloid is also found in the neuritic plaques. We, therefore, propose as a working hypothesis (Fig. 5) that CVA derives from an isotypic variant of a serum protein precursor (45) as e.g. the variant prealbumin in familial amyloidotic polyneuropathy FAP (57). The CVA damages capillary walls (22) causing seepage of β protein precursor, amongst other plasma substances, into the neuropil leading to the formation of the amyloid of the neuritic plaque (Fig. 5) via lysosomal (21,47) enzyme activity of microglia degrading the precursor of β protein (54,58). We suggest that β protein is also neurotoxic, blocking strategic receptors of specific cortical neurons, perturbing their environment and leading to PHF formation from neurofilament protein.

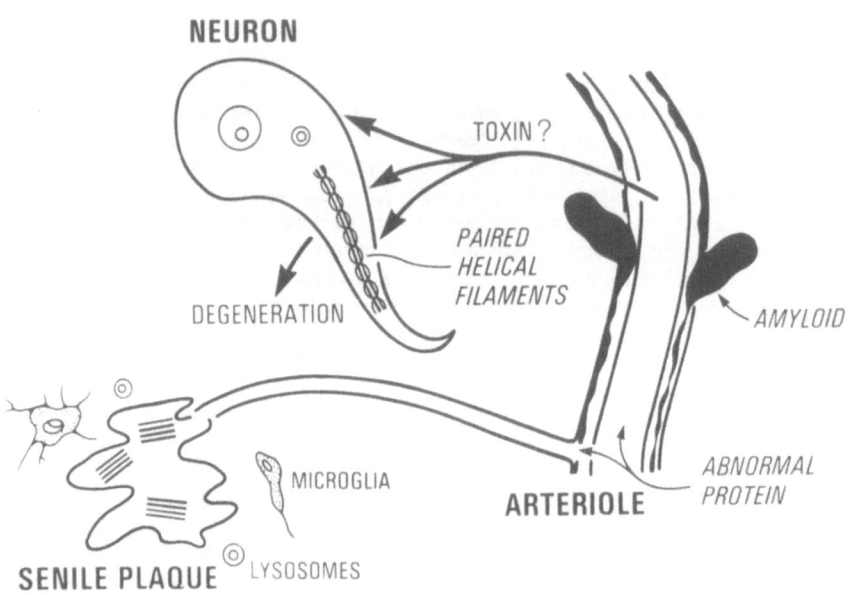

Figure 5: Diagrammatic representation of the pathogenesis of Alzheimer's disease: An abnormal β protein serum precursor is taken up specifically by cerebrovascular endothelial cells to be proteolytically cleaved by their lysosomal content to form amyloid fibrils. The amyloid fibril deposition breaks the blood-brain barrier and the (abnormal) serum protein(s) bind to neuronal cell membranes perturbing their environment. These neurons form abnormal neurofilaments (paired helical filaments) which cause the cell's death. Proteolytic cleavage by microglia of β protein, which has seeped through amyloid-affected capillary walls, produces the amyloid cores of the neuritic plaques.

One of the major objectives of this laboratory is to develop a bio-chemical assay by which Alzheimer's disease can be diagnosed. For the present its diagnosis is by eliminating all other possible causes of dementia. This is costly, time consuming and fraught with a 20% clinical error. If the formation of the cerebrovascular amyloid deposits in Alzheimer's disease and adult Down's syndrome is due to an abnormal serum protein precursor, this can be exploited to provide a relatively simple serum test. Such a test has already been devised for familial amyloidotic polyneuropathy (59). With the acquisition of OP1MS1 and its anticipated monoclonal antibody counterparts, we are hopeful that they will provide an affinity chromatographic technique for purification of the putative serum precursor of the β protein as well as the basis of a specific diagnostic radioimmunoassay for Alzheimer's disease.

In addition with this antibody it will now be possible to utilize molecular cloning technology to identify the genome involved in β protein synthesis and to characterize a suspected gene abnormality in Alzheimer's disease and adult Down's syndrome (60).

Acknowledgements

We wish to express our appreciation to Karen Rasmussen for technical assistance, Dennis Olshefsky for synthesizing the OP1 peptide, Drs. R.M. Peterson and H.L.Wolfinger, Jr., of the San Diego Regional Center for the Developmentally Disabled for Down's syndrome tissues, Margie Zajonc for her assistance in helping prepare the manuscript. This study was supported by a grant from the National Institutes of Health, AG 056683, the Weingart Foundation and a contribution from the National Alzheimer's Disease and Related Disorders Association.

References

1. Tomlinson, B.E., Blessed, G. & Roth, M. J. Neurol. Sci. 11, 205-242, 1970.
2. Burger, P.C. & Vogel, F.S. Am. J. Pathol. 73, 457-476, 1973.
3. Ellis, W.G., McCulloch, J.R. & Corley, C.L. Neurology 24, 101-106, 1974.
4. Jervis, G.A. Am. J. Psychiatry 105, 102-106, 1984.
5. Glenner, G.G. Banbury Report 15: Biological Aspects of Alzheimer's Disease, Katzman, R., Ed. Cold Spring Harbor Symposium, 137-146, 1983.
6. Alzheimer, A. Allg. Z. Psychiatrie, 64, 146-148, 1907.
7. Divry, P. J. Belge Neurol. 27, 643-657, 1927.
8. Divry, P. & Florkin, M. C.R. Soc. Biol. 97, 1808-1810, 1927.
9. Terry, R.D., Gonatas, N.K. & Weiss, M. Am. J. Pathol. 44, 269-297, 1964.
10. Kidd, M. Nature 197, 192-193, 1963.
11. Kidd, M. Brain 87, 307-320, 1964.
12. Wisniewski, H., Narang, H.K. & Terry, R.D. J. Neurol. Sci. 27, 173-181, 1976.
13. Glenner, G.G., Eanes, E.D., Bladen, H.A. et al. J. Histochem. Cytochem. 22, 1141-1158, 1974.
14. Anderton, B.H., et al. Nature 298, 84-86, 1982.
15. Miller C.C.J., Brion, J.P., Calvert, R. et al. EMBO J. 3, 269-275, 1985.
16. Selkoe, D.J. Ann. Neurol. 10, 429-436, 1981.
17. Bleag, P. & Masiness, C. Semaine Medicale (Paris), 12, 445-446, 1982.
18. Wisniewski, H.M. & Terry, R.D. Progress in Neuropathology, Vol.11, Zimmerman, H.M. ed., Grune and Stratton, New York, 1-26, 1973.
19. Ishii, T., Haga, S. & Shimizu, F. Acta Neuropathol. (Berlin) 32, 157-162, 1975.
20. Powers, J.M., Schlaeffer, W.W., Willingham, M.C., et al. (Abstract). J. Neuropathol. 39, 311, 1981.
21. Cohen, A.S., Said, S.I. & Terry, R.D. (Abstract) J. Neuropathol. 39, 310, 1981.
22. Glenner, G.G. Henry, J.M. & Fujihara, S. Ann. Pathol. 1, 105-108, 1981.
23. Friede, R.L. & Magee, K.P. Neurology 12, 213-222, 1962.
24. Morel, F. & Wildi, F. Proc. First Intl. Cong. Neuropath. 2, 347-374, 1952.
25. Fischer, O. Neurol. Psychiat. 3, 371-471, 1910.
26. Pantelakis, S. Psychiat. Neurologie 128, 219-256, 1954.
27. Surbeck, E.B. Acta Neuropathol. 1, 168-197, 1961.
28. Torack, R.M. Am. J. Pathol. 81, 349-366, 1975.
29. Gudmundsson, G., Hallgrimasson, J., Johasson, T.A., et al. Brain 95, 387-404, 1972.
30. Cohen, D.E., Feiner, H., Jensson, O., et al. J. Exp. Med. 158, 623-628, 1983.
31. Glenner, G.G., Harada, M. & Isersky, C. Prep. Biochem. 2, 39-51, 1972.
32. Harada, M., Iserksy, C., Cuatrecasas, P., et al. J. Histochem. Cytochem. 19, 1-15, 1971.
33. Eanes, E.D. & Glenner, G.G. J. Histochem. Cytochem. 16, 673-677, 1976.
34. Laemmli, U.D. Nature 227, 680-685, 1970.
35. Marglin, A. & Merrifield, R.B. Ann. Rev. Biochem. 39, 841-866, 1970.
36. Green, N., et al. Cell 28, 477-482, 1982.
37. Walter, G. & Doolitte, R.R. Genetic Engineering: Principles and Methods, Vol. 5 Satlow, J.K. and Hollaender, A., eds Plenum Press, New York, 61-91, 1983.

38. Fujihara, S. & Glenner, G.G. Lab. Invest. 44, 55-60, 1981.
39. Puchtler, H., Sweat, F. & Levine, M. J. Histochem. Cytochem. 10, 355-364, 1962.
40. Glenner, G.G. & Wong, C.W. Biochem. Biophys. Res. Commun. 122, 1131-1135, 1984.
41. Glenner, G.G. & Wong, C.W. Biochem. Biophys. Res. Commun. 120, 855-890, 1984.
42. Epstein, C.J. Banbury Report 15: Biological Aspects of Alzheimer's Disease, Katzman, R. Ed. Cold Spring Harbor Symposium, 169-182, 1983.
43. Heston, L.L. Science 196, 322-323, 1977.
44. Kidd, M., Allsop, D. & London, M. Lancet i, 278, 1978.
45. Allsop, D., London, M. & Kidd, M. (In Press).
46. Shirahama, T., Skinner, M., Westermark, P., et al. Am. J. Pathol. 107, 41-50, 1982.
47. Glenner, G.G. Medical Hypotheses 5, 1231-1236, 1979.
48. Glenner, G.G. Arch. Pathol. Lab. Med. 107, 218-282, 1983.
49. Wong, C.W., Quaranta, V. & Glenner, G.G. Proc. Natl. Acad. Sci. USA 82, 8729-8932, 1985.
50. Masters, C.L., Simms, G., Weinman, N.A., et al. Proc. Natl. Acad. Sci. USA 82, 4245-4249, 1985.
51. Masters, C.L., Multhaup, G. & Simms, G. EMBO Journal 4, 2757-2763, 1985.
52. Allsop, D.; personal communication; Selkoe, D.; personal communication; Wisniewski, H.; personal communication.
53. Scholz, W. Neurol. Psychiatr. 162, 694-715, 1938.
54. Glenner, G.G. New Engl. J. Med. 302, 1283-1292 and 1333-1343, 1980.
55. Glenner, G.G. J. Clin. Lab. Med. 98, 807-810, 1981.
56. Miyakawa et al. Virchows Arch. (Cell Pathol) 40, 121-129, 1982.
57. Dwulet, F.E. & Benson, M.D. Proc. Natl. Acad. Sci. USA 81, 694-698, 1984.
58. Glenner, G.G., Ein, D., Eanes, E.D., et al. Science 174, 712-714, 1971.
59. Benson, M.D. & Dwulet, F.E. J. Clin. Invest. 75, 71-75, 1985.
60. Maniatus, T., Fritsch, E.F. & Sambrook, J. Molecular Cloning: A Laboratory Manual. Cold Spring Harbor New York Press, 545, 1982.

VI.2   BIOCHEMISTRY OF CEREBRAL AMYLOID IN ALZHEIMER'S
       DISEASE, THE UNCONVENTIONAL SLOW VIRUS DISEASES AND
       ICELANDIC CEREBROVASCULAR AMYLOIDOSIS

David Allsop

Department of Biochemistry, University of Nottingham,
Medical School, Queen's Medical Centre,
Nottingham, England.

1. Introduction

It is estimated that 4-5% of the population over the age of 65 are severely demented (1); of these individuals approximately half suffer from
Alzheimer's disease (AD) (2), a progressive degenerative disease of the
brain, the aetiology of which is obscure, and for which there is no
form of effective treatment. The demonstration of abundant senile
plaques and neurofibrillary tangles (NFT) in a brain biopsy specimen is
the only means of obtaining an unequivocal diagnosis of this disease
during a patient's lifetime. These hallmark lesions are found mainly in
the neocortex (particularly the frontal and temporal lobes) and the
hippocampus; their clinical significance has been highlighted by showing
correlations between their numbers and (a) the extent of cognitive impairment (3,4) and (b) the characteristic decline in cholinergic function
(5,6) which is the best described, but not the only neurotransmitter-
-related abnormality (for recent reviews of neurotransmitter systems in
AD see refs. 7,8). Smaller numbers of plaques and NFT do occur in
normal aged individuals (3,4), and even in nondemented individuals at
presenile age (9).
    The classical senile plaque (Fig. 1a) can be up to 200 μm in diameter,
and consists of an extracellular stellate core of amyloid fibrils surrounded by an argyrophilic rim of dystrophic neurites and synapses
containing paired helical filaments (see below) and abnormal mito-
chondria (10,11). Microglial and astrocytic processes are also found in
this peripheral region (10,11). The plaque amyloid fibrils have been described as a pair of approximately 6 nm protofilaments arranged in the
form of a bifilar helix (12,13).
    In contrast, the NFT are intracellular fibrous bundles which can oc-
cupy most of the perinuclear cytoplasm of the affected neuronal cell
bodies, and frequently enter the cell processes. NFT exhibit all of the
staining properties of amyloid, including the characteristic Congophilia
with birefringence (Fig. 1b) but ultrastructurally they are composed of
paired helical filaments (PHF) which are pairs of 10 nm filaments arranged in the form of a double helix with a cross-over approximately
every 80 nm (14) (Fig. 1c). These resemble neither amyloid fibrils, nor
any normal fibrous component of the neuron, but since the protein in
isolated PHF is in cross-β configuration (15), there is no doubt that

243

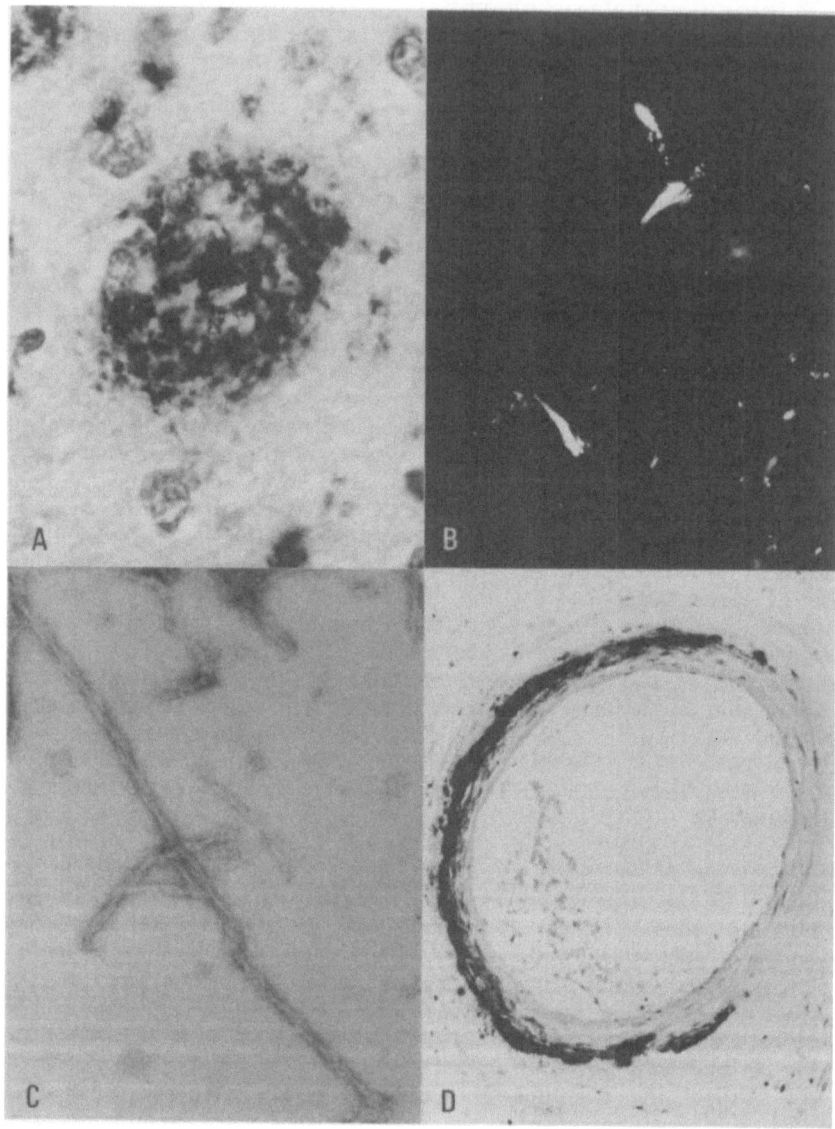

Figure 1: a. Classical senile plaque from a case of Alzheimer's disease stained by the indirect immunoperoxidase technique using a monoclonal antibody (1G10/2/3) (38) raised against a synthetic peptide consisting of residues 8-17 of an amino acid sequence reportedly common to plaque cores, cerebrovascular amyloid and PHF (see Fig. 2) (x 670). b. Preparation of isolated neuronal cell bodies (28, 31) from Alzheimer-affected cerebral cortex after Congo red staining and polarization microscopy showing characteristic flame-shaped neurofibrillary tangles (x 700). c. Isolated paired helical filaments negatively stained by uranyl acetate and observed under the electron microscope (16) (x 105,000). d. Cerebrovascular amyloid in Alzheimer's disease stained as in a (x 225).

these enigmatic structures should be considered as an intracellular form of amyloid. In negatively stained PHF preparations, each 10 nm filament can give the appearance of two 3.5-4.5 nm protofilaments, the whole PHF being apparently constructed from four protofilaments (16,17). According to Wisniewski (18) "ultrathin" sections of PHF in situ reveal the presence of a second set of protofilaments directly beneath these four, giving eight protofilaments in all. Crowther and Wischik (19) have recently analyzed PHF by image reconstruction techniques and conclude that these interpretations are not correct; each 10 nm filament being in fact a single stack of transversely oriented subunits, each of which possesses three domains: these authors conclude that the striated appearance alluded to above is explained by the lining up in an axial direction of the domains in adjacent subunits rather than the presence of four or more protofilaments.

In around 90% of cases of histopathologically confirmed AD, cerebral amyloid is also found in the walls of the cortical, subcortical, and often meningeal arterioles and capillaries (20,21) (Fig. 1d). Cerebrovascular amyloidosis, which has also been documented in the absence of dementia (21), is seldom accompanied by systemic amyloid deposition.

Cerebral amyloid deposition at one or more of these three sites is not restricted to AD. Plaques, some of which appear to differ in their morphology from any of the plaques seen in AD (22), and NFT are found in the majority of cases of Down's syndrome surviving to middle age (23). Amyloid plaques in the absence of NFT are found in varying numbers, most often in the cerebellar cortex, in the unconventional slow virus diseases Creutzfeldt-Jakob disease (CJD), Gerstmann-Straussler syndrome (GSS) and kuru in humans, and scrapie in animals (for key references see (24)). When present these plaques generally differ from those in AD in that they consist solely of a mass of amyloid with no surrounding dystrophic neurites. NFT alone occur in dementia pugilistica (the dementia of "punch drunk" boxers) (25) and in Guam-Parkinson dementia (26). Vessel amyloid may be found in all of these conditions, but its incidence is not well documented. Vessel amyloid with no significant numbers of plaques or NFT occurs in an inherited form of cerebral haemorrhage described in certain Icelandic families (27). The precise sequence of events leading to amyloid deposition is not clear for any of these conditions, but significant progress has recently been made in the biochemical characterization of some of the cerebral amyloids. To date three chemically distinct types of cerebral amyloid have been described: 1. The amyloid in AD and Down's syndrome which is formed from a circa 4 Kdalton protein of unknown origin and function, 2. Some amyloid plaques in the unconventional slow virus diseases which appear to be related to a 26-30 Kdalton protein associated with infectivity, 3. The amyloid in Icelandic hereditary cerebrovascular amyloidosis which is formed from the serum protein gamma-trace. These are discussed in the three sections below.

2.Biochemistry of cerebral amyloid in Alzheimer's disease

Due to difficulties in obtaining sufficiently pure preparations of the three forms of cerebral amyloid little progress was made in this area until the last few years. The isolation of plaque amyloid (in the form of intact plaque cores) form freshly frozen post-mortem brain tissue was first reported in 1983 (28); around this time methods were also developed for the isolation of PHF (29,30). Surprisingly, both plaque cores and PHF proved to be extremely insoluble in conventional SDS, urea or guanidine-containing protein solvents and this initially restricted their further characterization (28-31). Nevertheless, plaque core protein was shown to yield an unusual and reproducible amino acid composition which clearly excluded the well-characterized amyloids as major components of the plaque core (28,31); moreover, isolated PHF gave an intriguingly similar composition (Table I) (16,32). In 1984, a 4 Kdalton protein (termed "β-protein") was isolated from amyloid-laden meningeal vessels in AD and Down's syndrome (33,34), and the amino acid composition of this protein was strikingly similar to that of plaque core and PHF protein (Table I) (16,32) leading to the proposal that all three amyloids are deposits of the same, or a group of closely similar proteins (32).

TABLE I: AMINO ACID COMPOSITIONS (moles %) OF BULK PLAQUE CORES (APC), BULK PAIRED HELICAL FILAMENTS (PHF) AND PURIFIED β-PROTEIN FROM VESSEL AMYLOID (CVA) IN ALZHEIMER's DISEASE
[APC and PHF compositions are presented from two different research groups]

	APC(28)	APC(39)	PHF(16)	PHF(39)	CVA(33)
Asp	7.8	9.3	8.0	9.9	11.1
Thr	1.5	2.7	3.5	3.2	1.4
Ser	4.8	6.5	6.4	6.9	5.4
Glu	11.2	10.0	10.4	10.8	11.2
Pro	2.0	trace	7.9	3.0	trace
Gly	15.0	17.5	17.6	14.7	15.2
Ala	9.0	7.7	6.1	7.7	7.9
Cys	N.D.	1.0	N.D.	0.7	trace
Val	12.8	9.3	9.3	8.4	11.7
Met	1.9	1.8	1.1	0.7	2.5
Ile	6.7	4.8	5.1	3.2	3.9
Leu	6.6	7.0	6.3	6.5	6.3
Tyr	2.4	3.6	1.5	1.9	2.1
Phe	5.4	5.5	3.4	5.9	7.0
His	5.2	4.3	3.6	6.4	5.9
Lys	5.3	5.4	6.6	7.5	5.4
Arg	2.3	4.4	3.0	2.9	2.9
Trp	N.D.	N.D.	N.D.	N.D.	N.D.

Beta-protein has been sequenced up to residue 28 (35) (Table II) and this sequence shows no homology with any known protein (33). It has become apparent that more than 90% of the protein in plaque core and PHF preparations is soluble in formic acid, and this has resulted in the identification of similar 4 Kdalton proteins from amyloid plaque cores in

AD and Down's syndrome (36) and PHF in AD (37). These 4 Kdalton proteins will be referred to as APC-A_4 and NFT-A_4 respectively, following the terminology of Masters et al (36,37). Under certain conditions the A_4 monomers aggregate to form dimers (A_8), tetramers (A_{16}) or hexadecamers (A_{64}). In support of the "common protein" proposal the N-terminal amino acid sequences of bulk cores, APC-A_8/A_{16}, bulk PHF and NFT-A_8 were identical to the β-protein sequence apart from a few limited substitutions (Table II); wether these are genuine, or whether they are due to misinterpretation of the sequenator data, is an important point that should be further investigated. Due to lack of quantitative data it is not possible to determine what proportion of the bulk preparations the sequenced material represents. However, the similarity of the amino acid compositions of APC-A_4 and NFT-A_4 to the bulk preparations strongly suggests (but does not prove) that these low molecular weight components are representative of the whole preparations, and not minor contaminants.

TABLE II: N-TERMINAL AMINO ACID SEQUENCES DERIVED FROM VESSEL AMYLOID β-PROTEIN (CVA)(33), PLAQUE CORE PROTEIN (APC)(36) AND PAIRED HELICAL FILAMENT PROTEIN (PHF)(37) IN ALZHEIMER's DISEASE

	1	2	3	4	5	6	7	8	9	10	11	12	13	14
CVA	Asp-Ala-Glu-Phe-Arg-His-Asp-Ser-Gly-Tyr-Gln-Val-His-His-
APC											-Glu-
PHF											-Glu-

	15	16	17	18	19	20	21	22	23	24	25	26	27	28
CVA	Gln-Lys-Leu-Val-Phe-Phe-Ala-Glu-Asp-Val-Gly-Ser-Asn-Lys-
APC												-Ser-Ala-
PHF	Gln-/

The protein biochemical data on plaque and vessel amyloid have been fully substantiated by immunohistochemical studies with polyvalent (35,37) and monoclonal antibodies (38) to synthetic peptides corresponding to various parts of the sequences given in Table II. Figures 1a and 1d show immunoperoxidase staining of plaque and vessel amyloid using a monoclonal antibody (1G10/2/3) raised to a peptide consisting of residues 8-17 of the plaque core protein sequence (38). In the case of PHF, the immunohistochemical studies have been less conclusive and more difficult to interpret. In common with two other anti-peptide antibodies (35,37) 1G10/2/3 does not stain NFT in tissue sections (38). Furthermore Selkoe and co-workers (39) reported that an antiserum to the 8 Kdalton protein isolated from a PHF preparation labelled vessel and plaque amyloid but not NFT. However, these same workers have found that an anti-PHF antiserum can be used to stain plaque cores (40), and Masters et al (37) reported that an antiserum to residues 1-11 of the plaque core protein sequence and an antiserum to the APC-A_8/A_{16} species also labelled NFT. Thus it appears that at least part of the plaque core protein sequence forms an exposed epitope in NFT. Some plaque core protein epitopes may be concealed in NFT due to protein conformational differences between plaque amyloid fibrils and

PHF, and/or due to steric hindrance resulting from the decoration of PHF fibrils with partially degraded filamentous material (see below). Further work is required to clarify these points. The data discussed above must be reconciled with the fact that certain antibodies to neurofilament proteins label NFT, which has reinforced the belief that PHF are formed from abnormal neurofilaments or fragments of neurofilaments (41-46). Mammalian neurofilaments consist of three subunit proteins with apparent molecular weights of 200 Kdalton (NF-H), 150 Kdalton (NF-M) and 68 Kdalton (NF-L). These all possess a central α-helical rod region of 310 residues flanked by hypervariable non-helical head and tail domains in accord with the common structural organization of intermediate (10 nm) filaments (47). The carboxy-terminal tail regions of NF-H and NF-M are thought to form side arms which connect adjacent filaments (47). The complete amino acid sequence of porcine NF-L is known (48), but only partial sequences are available for NF-M (49) and NF-H (47). The 4 Kdalton common protein shows no homology with these known sequences. However, all of the neurofilament monoclonal antibodies that label NFT are (where the location of the epitope is known) directed against epitopes on the carboxy-terminal tail extensions of either NF-M or NF-H (42-44), which are the unsequenced regions. Therefore the possibility that NFT-A_4 is a proteolytic fragment of these regions cannot at the moment be discounted but the present author considers this unlikely for the following reasons: 1. The anti-neurofilament antibodies that recognize in situ NFT fail to label "ghost tangles" (i.e. naked NFT in tissue sections, where the surrounding cell has completely degenerated) (45), 2. Most of these antibodies fail to label the majority of PHF after isolation by SDS extraction (42,43), 3. Anti-PHF antibodies do not recognize any neurofilament components (30), 4. Monoclonal antibody 1G10/2/3 (see above) (38) cannot be used to stain neurofilaments (Lowe, J.S., Allsop, D., Landon, M. and Kidd, M., unpublished observation), 5. After immunogold labelling of SDS-treated isolated PHF with anti-neurofilament antibodies it is apparent that the paired-helical shaft of the PHF is not labelled with gold particles; instead, the colloidal gold mainly appears to be located on amorphous material adhering to the shaft (42,43,46). Thus some isolated PHF appear to be "decorated" with neurofilament-like immunoreactive material that is not removed by SDS treatment. In the light of this latter observation in particular, and with the knowledge that the neurofilament side arms are known to be more resistant to proteolysis than the α-helical rod regions (50), it is proposed that the neurofilament immunoreactivity of NFT is due to an association between PHF per se and the proteolytic remnants of neurofilament proteins. These proteins are synthesized in the neuronal cell bodies and transferred in an anterograde direction by the process of slow axoplasmic transport (51). The presence of large bundles of PHF in the cytoplasm is likely to interfere with this transport system which may lead to proteolysis of newly-synthesized neurofilament protein. Neurofilaments are known to be susceptible to an endogenous calcium-activated protease (52). Poly-ribosomes have been found in association with PHF (53,54); and Perry et al (46) have noted that anti-neurofilament antibodies stain granular material within NFT that could "represent degradation products of poly-ribosomes"; this staining may be due to the synthesis of neurofilament protein on these ribosomes.

Antibodies to microtubule-associated protein 2 (MAP-2) (which pro-vides a site of interaction between microtubules and neurofilaments) (55) and tau (a further microtubule-associated protein) (40) also la-belled NFT in situ; only the latter antibodies labelled PHF purified by SDS extraction but, significantly, they again did not label "ghost" tan-gles (40).

Thus the available evidence suggests that NFT are complex hetero-geneous structures containing PHF per se and, in addition, neuro-filament, MAP-2, and tau-like immunoreactive material. Some of this material seems to be tightly associated with PHF and is retained after SDS extraction. In view of this, anti-PHF antibodies are unlikely to be specific for PHF per se, and it is not surprising that these antibodies possess some anti-tau activity (40). The "ghost" tangles mentioned above are most likely naked PHF which are essentially free of any asso-ciated filament-related material.

The site of synthesis of the common 4 Kdalton protein, and the mechanism of its distribution into the three sites of amyloid deposition, is at present unknown. Three possible interrelationships are outlined in Figure 2.

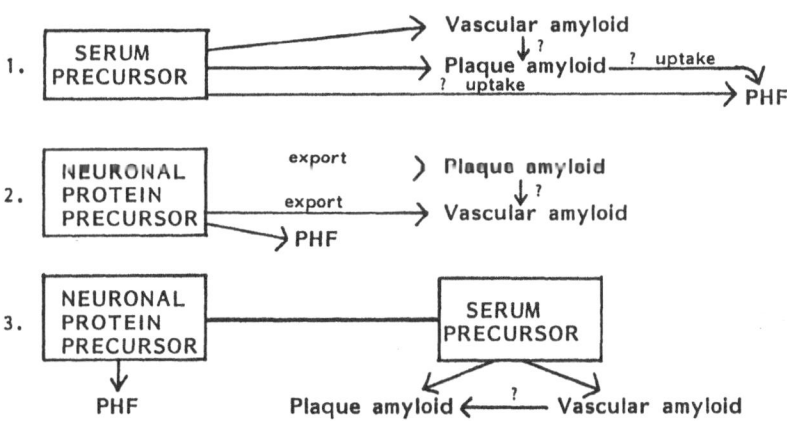

Figure 2: Possible interrelationships between the three sites of cerebral amyloid deposition in Alzheimer's disease.

In the first of these, β-protein arises from an amyloidogenic serum precursor, analogous to amyloid derived from IgG light chains, SAA protein, prealbumin, and gamma-trace. In this case it is necessary to explain why amyloid is found only in the vessels of the brain, and not in the peripheral vessels. Glenner (56) has suggested that this might be due to differences in the lysosomal complements of proteolytic enzymes at these sites. Plaque amyloid then arises as a result of a breakdown in the blood-brain barrier due to the weakening of amyloid--infiltrated vessel walls, but it is difficult to conceive how the protein could enter the neurons to form NFT. One possibility (32) is that the endings of the affected neurons have the capacity to take up the protein by pinocytosis in a similar way to the process of ferrugination (57) or the well-known capacity of neurons to take up and retrogradely transport various exogenous substances (51). If a serum precursor to β-protein is identified it should be possible to carry out experiments with neurons in culture to test the validity of this hypothesis. The presence of such a precursor could also permit the development of a serum test to aid to the diagnosis of AD (56).

In the second possibility, the common protein precursor is synthesized within neurons and is then deposited in the plaques and also in the vessel walls as described recently by Masters et al (37).

Finally, it is not impossible for the precursor to be synthesized within neurons (forming PHF), and also to be present in the serum (independently giving rise to vessel and possibly plaque amyloid). Studies already in progress using antisera to the common protein should soon produce some answers to these questions, which are central to our understanding of the pathogenesis of AD; also the availability of amino acid sequence data will permit gene probes to be constructed, and the powerful techniques of molecular biology can then be applied to this problem.

3. Cerebral amyloid in the slow virus diseases

These diseases are clearly transmissible, but the nature of the infectious agent remains elusive (for recent reviews on the nature of the agent see 58,59). Subcellular fractions enriched for scrapie infectivity, prepared by two different procedures (60,61), have been found to contain a predominant proteinase K-resistant protein ("prion protein" or PrP) with an apparent molecular weight of 26-30 Kdalton and rod-like structures, referred to as either "prion rods" (60) or "scrapie associated fibrils" (61). Recently similar observations were made with fractions enriched for CJD infectivity (62). Whether these rod-like structures are a form of infectious agent, or whether they arise as a pathological response to infection, or during the preparative procedures, and fortuitously co-purify with an as yet undetected agent remains to be established. Antibodies to PrP have been shown to decorate these rods (63), which are therefore presumed to be aggregates of PrP, and the rods exhibit the characteristic green birefringence of amyloid after Congo red staining (64). This had led to the proposal that the plaque amyloid fibrils are paracrystalline arrays of the infectious agent; this hypothesis has also been extended to AD which has not been successfully transmitted to animals (65). PrP is encoded on a host gene and appears to arise by proteolytic processing of a larger precursor protein (66,67), which is certainly reminiscent of some amyloids. The PrP gene is transcribed and translated in a variety of tissues in both normal and infected animals, but in normal animals the gene product is susceptible to proteinase K; the proteinase K-resistant PrP species can be isolated from infected animals only (66). The implications of this for the nature of the infectious agent have been discussed by others (68,69).

As far as AD is concerned, the amino acid sequence of the common 4 Kdalton protein shows no homology with the sequence deduced from the PrP gene. Furthermore, scrapie associated fibrils have not been found in AD (70), and the antibodies to PrP did not label any of the forms of cerebral amyloid (71). Thus the above hypothesis is unlikely to be correct for AD, and it now seems improbable that a slow viral agent is involved in the etiology of this disease.

Anti-PrP antibodies did, however, label some (but not all) plaques in scrapie and CJD in rodents, and similarly in GSS and CJD in humans (71-72). In a recent study (Roberts, G., Allsop, D., Landon,M., Kidd, M., Prusiner, S.B., Crow, T.J. and Brown, R., unpublished results) monoclonal antibody 1G10/2/3 (38) (see above) also labelled some plaques in 5 out of 14 brains from patients with CJD, and similarly in one kuru brain; double labelling with both anti-PrP and 1G10/2/3 showed very little co-localization in the CJD brains, and co-localization in 10-15% of plaques in the kuru brain. These results indicate that two distinct types of plaque, composed of different amyloids, can co-exist in the human slow viral disease; one of these seems to be related to PrP, and the other is similar to the Alzheimer plaque: a minority of plaques are apparently hybrids. Any cerebrovascular amyloid present was labelled with 1G10/2/3 only, and so is likely to be formed from β--protein.

Isolation and characterization of the amyloid (both plaque and vessel) is required to confirm these conclusions, and it is also important to establish whether the Alzheimer-type amyloid is deposited as a result of slow viral infection, and so plays a role in the pathogenesis of these diseases, or whether this merely represents amyloid associated with "normal" aging.

4. Icelandic cerebrovascular amyloidosis

Cerebrovascular amyloidosis resulting in fatal cerebral haemorrhage occurs in certain Icelandic families, where it exhibits an autosomal dominant mode of inheritance (27). Amyloid fibrils isolated from the leptomeningeal blood vessels of three such cases proved to yield a protein of molecular weight 11,500 dalton, the N-terminal sequence of which was homologous to the serum protein gamma-trace, commencing at residue 11 of this protein (73). Gamma-trace is a small basic protein of molecular weight 13,260 dalton (calculated from the complete amino acid sequence (74)) that is also present in cerebrospinal fluid (CSF) (74). This protein is quite distinct from β-protein in AD and is thought to function as a cysteine proteinase inhibitor; the alternative name of cystatin C, which reflects homology with other cystatins, has been proposed (75). The isoelectric point of gamma-trace from patients afflicted with this inherited condition was identical to that of normal gamma-trace suggesting that the primary defect is not in the protein itself (76). Alternative possibilities involve the defective transport of this protein into the CSF (77), or abnormal catabolic metabolism (74) both of which could explain the reduced levels of gamma-trace in the CSF of these patients (76).

Acknowledgements

The author wishes to thank Dr. M. Landon and Dr. M. Kidd for helpful discussions and advice; Dr. J.S. Lowe and Mrs. A. Tomlinson for help with some of the figures; and most of all, The Wellcome Trust for financial support.

References

1. Wang, H.S. In Aging and Dementia, Smith, W.L. and Kinsbourne, M., Eds. Spectrum, New York, 1-24, 1977.
2. Plum, F. Nature 279, 372-373, 1979.
3. Blessed, G., Tomlinson, B.E. & Roth, M. Br. J. Psychiat. 114, 797-811, 1968.
4. Wilcock, G.K. & Esiri, M.M. J. Neurol. Sci. 56, 343-356, 1982.
5. Perry, E.K., Tomlinson, B.E., Blessed, G., et al. Br. Med. J. 2, 1457-1459, 1978.
6. Wilcock, G.K., Esiri, M.M., Bowen, D.M., et al. J. Neurol. Sci. 57, 407-417, 1982.
7. Perry, E.K. Br. Med. Bull. 42, 63-69, 1986.
8. Rossor, M. & Iversen, L.L. Br. Med. Bull. 42, 70-74, 1986.
9. Ulrich, J. Gerontology 28, 86-90, 1982.
10. Kidd, M. Brain 87, 307-320, 1964.
11. Terry, R.D., Gonatas, N.K., & Weiss, M. Am. J. Pathol. 44, 269-297, 1964.
12. Narang, H.K. J. Neuropathol. Exp. Neurol. 39, 621-631, 1980.
13. Merz, P.A., Wisniewski, H.M., Somerville, R.A., et al. Acta Neuropathol. 60, 113-124, 1983.
14. Kidd, M. Nature 197, 192-193, 1963.
15. Kirschner, D.A., Abraham, C., Selkoe, D.J. Proc. Natl. Acad. Sci. USA 83, 503-507, 1986.
16. Allsop, D., Landon, M. & Kidd, M. In Amyloidosis. Glenner, G.G., Osserman, E., Benditt, E.P., Calkins, E., Cohen, A.S., Bucker Franklin, D., Eds. Plenum Press, New York, 723-732, 1986.
17. Wisniewski, H.M., Merz, P.A. & Iqbal, K. J. Neuropathol. Exp. Neurol. 43, 643-656, 1984.
18. Wisniewski, H.M. & Wen, G.Y. Acta Neuropathol. 66, 173-176, 1985.
19. Crowther, R.A. & Wischik, C.M. EMBO J. 4, 3661-3665, 1985.
20. Glenner, G.G., Henry, J.H. & Fujihara, S. Ann. Pathol. 1, 120-129, 1981.
21. Mandybur, T.I. J. Neuropathol. Exp. Neurol. 45, 79-90, 1986.
22. Allsop, D., Kidd, M., Landon, M., et al. J. Neurol. Neurosurg. Psych. (In Press).
23. Wisniewski, K.E., Wisniewski, H.M. & Wen, G.Y. Ann. Neurol. 17, 278-282, 1985.
24. Salazar, A.M., Brown, P., Gajdusek, D.C., et al. In Alzheimer's Disease; The Standard Reference. Reisberg, B., Ed. Free Press, London and New York, 311-318, 1983.
25. Wisniewski, H.M., Narang, H.K., Corsellis, J.A.N., et al. J. Neuropathol. Exp. Neurol. 35, 367, 1976.
26. Wisniewski, K.E., Jervis, G.A., Moretz, R.C., et al. Ann. Neurol. 5, 288-294, 1979.
27. Gudmundsson, G., Hallgrimsson, J., Jonasson, T.A., et al. Brain, 95, 387-404, 1972.
28. Allsop, D., Landon, M. & Kidd, M. Brain Res. 259, 348-352, 1983.
29. Selkoe, D.J., Ihara, Y. & Salazar, F.J. Science 215, 1243-1245, 1982.
30. Ihara, Y., Abraham, C. & Selkoe, D.J. Nature 304, 727-730, 1983.

31. Kidd, M., Allsop, D. & Landon, M.   In Modern Approaches to the Dementias, Part 1, Etiology and Pathophysiology. Interdiscipl. Topics Geront., Vol. 19, Clifford R.F., Ed. Karger, Basel, 114-126, 1985.
32. Kidd, M., Allsop, D. & Landon, M. Lancet i, 278, 1985.
33. Glenner, G.G. & Wong, C.W. Biochem. Biophys. Res. Commun. 120, 885-890, 1984.
34. Glenner, G.G. & Wong, C.W. Biochem. Biophys. Res. Commun. 122, 1131-1135, 1984.
35. Wong, C.W., Quaranta, V. & Glenner, G.G. Proc. Natl. Acad. Sci. USA 82, 8729-8732, 1985.
36. Masters, C.L., Simms, G., Weinman, N.A., et al. Proc. Natl. Acad. Sci. USA 82, 4245-4249, 1985.
37. Masters, C.L., Multhaup, G. & Simms, G. EMBO J. 4, 2757-2763, 1985.
38. Allsop, D., Landon, M., Kidd, M., et al. Neurosci. Lett. (In press).
39. Selkoe, D.J., Abraham, C.R., Podlisny, M.B., et al. J. Neurochem. 46, 1820-1834, 1986.
40. Kosik, K.S., Joachim, C.L. & Selkoe, D.J. Proc. Natl. Acad. Sci. USA 83, 4044-4048, 1986.
41. Anderton, B.H., Breinburg, D., Downes, M.J., et al. Nature 298, 84-86, 1982.
42. Miller, C.C.J., Brion, J.P., Calvert, R., et al. EMBO J. 5, 269-276, 1986.
43. Miller, C.C.J., Haugh, M., Anderton, B.H. Trends Neurol. Sci. 9, 76-81, 1986.
44. Cork, L.C., Sternberger, N.H., Sternberger, L.A., et al. J. Neuropathol. Exp. Neurol. 45, 56-64, 1986.
45. Rasool, C.G., Abraham, C., Anderton, B.H., et al. Brain Res. 310, 249-260, 1984.
46. Perry, G., Rizzuto, N., Autilio-Gambetti, L., et al. Proc. Natl. Acad. Sci. USA 82, 3916-3920, 1985.
47. Geisler, N., Fischer, S., Vandekerckhove, J., et al. EMBO J. 4, 57-63, 1985.
48. Geisler, N., Plessmann, U. & Weber, K. FEBS Lett. 182, 475-478, 1985.
49. Geisler, N., Fischer, S., Vandekerckhove, J., et al. EMBO J. 3, 2701-2706, 1984.
50. Geisler, N., Kaufmann, E., Fischer, S., et al. EMBO J. 2, 1295-1302, 1983.
51. Grafstein, B. & Forman, D.S. Physiol. Rev. 60, 1167-1283, 1980.
52. Nixon, R.A., Brown, B.A. & Marotta, C.A. J. Cell Biol. 94, 150-158, 1981.
53. Hirano, A., Dembitzer, H.M., Kurland, L.T., et al. J. Neuropathol. Exp. Neurol. 27, 167-182, 1968.
54. Metuzals, J., Montpetit, V. & Clapin, D.F. Cell Tissue Res. 214, 455-482, 1981.
55. Kosik, K.S., Duffy, L.K., Dowling, M.M., et al. Proc. Natl. Acad. Sci. USA 81, 7941-7945, 1984.
56. Glenner, G.G. Human Pathol. 16, 433-435, 1985.
57. Blackwood, W., McMenemey, W.H., Meyer, A., et al. In Greenfield's Neuropathology, 2nd Edition. Arnold, London, 35-36, 1963.
58. Carp, R.I., Merz, P.A., Kascsak, R.J., et al. J. Gen. Virol. 66, 1357-1368, 1985.
59. Kimberlin, R.H. Trends Biochem. Sci. 7, 392-394, 1982.
60. Bolton, D.C., McKinley, M.P. & Prusiner, S.B. Science 218, 1309-1311, 1982.
61. Diringer, H., Gelderblom, H., Hilmert, H., et al. Nature 306, 476-478, 1983.
62. Bendheim, P.E., Bockman, J.M., McKinley, M.P., et al. Proc. Natl. Acad. Sci. USA 82, 997-1001, 1985.
63. Barry, R.A., McKinley, M.P., Bendheim, P.E., et al. J. Immunol. 135, 603-613, 1985.
64. Prusiner, S.B., McKinley, M.P., Bowman, K.A., et al. Cell 35, 349-358, 1983.
65. Prusiner, S.B. New Eng. J. Med. 310, 661-663, 1984.
66. Oesch, B., Westaway, D., Walchli, M., et al. Cell 40, 735-746, 1985.
67. Chesebro, B., Race, R., Wehrly, K., et al. Nature 315, 331-333, 1985.
68. Harris, T. Nature 315, 275, 1985.
69. Robertson, H.D., Branch, A.D. & Dahlberg, J.E. Cell 40, 725-727, 1985.
70. Merz, P.A., Rohwer, R.G., Kascsak, R., et al. Science 225, 437-440, 1984.
71. Kitamoto, T., Tateishi, J., Tashima, T., et al. Ann. Neurol. (In Press).
72. DeArmond, S.J., McKinley, M.P., Barry, R.A., et al. Cell 41, 221-235, 1985.
73. Cohen, D.H., Feiner, H., Jensson, O., et al. J. Exp. Med. 158, 623-628, 1983.
74. Grubb, A. & Lofberg, H. Proc. Natl. Acad. Sci. USA 79, 3024-3027, 1982.
75. Barrett, A.J., Davies, M.E. & Grubb, A. Biochem. Biophys. Res. Commun. 120, 631-636, 1984.
76. Grubb, A., Jensson, O., Gudmundsson, G., et al. New Eng. J. Med. 311, 1547-1549, 1984.
77. Hochwald, G.M. & Thorbecke, G.J. New Eng. J. Med. 312, 1127-1128, 1985.

VI.3 AMYLOID OF THE ISLETS OF LANGERHANS AND ITS
CONNECTION WITH DIABETES MELLITUS

Per Westermark

Department of Pathology, University Hospital,
S-751 85 Uppsala, Sweden.

1. Introduction

Among the microdepositions of amyloid occurring in connection with aging are those found in the islets of Langerhans and in the brain most interesting due to their relation to two common and very important diseases, namely type II (non-insulin dependent) diabetes mellitus and senile dementia of Alzheimer's type. In both one can expect that clarification of the pathogenesis of the amyloid deposits and their chemical natures will give important knowledge to our understanding of these diseases.

Early in this century, Opie (1) described a hyalinization of the islets of Langerhans in diabetes mellitus. It was not until the more constant use of Congo red stain in combination with polarized light that this substance really was regarded as a local form of amyloid (2). Although deposition of amyloid in the islets is the most constantly appearing pancreatic alteration in type II diabetes, it has not attracted any major interest among most scientists working with diabetes. The reason of this is difficult to understand but one explanation may be the fact that islet amyloid does not occur among most laboratory animals.

2. Frequency of islet amyloid

Islet amyloid is typical of type II diabetes mellitus and is rare in type I (insulin dependent) diabetes. Several studies on the frequency of islet amyloid have been performed and the results in these differ greatly (2-6). The reason for this is probably that small deposits are easily overlooked and that many investigators have used routine stainings such as hematoxylin-eosin. Furthermore, the affinity for Congo red varies and a rather faint staining is seen in many cases. Finally, the found frequencies depend on which part of the pancreas is studied. The body and the tail contain more amyloidotic islets than the head of the pancreas (6-8). If several sections are studied, amyloid depositions are found in virtually all pancreases from patients with type II diabetes (5,6). Most of these patients have deposits in 25-75% of their islets (6,8). The amount of amyloid in each island increases when the number of involved islets rises (8,9).

As seen in Table I, amyloid deposits occur in the islets of non--diabetic persons as well, but more frequently (2-6). There is a striking difference between the two groups in the mean percentage of islets with amyloid.

TABLE I: THE PERCENTAGE OF PANCREATIC ISLETS WITH AMYLOID DEPOSITS IN DIABETIC AND NON-DIABETIC OLD PERSONS [materials from references 6 and 10]

	No. of patients with islet amyloid	Mean age (years)	Mean frequency (%) of islets with amyloid	
			Caput	Cauda
Non-diabetics (n=27)	16 (59%)	75.4	2.9	7.1
Diabetics (n=23)	22 (96%)	72.6	37.3	65.9

Even if patients without any islet amyloid are excluded, a great difference between diabetic and non-diabetic patients persists (Table II). The connection of islet amyloid with diabetes is therefore absolutely clear.

TABLE II: THE PERCENTAGE OF PANCREATIC ISLETS WITH AMYLOID DEPOSITS IN THE SAME PATIENTS AS IN TABLE I, BUT EXCLUDING PERSONS IN WHOM NO ISLET AMYLOID WAS DETECTED

	Mean frequency (%) of islets with amyloid	
	Caput	Cauda
Non-diabetics (n=16)	4.8	12.0
Diabetics (n=22)	39.1	68.9

3.Morphology

The amyloid of the islets has the same tinctorial properties as other amyloid. It is composed of fine fibrils as all amyloids, but the fibrils are stuck together more tightly compared to most types of amyloid although ordinary fibrils also occur. The fibrils also tend to be thinner and more wavy than is usually seen (11). The amyloid is strictly confined to the islets and is not seen in the exocrine parenchyma. Electron microscopic studies have revealed a close contact between β-cells and amyloid (Fig. 1). Bundles of fibrils have been seen running into pockets of these cells in a manner resembling fibrils in contact with reticulo-endothelial cells in experimental amyloidosis (12). This finding has led to the suggestion that the islet amyloid might be a product of islet β-cell.

The number of islet β-cells is reduced in type II diabetes, although not in the same extent as in type I diabetes (5,13,14). The proportion of β-cells compared to other islet cells decreases when islet amyloid develops (5). If it is taken into consideration that many β-cells show mor-

phological signs of lesions when in contact with amyloid, the total number of β-cells in type II diabetes is also greatly reduced (6). This fact
is often forgotten when the β-cell volume in diabetes mellitus is discussed.

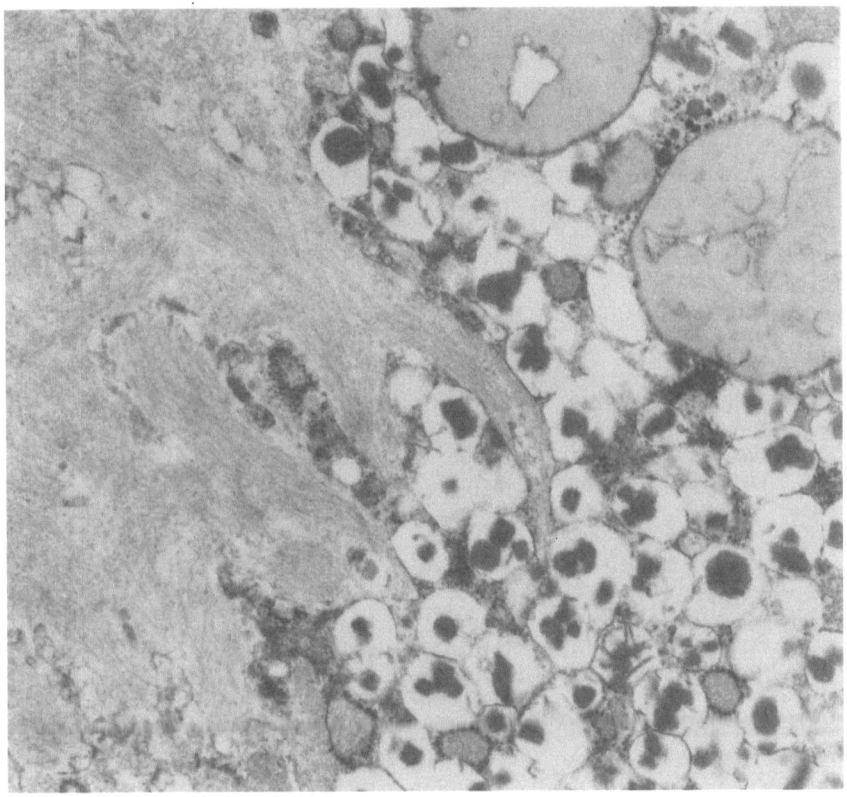

Figure 1: Islet β-cell in contact with amyloid. Parallel bundles of fibrils are seen in
the periphery of the cell and there is no visible basement membrane. The organization of
the fibrils indicates that they form in close contact with the β-cell. The recent
elucidation of the chemical structure of the fibrils makes it more probable that they
penetrate into the cell rather than being secreted from it, it contrary to what has been
believed previously. Magnification: x 35,500.

4. The nature of islet amyloid and its pathogenesis

The restriction of the amyloid to the islets and its connection with
diabetes led to the suspicion that the amyloid might be derived from
insulin (15) although many other suggestions have been given. Pearse
et al (16) when studying amyloid in endocrine tumours and among them
insulinomas, suggested that the insulinoma and islet amyloid is derived
from the proinsulin C-peptide, since they were unable to demonstrate

tryptophan or tyrosine histochemically. However, while studies of islet amyloid had confirmed lack of tryptophan, tyrosine has later been shown to be an ingredient of islet amyloid. Immunohistochemical studies with antisera to different known amyloid fibril proteins have given negative results (17). On the other hand amyloid P-component is constantly present in the amyloid of the pancreatic islets (18).

The finding that insulin can be converted to amyloid-like fibrils (19) encouraged us (and others) to make immunohistochemical studies on islet amyloid with different antisera to insulin. These studies have mainly given negative results, except when an antiserum was used, that had been obtained by immunization with a B-chain rich fraction of insulin (20). Absorption of the antiserum with insulin B-chain prior to incubation abolished this reaction. The reaction with antiserum to the B-chain rich insulin fraction was, although definite, much weaker than with the β-cells, probably indicating that insulin B-chain only constitutes a small part of the islet amyloid (Fig. 2). Insulin fibrils can easily be con-

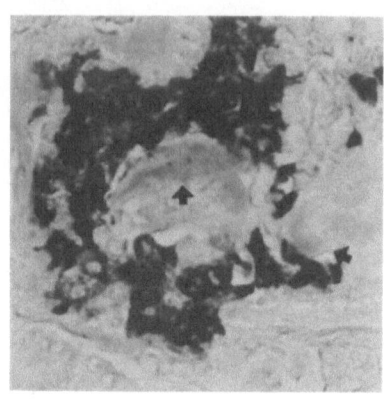

Figure 2: Immunohistochemical reaction of islet (insulin producing) β-cells (black) and amyloid (arrows) with an antiserum to a β-chain-rich insulin preparation. The reaction of the antiserum with the amyloid is much weaker than with the cells (x 500).

verted to native insulin by treatment with alkali (21). Alkali treatment of purified islet amyloid released only small amounts of immunoreactive insulin (15). Islet amyloid can be obtained in a fairly pure form, estimated on Congo red stained smears. When purification is performed according to Pras et al, most of the islet amyloid is not water-extractable (22). The pelleted amyloid-containing material can then be treated with pepsin followed by stirring in guanidine since the islet amyloid is mainly resistant to this treatment. The amino acid composition of islet amyloid obtained in this way was similar to that of amyloid from an insulinoma (23) but differed considerably from that of proinsulin or any of its component chains.

All these difficulties in the demonstration of an insulin related molecule in the islet amyloid seem now to get their explanation. N-terminal amino acid sequence analysis of a major peptide purified from the amyloid of an insulinoma has given the partial amino acid sequence

Lys-X-Asn-X-Ala-X-Ser-Ala-X-Gln-Arg-,

which is different from any part of human preproinsulin (23).

5. Conclusion

The amyloid of the islets of Langerhans seems to contain two fibrillar proteins, one major, previously probably unknown peptide (23) and one minor insulin-related peptide (20). The pathogenesis is still obscure but might be clarified when the function of this newly described peptide is understood. The amyloid does not seem to cause the diabetic disease, but reflects some disturbed mechanism in the β-cell. Understanding of this abnormality might give valuable information about the pathogenesis in type II diabetes.

Acknowledgements

Studies reviewed in this paper were in part supported by the Swedish Medical Research Council and the Research Fund of King Gustaf V.

References

1. Opie, E.L. J. Exp. Med. 5, 397-428, 1900.
2. Ehrlich, J.C. & Ratner, I.M. Am. J. Pathol. 38, 49-59, 1961.
3. Bell, E.T. Am. J. Pathol. 35, 801-805, 1959.
4. Melato, M., Antonutto, G. & Ferronato, E. Beitr. Pathol. 160, 73-81, 1977.
5. Westermark, P. & Grimelius, L. Acta Path. Microbiol. Scand. (A) 81, 291-300, 1973.
6. Westermark, P. & Wilander, E. Diabetologia 15, 417-421, 1978.
7. Clark, A., Holman, R.R., Matthews, D.R., et al. Diabetologia 27, 527-528, 1984.
8. Westermark, P. Upsala J. Med. Sci. 77, 91-94, 1972.
9. Maloy, A.L., Longnecker, D.S. & Greenberg, E.R., Hum. Pathol. 12, 917-922, 1981.
10. Westermark, P. Virchows Arch. Abt. A. 354, 17-23, 1971.
11. Westermark, P. Virchows Arch. Abt. A. 373, 161-166, 1977.
12. Westermark, P. Virchows Arch. Abt. A. 359, 1-18, 1973.
13. Maclean, N. & Ogilvie, R.F. Diabetes 4, 367-376, 1955.
14. Gepts, W. Endokrinologie 36, 185-211, 1958.
15. Westermark, P. Histochemistry 38, 27-33, 1974.
16. Pearse, A.G.E., Ewen, S.W.B. & Polak, J.M. Virchows Arch. Abt. B. 10, 93-107, 1972.
17. Cornwell, G.G. III, Natvig, J.B., Westermark, P., et al. J. Immunol. 120, 1385-1388, 1978.
18. Westermark, P., Skinner, M. & Cohen, A.S. Scand. J. Immunol. 4, 95-97, 1975.
19. Glenner, G.G., Eanes, E.D., Bladen, H.A., et al. J. Histochem. Cytochem. 22, 1141-1158, 1974.
20. Westermark, P. & Wilander, E. Diabetologia 24, 342-346, 1983.
21. Waugh, D.F. J. Am. Chem. Soc. 70, 1850-1857, 1948.
22. Westermark, P. Acta Path. Microbiol. Scand. (C) 83, 439-446, 1975.
23. Westermark, P., Wernstedt, C., Wilander, E., et al. (Manuscript submitted).

VI.4 SENILE AMYLOID AFFECTING THE HEART

Knut Sletten[1] and Per Westermark[2]

Department of Biochemistry, University of Oslo,
Oslo, Norway[1],
Department of Pathology, University Hospital,
S-751.85 Uppsala, Sweden[2].

1.Introduction

Cardiovascular deposits of amyloid are common and their frequency increases with age. The amyloid depositions are usually small and invisible without microscope and in most patients of no clinical significance. Exceptions do occur, however. There are several chemically different forms of amyloid which mainly involve the heart or the cardiovascular system.

2.Isolated atrial amyloid (IAA) deposits

This is the most common amyloid form affecting the heart. The amyloid is limited to the atria, especially the auricles, where thin deposits face the muscle cells (1). Atrophy of muscle cells does not occur and the clinical significance of the deposits is uncertain. No significant increase in atrial fibrillation in patients with IAA compared to age--matched controls has been found (2). The nature of the amyloid in IAA is unknown. It differs histochemically and immunochemically from characterized forms of amyloid (1,2). It is probably different from the amyloid that often occurs in the valves of the heart (3) and from the senile aortic amyloid (4).

3.Senile systemic amyloidosis (SSA)

This form of amyloidosis has previously been referred to as senile cardiac amyloidosis since the most obvious alterations often are found in the heart. However, like in other systemic amyloidoses, deposits occur in most organs and senile systemic amyloidosis (SSA) is therefore a better name (5).

3.1 Prevalence

SSA is the most common form of systemic amyloidosis although it is rarely seen before the age of 80 (1), above which age it has been found in approximately 25% of patients in autopsy studies (1,2). There is no sex difference although massive infiltration seems to be more common in men (5).

3.2 Distribution and histological characteristics

3.2.1 Heart

In most cases, the heart involvement is restricted to small and medium-sized vessels. A patchy infiltration between muscle cells often occurs, sometimes without conspicuous affection of intramural vessels. Muscle cells between the deposits tend to atrophy. The heart weight is not affected in most patients (2,6-8). However, in a few patients the amount of amyloid is large, resulting in cardiomegaly. Such hearts can weigh up to 950 grams and have a macro- and microscopical appearance indistinguishable from hearts in AL-amyloidosis. This pronounced form of SSA seems to be more common in men (5). Amyloid deposits in SSA are found in all parts of the heart including the atria and the pericardial fat tissue.

3.2.2 Lung

Heavy deposits in the heart are usually accompanied by significant amyloid infiltration in the lungs, where amyloid is seen in vessel walls and often in a droplet-fashion in the alveolar walls (5). The last mentioned deposits are sometimes very pronounced.

3.2.3. Other organs

Besides the heart and the lungs, the amounts of amyloid in SSA are fairly small. However, also in many patients with very slight degree of the disease, deposits do occur in most organs in the body, except for the central nervous system. Deposits in the spleen are limited to the vessels, whereas in the kidneys, in addition to the vessels, amyloid is found in the medulla. The glomeruli are spared in contrary to other systemic amyloidoses (2,5).

3.3 Amyloid protein in SSA

Structural studies have been performed on the low molecular-weight subunit protein (protein ASc_1) (9). N-terminal analysis revealed a blocked N-terminus. However, it is impossible to exclude the possibility that a certain amount of the protein has a very ragged N-terminal end. A peptic digestion of the protein, followed by different purification procedures, resulted in four peptides that were characterized by Edman degradation. The peptides were found to correspond to positions 70-90, 96-107, 109-115, 121-127 and were completely homologous to those in prealbumin (10). Determination of the amino acid composition revealed a slightly higher content of aspartic acid, glutamic acid, isoleucine, leucine and arginine and the presence of methionine (9). Treatment of the purified prealbumin-like component of ASc_1 (see below) with cyanogen bromide revealed no cleavage at position 30 (unpublished result).

This indicates, that the amyloid protein in SSA contains no methionine in position 30, as has been found in prealbumin isolated from patients with familial amyloidotic polyneuropathy.

Electrophoretical studies of dissolved amyloid fibrils in SSA have shown that protein ASc_1 is heterogeneous in size (11). One component behaves like human prealbumin in SDS-PAGE, while the major component (designated the 13 Kdalton component) is smaller and with a molecular weight probably less than 13 Kdalton. Even smaller components exist. In Western blot analysis, only the prealbumin-like component reacts with anti-prealbumin antibodies (11). The proportions between the components vary, but the amount of the prealbumin-like component seems always to be smaller than that of the 13 Kdalton component. Western blot analysis of reduced fibril proteins treated with (^{14}C)-iodoacetamide revealed free thiol groups in the prealbumin-like component but not in the 13 Kdalton component (11). This may indicate that the 13 Kdalton component lacks the N-terminal part of prealbumin.

3.4 Antigenic properties

In double immunodiffusion, degraded amyloid fibril (DAM) solutions of SSA do not give any lines when tested against prealbumin antibodies and antiserum to SSA does not react with purified human prealbumin (12). The same pattern of reactivity is obtained when purified ASc_1 is used. The purified prealbumin-like component of ASc_1, when separated from the 13 Kdalton component, reacts with anti-human-prealbumin antibodies and gives one line of identity with purified human prealbumin (Johansson and Westermark, unpublished result). In immunofluorescence, the deposits in SSA show a reaction with both anti-ASc_1 and anti-prealbumin antibodies (12). The reason for this pattern of reactivity is not fully understood, but the 13 Kdalton component seems to inhibit precipitation of the prealbumin like component with antiserum to prealbumin.

3.5 Pathogenesis

The pathogenesis in SSA is obscure. There is no evidence for a mutant form of prealbumin. A significantly lower plasma concentration of prealbumin is found in patients with SSA compared to age-matched control patients (13). This may indicate that an altered prealbumin metabolism is involved in the pathogenesis. There is no explanation why different organs are involved in familial amyloidotic polyneuropathy as compared to senile systemic amyloidosis, both of which have deposits of prealbumin nature.

3.6 Clinical significance

In most cases the clinical significance probably is small. An increased frequency of atrial fibrillation may occur (7) although the reports are

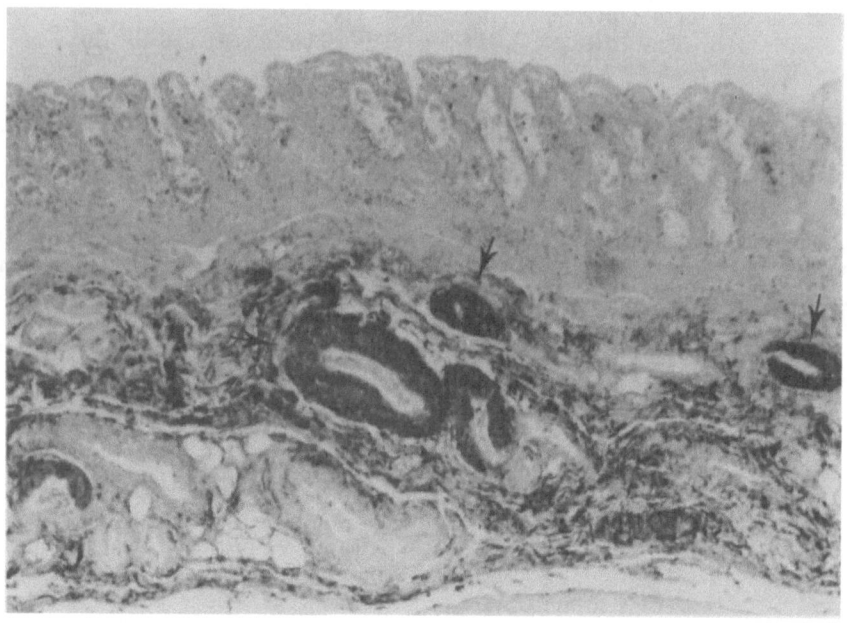

Figure 1: Rectal tissue from a patient with SSA. There are several submucous vessels with heavy deposits of amyloid (arrows). Anti-ASc$_1$ antiserum, peroxidase-anti-peroxidase method. Magnification: x 80.

divergent (2,8). In those patients in whom heavy engagement of the heart occurs, the disease has probably the same serious prognosis as AL-amyloidosis. The effect of the lung involvement has not yet been evaluated. It is a general conception that SSA only can be identified at autopsy. This is, however, wrong and the diagnosis is often possible to obtain by rectal or subcutaneous fat biopsy (2,5) (Fig. 1). One should also remember that amyloid-positive rectal or subcutaneous fat biopsies in old persons can mean benign SSA and not necessarily a serious AL, AA or AF amyloidosis.

Acknowledgements

The studies reviewed in this paper were in part supported by the Swedish Medical Research Council and the Research Fund of King Gustaf V.

References

1. Westermark, P., Johansson, B. & Natvig, J.B. Scand. J. Immunol. 10, 303-308, 1979.
2. Cornwell III, G.G., Murdoch, W.L., Kyle, R.A., et al. Am. J. Med. 75, 618-623, 1983.
3. Goffin, Y.A., Murdoch, W.L., Cornwell III, G.G., et al. J. Clin. Pathol. 36, 1342-1349, 1983.
4. Cornwell III, G.G., Westermark, P., Murdoch, W.L., et al. Am. J. Pathol. 108, 135-139, 1982.
5. Pitkänen, P., Westermark, P. & Cornwell III, G.G. Am. J. Pathol. 117, 391-399, 1984.
6. Buerger, L. & Braunstein, H. Am. J. Med. 28, 357-367, 1960.
7. Hodkinson, H.M. & Pomerance, A. Q. J. Med. 46, 381-387, 1977.
8. Wright, J.R. & Calkins, E. J. Am. Geriatr. Soc. 23, 97-103, 1975.
9. Sletten, K., Westermark, P. & Natvig, J.B. Scand. J. Immunol. 12, 503-506, 1980.
10. Kanda, Y., Goodman, D.S., Canfield, R.E., et al. J. Biol. Chem. 249, 6796-6805, 1974.
11. Felding, P., Fex, G., Westermark, P., et al. Scand. J. Immunol. 21, 133-140, 1985.
12. Cornwell III, G.G., Westermark, P. & Natvig, J.B. Immunology 44, 447-452, 1981.
13. Westermark, P., Pitkänen, P., Benson, L., et al. Lab. Invest. 52, 314-318, 1985.

VI.5 AMYLOID ARTHROPATHY

Lawrence M. Ryan

Medical College of Wisconsin,
Department of Medicine, Rheumatology Section,
Milwaukee County Medical Complex,
Milwaukee, Wisconsin 53226, U.S.A.

1. Introduction

Articular and periarticular deposition of amyloid occurs in a variety of settings producing diverse clinical manifestations. A brief summary follows. For the purpose of taxonomy, various clinical divisions will be distinguished based on clinical features and associated conditions.

2. Amyloid arthropathy resembling rheumatoid arthritis

Many patients, primarily with myeloma-associated amyloidosis, have developed symmetrical macroscopic amyloid deposition in and about joints which mimics rheumatoid arthritis (1-4). This has been termed amyloid arthropathy as the infiltration of tissues with amyloid appears to cause the symptoms and signs noted in these patients. This arthropathy may antedate the recognition of myeloma. Diagnostic confusion with rheumatoid arthritis (RA) stems from features shared commonly by RA and amyloid arthropathy: articular pain, morning stiffness, articular swelling, symmetrical joint involvement, involvement of both large and small joints, as well as subcutaneous nodule formation. However, joints involved in amyloid arthropathy are neither warm nor red and are non--tender or minimally tender. Fingers, knees, wrists and shoulders are the most common sites. Flexor tendon contractures in the palms are frequent. Approximately one-third of patients will concomitantly have a carpal tunnel syndrome. Shoulder involvement with massive deposition leads to the "shoulder pad sign" based upon the resemblance of affected patients to football players wearing shoulder pads (5,6). Since nodular rheumatoid arthritis is nearly invariably accompanied with a positive latex test for rheumatoid factor, the absence of rheumatoid factor in these patients is often an important clue that the disease is not RA. Additionally, roentgenograms fail to show erosions as might be expected in RA. However, radiographs are frequently abnormal and often show diffuse osteoporosis (as might be expected in other patients with multiple myeloma) and/or lytic periarticular bone lesions which represent intraosseous accumulations of amyloid. Joint fluid is viscous. Synovial fluid white counts are generally less than 2,000 per mm^3. Congo red staining of synovial fluid pellets may disclose characteristic material under polarized light. False positive stains are infrequent. Macroscopic nodules are present in the synovium of these patients (7). The deposits are located at the surface of the synovium or in the subsynovial layer. Amyloid also occurs in articular cartilage of some of these patients (8). Coexistent extra-articular involvement is the rule in this classic form of amyloid arthropathy.

3. Amyloid in intervertebral discs

Much more frequent than the rheumatoid-like arthritis described above is the deposition of amyloid in intervertebral discs. Rarely this occurs in primary systemic amyloidosis where the discs may become calcified (9). Usually, however, disc deposits are seen in the absence of clinical evidence for primary amyloidosis, secondary amyloidosis or multiple myeloma (10). The avascular, fibrocartilagenous annulus fibrosis of the disc is the preferential site of deposition. In autopsy specimens a significant positive correlation between frequency of deposition and age was observed, increasing from 12.5% in the third decade to 87.5% in the seventh decade. Deposits were generally $KMnO_4$-resistant suggesting that they were not AA amyloid. The relationship of amyloid to antemortem symptoms, radiographic changes, gross appearance of the discs, or routine histologic appearance has not been addressed. Chemical or immunologic definition of the amyloid type is absent. Interestingly, age related deposition of amyloid in the intervertebral discs of an AKR strain of mice inbred for accelerated senescence has been reported (11). These mice also have microscopic amyloid deposits in peripheral joints.

4. Amyloid in osteoarthritic joints

Christensen and Sorensen first reported detection of amyloid in the joint capsules in 7 of 43 specimens obtained at the time of hip replacement for severe osteoarthritis (12). Mohr confirmed this finding and postulated it to be an age related phenomenon without clinical relevance (13). Ladefoged and Christensen found amyloid in 43% of hip capsules in unselected autopsies and an even higher prevalence (93%) in joint cartilage (14). The amount of amyloid was estimated histologically and was found to correlate positively with the age of the subject. In a larger study superficial cartilage deposits of amyloid were found in 75 of 116 femoral heads (65%) obtained during surgery for osteoarthritis (15). These deposits are primarily microscopic as opposed to the dense infiltration noted in the myeloma-associated amyloid arthropathy. Amyloid in periarticular structures and on cartilage surfaces also are frequent in the aforementioned inbred strain of AKR mice developed as a model of premature senescence (16). In this model the presence of amyloid correlated with age and occurred more frequently in AKR senescent mice than in control AKR litters. In both the human and mouse studies the presence of amyloid is clearly age related and may be related to the coexistent osteoarthritis.

5.Amyloid in calcium pyrophosphate dihydrate deposition disease

In 1976 an abstract by Kaplinski et al described a patient with amyloid and pseudogout (17). In 1978 we reported five patients with articular amyloid deposits, four of whom had roentgenographic chondro-calcinosis (18,19). Four of the five patients had diffusely swollen hands with pitting edema and palmar tendon thickening. Three also had carpal tunnel syndrome. Teglbjaerg et al found amyloid in synovial specimens from 14 of 15 patients with crystal proven calcium pyrophosphate di-hydrate (CPPD) deposition disease (20). In two studies the amyloid deposits were described as being in close proximity to CPPD crystals (21,22). We have speculated that amyloid deposits may stimulate local inorganic pyrophosphate (PPi) production and may bind the PPi much as amyloid binds diphosphonates which are analogues of PPi. Either pyro-phosphate or diphosphonate can be used as a scanning agent for amyloid as a result of this binding property (23). Nonetheless, both CPPD deposition and articular amyloid deposition occur with increased frequency in an aging population and their concurrence may result from chance alone.

6.Articular amyloid in renal failure/hemodialysis

Carpal tunnel syndrome is increasingly recognized as a complication of long term hemodialysis. In the majority of these patients treated surgi-cally, amyloid has been present in the excised tissue (24). Eighteen patients with end stage renal failure who were treated with hemodialysis had proven synovial amyloid deposits particularly in the flexor teno-synovium of the fingers. All patients had carpal tunnel syndrome which was bilateral in 14. Four patients had clinically evident finger flexor tenosynovitis and two had destructive hip arthropathy. Juxta-articular cystic radiolucencies were prevalent especially in the carpal bones (6/19), hips (5/19) and tibial plateaus (2/19). In similar patients these lucencies have been found to contain amyloid or amyloid laden synovium (25). In these hemodialysis patients, the deposits are composed primarily of β_2-microglobulin. The etiopathogenesis of such infiltration is uncertain.

In addition to the well described amyloid arthropathy of multiple myeloma, we have reviewed several other forms which occur in the ab-sence of myeloma. Future studies will help define the relationship of amyloid to degenerative processes, to crystal deposition and to chronic renal failure.

References

1. Magnus-Levy, A. Acta Med. Scand. 95, 217-280, 1938.
2. Goldberg, A., Brodsky, I. & McCarty D. Am. J. Med. 37, 653-658, 1964.
3. Gordon, D.A., Pruzanski, W., Ogryzlo, M. & Little, H.A. Am. J. Med. 55, 142-154, 1973.
4. Wiernik, P.H. Medicine 51, 465-479, 1972.
5. Katz, G.A., Peter, J.B, Pearson, C.M. & Adams, W.S. New Engl. J. Med. 288, 354-355, 1973.
6. Lakhanpal, S., Li, C.Y., Gertz, M.A., et al. Arthritis Rheum. 29(4, Suppl.), S49, 1986.
7. Cohen A.S.. & Canoso, J.J. Clin. Rheum. Dis. 1, 149-161, 1975.
8. Bywaters, E.G.L. & Dorling, J. Ann. Rheum. Dis. 29, 294-306, 1970.
9. Christensson, T. Ann. Int. Med. 85, 614-616, 1976.
10. Takeda, T., Sanada, H., Ishii, M., et al. Arthritis Rheum. 27, 1063-1065, 1984.
11. Shimizu, K., Ishii, M., Yamamuro, T., et al. Arthritis Rheum. 25, 710-712, 1982.
12. Christensen, H.E & Sørensen, K.H. Acta Pathol. Microbiol. Scand. (A)80, Suppl. 233, 128-131, 1972.
13. Mohr, W. Z. Rheumatol. 35, 412-417, 1976.
14. Ladefoged, C. & Christensen, H.B. Acta Pathol. Microbiol. Scand. (A) 88, 55-58, 1980.
15. Ladefoged, C. Acta Orthop. Scand. 53, 581-586, 1982.
16. Shimizu, K., Kasai, R., Yamamuro, T., et al. Arthritis Rheum. 24, 1540-1543, 1981.
17. Kaplinski, N., Biran, D. & Frankl O. Harefuah 91, 28-29, 1976.
18. Ryan, L.M. & Bernhard, G.C. Arthritis Rheum. 21, 587-588, 1978.
19. Ryan, L.M., Liang, G. & Kozin, F. J. Rheum. 9, 273-278, 1982.
20. Teglbjaerg, P.S., Ladefoged, C., Sørensen, K.H. & Christensen, H.E. Acta Pathol. Microbiol. Scand. (A) 87, 307-311, 1979.
21. Egan, M.S., Goldenberg, D.L., Cohen, A.S. & Segal, D. Arthritis Rheum. 25, 204-208, 1982.
22. Sørensen, K.H., Teglbjaerg, P.S., Ladefoged, C. & Christensen H.E. Acta Orthop. Scand. 52, 129-133, 1981.
23. Yood, R.A., Skinner, M., Cohen, A.S & Lee, V.W. J. Rheum. 8, 760-766, 1981.
24. Bardin, T., Kuntz, D., Zingraff, J., et al. Arthritis Rheum. 28, 1052-1058, 1985.
25. Huaux, J.P., Noel, H. Malghem, J., et al. Arthritis Rheum. 28, 1075-1076, 1985.
26. Bardin, T., Kuntz, D., Noel, L.H., et al. Arthritis Rheum. 29 (4, Suppl.), S11, 1986.

VI.6 PERIPHERAL ANGIOPATHY

Thos. J. Muckle

Department of Pathology,
Faculty of Medicine, McMaster University;
Hamilton, Ontario, Canada L8N 3Z5.

1.Introduction

The extracerebral peripheral blood vessels of the elderly may be affected directly by amyloid deposition in a number of ways (Table I).

TABLE I: EXTRACEREBRAL PERIPHERAL AMYLOID ANGIOPATHIES OCCURRING IN
THE ELDERLY

A. SENILE PROPER
   1.Senile Systemic Amyloidosis
   2.Senile Aortic Amyloidosis
   3.Senile Amyloidosis of the Aortic Branches and Pulmonary Artery
   4.Senile Amyloidosis of the Temporal Artery
   5.Microdeposits

B. INCOMPLETELY DEFINED
   6.Small Artery Amyloidosis Ischemia Syndrome

C. INCIDENTALLY ASSOCIATED
   7.Myelomatous Amyloid Angiopathy
   8.Primary Amyloid Angiopathy - primary ("myeloma") pattern
   9.Primary Amyloid Angiopathy - secondary pattern
   10.Classical Secondary Amyloid Angiopathy
   11.Genetic Amyloid Angiopathy

However, it is usual to confine the designation "senile" to those forms of amyloidosis which differ from the others in three particulars, (i) they do not occur much before middle age, after which the prevalence and quantity of their deposits increases with age; (ii) within this temporal limitation they are relatively common in the general population; and (iii) they exhibit restriction of anatomical distribution of the deposits. In this way the strictly senile amyloidoses are demarcated from examples of other forms which may just happen to occur in the senium, for the elderly are not immune from regular secondary amyloidosis, while myelomatous and the sporadic primary systemic forms occur with peak age frequency in the sixth and seventh decades (1). Senile amyloidosis of the peripheral vasculature therefore does not include manifestation in incidentally elderly subjects of that involvement of the blood vessels which is so notable a feature of the secondary, sporadic primary, myelomatous, and some hereditary systemic amyloidoses. Also excluded from the senile category are those examples of vasculopathy sometimes occurring in hereditary and myelomatous amyloidosis where the affliction of the vessel wall is essentially neuropathic and not due directly to deposition of amyloid.

271

2.Senile Systemic Amyloidosis (SSA)

This entity, previously entitled Senile Cardiac Amyloidosis (2), was first clearly distinguished from other cardiovascular forms by Westermark and colleagues (3) upon the basis of its unique amyloid fibril protein ASc_1. The distribution of deposits throughout the body, as determined by immunoperoxidase technique using specific antibody to ASc_1, was widespread in the vascular bed and also showed sparse circumscribed foci of apparently nonvascular deposition. The location of SSA deposits was in close relation to muscle cells including the myocardium, myocytes of small blood vessels throughout the body, and nonvascular muscle tissue in tongue and rectal wall. Such light microscopically evident close association of senile amyloid deposition to cardiac, vascular and other muscle tissue has been confirmed in great detail at the electronmicroscopic level (4). Possibly nonvascular deposits occurred fairly extensively in the lung, and to a lesser degree in the renal papillae, adipose tissue, within the substance of small peripheral nerves and around some bronchial glands. Characteristically, parenchymatous involvement of the type seen in non-senile systemic amyloidosis did not occur, so that glomeruli, hepatic sinusoids, and splenic pulp remained free from amyloid.

The pattern of this extensive deposition strongly recalls substantial portions of the pictures described in numerous older and some more recent (5-8) accounts of senile amyloidosis. If one substracts from these older descriptions the now recognized individual senile entities such as occur in the brain, the islets of Langerhans, seminal vesicles, and possibly the parenchymatous microdeposits of Ravid et al (9) it would seem that SSA would account for most if not all the deposits seen and described in such reports.

Deducing relative frequencies from the nonantigenically specific reports as well as the immunologically defined description (3), it is clear that the prevalence of SSA is very high indeed beyond the age of seventy or so. In the original report of Pitkänen et al (3), tissues from twenty-six different locations in thirteen patients showed 100% prevalence in fourteen locations, with 50% or better prevalence in a further eight locations. Most of these deposits were vascular and fairly small. Locations with a lesser frequency included subcutaneous fat with 43%, spleen with 18%, whereas none were found in the brain in spite of the presence of obvious Congophile angiopathy.

From isolation and immunological studies (2,10-13) there now seems little doubt that the amyloid fibril protein ASc_1 (Amyloid fibril protein from Senile cardiac amyloidosis number 1) is peculiar to SSA. This protein shows close antigenic similarity (11) and substantial amino acid sequential homology (14) to prealbumin. Curiously enough, although cross-reaction and cross-blocking is evident in histological immunofluorescence and immunoperoxidase preparations, neither prealbumin nor ASc_1 in fluid form crossreact with each others' antibodies at least in immunodiffusion (11,12). Presumably this reflects conformational antigenic differences between the free and the bound form of the proteins. Recent collateral evidence suggesting that circulating prealbumin contributes to SSA deposits comes from the demonstration of depressed serum prealbumin levels in affected subjects (15). Interestingly, the patients with SSA had mildly raised serum SAA levels while SAA and prealbumin levels in the blood showed a negative correlation; an alternative explanation for this finding of course is simply that so many old people have foci of low grade inflammation (16).

3. Senile Aortic Amyloidosis - General Comments

Older publications of pathological studies of senile amyloidosis reported low prevalence rates for aortic amyloid deposition in the aged, almost certainly because of lack of sensitivity (along with lack of specificity) of the staining and microscopic techniques which were employed. Thus Buerger and Braunstein (17) found only one aorta affected out of thirty-eight examined from subjects mostly over eighty (and almost all over seventy) years of age. Since then inspection for ultraviolet fluorescence (18) in sections stained by the alkaline Congo red method (19) with appropriate controls has provided levels of both sensitivity and specificity which render detection of microdeposits of amyloid reliable as well as simple. In this way small deposits which previously would have gone undetected become obvious, so that nowadays the aorta is recognized as one of the commonest sites for senile amyloid deposition.

There now appears to be good ground for differentiating three forms of senile amyloidosis of the aorta. These occur anatomically separate in the adventitia, the media, and the intima but are distinguished by more than merely location. Thus while all appear to be asymptomatic, demographically truly senile forms of amyloidosis, and exhibit identical histochemical reactions including permanganate resistance and tryptophane positivity, differences of prevalence and of fibril protein antigenic constitution have been defined. In some of the previously published accounts the data were not broken down sufficiently for distinction between these three types, but latter descriptions have been detailed enough to allow recognition of the subvarieties.

4. Senile Aortic Amyloidosis - Adventitial (SSA, SAoAdA)

Senile amyloidosis of the aortic adventitia appears to be exclusively a manifestation of Senile Systemic Amyloidosis (SSA), as shown by immunohistochemistry (3). In this report adventitial deposits reacting immunologically as the specific prealbumin-like amyloid fibril protein ASc_1 of SSA were found in the adventitia and vasa vasorum, diffusely in the former and focally in the latter, of six out of eight aortas from subjects over 74 years of age. This high detection rate may have achieved only through the sensitivity of immunohistochemistry, since other studies have described much lesser frequency. In a much more extensive study (6), but using neither immunohistochemistry nor ultraviolet fluorescence, aortic adventitial amyloid was found in only 1.9% of the 154 cases examined, a rate less than one-ninth that of SAoMA and SAoIA together in the same series of aortas. Even Schwartz (20) describes this form as uncommon but also as affecting particularly the vasa vasorum of the adventitia. Other detailed accounts, some using the highly sensitive (18,21) Congo red ultraviolet fluorescence, either stated failure to detect adventitial amyloid at all (5,7,22) or simply made no mention of having noticed any such deposits (4,24-26). Aortic adventitial SSA deposits, like their counterparts elsewhere, histochemically show permanganate resistance (5,6) and are positive for tryptophane (5,6,13).

5.Senile Aortic Amyloidosis - Medial (SAoA, SAoMA)

The prevalence of this form is clearly high among the aged (Table II) and there is good evidence that not only the frequency but also the quantity increases with increasing age (7,23,25). There appear to be no gender differences of prevalence.

TABLE II: PREVALENCE OF SENILE AORTIC MEDIAL AMYLOID; A REVIEW OF THE LITERATURE

References	Decade						Detection Methods
	40-49	50-59	60-69	70-79	80-89	90+	
Iwata 1978 (22)[#] [*]	!——51%——!		82%	90%	!——95%——!		CR Fluor.
Cornwell 1982 (5) [*]	-	-	-	!——100%——!			CR Fluor.
Cornwell 1983 (24) [*]	-	-	-	-	!——100%——!		CR Fluor
Pitkänen 1984 (3) [*]	-	-	!— - —! !——100%——!				CR Pol.
Storkel 1983 (7)	-	-	32%	45%	59%	75%	CR Pol.
Battaglia 1978 (23)[#]	57%	63%	-	-	-	-	CR Pol.
Ishii 1983 (6)[#]	-	-	4%	16%	29%	25%	CR Pol.
Wright 1969 (26)[#]	10%	-	10%	40%	70%	33%	CR Pol. ThioF etc.
Wright 1974 (25)[#]	-	-	!——66%——! !——70%——!				CR Pol. ThioF etc.
Schwartz 1970 (20)[#]	!—— - ——! !——100%——!						ThioF

Senile aortic amyloid including intimal but predominantly medial deposition.
* Age groups prevalence of senile aortic medial amyloid.
CR=Congo red; Fluor.=fluorescence microscopy; Pol.=polarization microscopy.

By light microscopy these deposits appear as specks, streaks or sometimes nodules located most frequently in the inner media (5-7,20,22,23,25,26), the streaks being orientated parallel to the direction of the smooth muscle cells (5,24) between the elastic lamellae (6,22,25). Ultrastructurally, the fibrils lie in "complete disorder" (5) closely investing the membranes of the smooth muscle cells but always extracellular, and with no particular relationship to the elastic laminae (7). This very close investment of smooth muscle cell walls may account for what by ordinary light microscopy appears to be intracellular location (5,23). There is no indication of whether the long axis of birefringence of the amyloid deposits is exactly longitudinal, or to a degree diagonal or transverse to the long axis of the aorta. The dif-

ferent segments along the length of the aorta may be unequally susceptible to this form of amyloid deposition. Thus the density of deposits
in the thoracic aorta has been reported as greater than in the
abdominal aorta (22,23) although one report found them to be equal
(25). No explanation for the discrepancy between these two reports is
evident. However, the inequality between the thoracic and abdominal
segments has been cited as part of the evidence for lack of association
of SAoMA (as opposed to SAoIA) with atherosclerosis of the aorta
(6,22,23,25,26) which is, of course, usually so much more marked in
the abdominal part. One report (25) took the dissociation even further,
since in this series the oldest people showed more SAoMA than the less
elderly group, but no more atherosclerosis.

Deposits of SAoMA, like the other aortic forms, are permanganate
resistant (5,6,23,24,27) and tryptophane positive (5,6,22-24,27).
Antigenically SAoMA depositis show no reaction with antisera specific
for the prealbumin-like fibril protein typical of SSA designated ASc_1 or
prealbumin itself (3,5) nor yet AA, $AL_\lambda IV$, $AL_\lambda VI$, or AEt (5).

6. Senile Aortic Amyloidosis - Intimal (SAoIA)

Data on SAoIA are scarce indeed, since in most reports this variant
appears to have been accepted, if considered separately at all, as differing from SAoMA only in location. Yet there are convincing indications
that SAoIA is a distinct and possibly unique entity related to atherosclerosis.

First, SAoIA shows close spatial association with atheromatous lesions,
being located either at the base of early fibrous plaques (6,22,25,26,28)
or in immediate juxtaposition to the cholesterol accumulations within advanced lesions (22,25,28). Second, the statistical association of the two
lesions is very high. Using Iwata's (22) data for atheroma grade of +
and +++ versus intimal and medial location of amyloid deposits, Chi^2 =
52.83, a very high figure for biological situations (p $\ll$ 0.0005). This
illustrates not only the association of SAoIA with atheroma, but recipro-
cally the negative association of atheroma with SAoMA. In these respects, the two locational forms of aortic amyloidosis would appear to be
distinct. Notwithstanding all of the above, SAoIA has also been reported as occurring occasionally in the absence of visible atheroma (20).

The overall prevalence of intimal amyloid deposits in the aorta has
been given as 7.8% (6) and 13.2% (22), but these two reports were
published separately so that the different rates in the two series are
not corrected for either prevalence of atherosclerosis or gender and age
discrepancies. Nevertheless, these percentages clearly indicate that
SAoIA is much less common than SAoMA. Wright and Calkins (25) and
Schwartz and Wolfe (28) describe SAoIA as much less frequent than
SAoMA, while the first two reports (6,22) calculated the intimal form to
be little more than respectively half and one-quarter as common as the
medial form. Tending to confirm this are four reports in which there is

no mention of detection of SAoIA at all (5,7,23,24) even though sensitive techniques were employed. To date, deposits of SAoIA appear to be histochemically indistinguishable from SAoMA, exhibiting permanganate resistance (6) and Adams (29) tryptophane positivity (6,22). Immunohistological data do not appear to be available at the present time.

7. Pulmonary Artery and Large Branches of the Aorta

Senile amyloidosis in the walls of these blood vessels has been almost entirely neglected. Apart from occasional accounts of single cases in the early literature, which lack convincing evidence that the deposition was actual senile as opposed to myelomatous or systemic in type, there seem to be extant only two considerations of anything more than anecdotal character. Schwartz (20) commented that senile amyloid deposits in these vessels were uncommon but similar to those found in the aorta. Ishii (6) described eleven examples of senile mural deposition in pulmonary elastic arteries among 194 cases examined (= 5.7%), in prevalence contrast to an overall rate of 19.5% for the aorta. These forms would appear therefore to be less frequent and extensive than deposition in the aorta itself, but much more work is needed for any valid conclusions.

8. Senile Amyloidosis of the Temporal Artery (SATA)

The features of this form of angiopathy are typical of the senile amyloidoses. SATA does not appear to occur below the age of 30 to 40 years; its prevalence and the size and extent of the deposits then rise progressively with increasing age so that the frequency approaches 100% by the tenth decade (Table III).

TABLE III: SENILE AMYLOIDOSIS OF THE TEMPORAL ARTERY

Decade group	n	Prevalence %	Grade (0-4)
40-49	6	0	0.00
50-59	18	28	0.39
60-69	41	56	0.65
70-79	42	69	1.21
80-89	13	77	1.58
90-99	2	100	3.00

$$r= 0.981 \qquad 0.989$$
$$2p= <0.001 \qquad <0.001$$

The deposits show restriction of distribution, macroanatomically occurring almost exclusively in the temporal arteries and microscopically being limited to the substance, surface and fenestrations of the internal elastic lamina. The amyloid is Adams (29) positive for tryptophane (30) and, upon the basis of permanganate resistance (30) and immuno-histology (31), does not appear to include amyloid fibril proteins AA, AL_λ, AL_κ, or ASc_1. Ultramicroscopically the fibrils are typical and measure approximately 70 Å across (30). None of the characteristics of SATA differ by gender, the deposits are never massive, and there is no evidence of associated symptomatology.

SATA was originally reported as a new form of senile amyloidosis in 1972 (32) and its histochemical and ultrastructural characteristics de-scribed in 1980 (30). Apart from these communications, amyloidosis of the vascular internal elastic lamina appears to have gone largely unno-ticed, probably because of the combination of the lack of associated clinical manifestations and the meager dimensions of the deposits. Schwartz (33) in 1970 published a single photograph of what looks exactly like SATA, but in a coronary artery. Meretoja and Teppo (34) described minimal amyloid involvement of the lamina elastica interna of femoral and thyroid capsular veins in three cases of the "Meretoja syndrome" (35) type of genetic amyloidosis. Finally, there is a report of sixteen temporal artery biopsies from elderly people in which SATA was present in all ten with giant cell arteritis (GCA) but in none of the six without GCA (36). My own experience with one hundred and twenty-two temporal artery specimens has shown no relationship between the occurrence of SATA and GCA (Chi^2 = 0.13 - a very low figure indeed, p = > 0.7). No quantitative relationship was evident either, and SATA showed no significant association with intimal fibrosis, mural cal-cification, or thrombosis of the lumen. There was, however, a moderate positive grade correlation between SATA and fragmentation of the internal elastic lamina (r + 0.53, 2p = <0.001).

Two aspects of SATA require further attention. Its apparent regional exclusivity should be challenged by an extensive survey of the other peripheral arteries of similar size in old people. As well, the chemical nature of its constituent fibrils has not yet been defined; this could represent a new senile amyloid protein, or even turn out to be no more than that of elastic microfibrils; only isolation and sequential amino acid analysis of these fibrils will tell.

9.Microdeposits

The occurrence of miniscule deposits of amyloid in a wide variety of locations in the body has been reported as increasing in prevalence with age in the elderly (6,9). Since the first study was published in 1967 much further work has been done on senile amyloidosis, and in retrospect it appears probable that the concept of microdeposits (9) represented an amalgam of separate subvarieties of senile amyloidosis, several of which are now defined as separate entities.

With particular respect to extracerebral vascular involvement, micro-deposits have been noted in pulmonary alveolar septae, and small arterial vessels and capillaries throughout the body, but not in such structures as hepatic or splenic sinusoids, or renal glomerular capillaries (6,7,9). Although it is not possible to be certain in retrospect, the details of these vascular descriptions closely parallel the characteristics of senile systemic amyloidosis (3), and the more widespread angiopathy described latterly (3,6,7) may simply reflect more sensitive detection procedures.

10. Small Artery Amyloidosis Ischemia Syndrome (SAAIS)

Of all the tissues subject to systemic amyloid deposition small peripheral arteries and arterioles are frequently the most consistently and earliest involved. In myelomatous and most primary examples small veins are often equally affected as well, whereas in the classical secondary condition it are the sinusoids and capillaries of parenchymatous and mucosal organs which also show amyloid deposits. Although so common, such involvement is hardly ever enough to cause functional vascular insufficiency beyond perhaps some impairment of the arteriolar vasodilatory flare element of the triple response in the skin, and the occasional example of Yamada Type II (large myelinated fibre loss) ischemic neuropathy (37). Very rarely, however, patients do present with major ischemic symptoms and signs which turn out to be due to amyloid deposition in the walls of small arteries and arterioles sufficiently massive to have caused severe stenosis or even occlusion.

A selection of fifty reasonably well-documented such cases published during the past five decades includes thirteen featuring clearly defined plasma cell dyscrasia (38-47), thirty-six putative primary cases (28,40,46-57) and one familial cardio-neuropathic example (40). In all cases the affected vessels were small arteries and arterioles of the dimensions of the intramural branches of the coronary arteries. In most cases the vasculopathy was generalized throughout the body even when the symptoms had been localized. In a few cases the pathology appears to have been localized as well. The list of ischemic consequences comprises twenty-one of myocardial infarction and sixteen of angina pectoris (with little or no atherosclerosis), assorted other ischemic lesions in different organs including a gangrenous leg, seven of intermittent claudication (39,47,48,57) and one of a myopathy closely resembling upper limb girdle muscular dystrophy (52). In two fascinating reports (47,53) comprising five cases the abnormal vascular dynamics were investigated in great detail. The nature of the amyloid protein in SAAIS remains uncertain. Permanganate resistant Congo red staining of the deposits was described in one myelomatous case (43), and lack of immunofluorescence with antisera to immunoglobulin gamma, mu, alpha, delta, kappa and lambda chains in another (42). Apart from these two isolated statements none of the reports include mention of permanganate resistance, antigenic constitution, or tryptophane reactivity of the amyloid in the blood vessel walls. These data are summarized in Table IV.

TABLE IV: PERMANGANATE RESISTANCE, TRYPTOPHANE CONTENT, AND KNOWN ANTIGENIC FEATURES OF THE MAJOR EXTRACEREBRAL SENILE AMYLOID PERIPHERAL ANGIOPATHIES

	SSA(SCA)	SAoAdA (SSA)#	SAoMA (SAoA)	SAoIA	SATA
$KMnO_4$	R (5)	R (6)	R (5,6,23,24)	R (6)	R (30)
TRP	+ (5,13)	+ (6)	+ (5,6,22-24)	+ (6,22)	+ (30)
ASc_1*	+ (2,5,10,11,13,24)	+ (3)	- (3,5)	n.a.	- (31)
PreAlb	+ (5,11,24)	n.a.	- (5)	n.a.	n.a.
AA	- (2,10-13)	- (3)	- (5)	n.a.	- (31)
AL_λ**	- (2,10,11)	n.a.	- (5)	n.a.	- (31)
AL_κ	n.a.	n.a.	n.a.	n.a.	- (31)
AEmct	- (10,11)	n.a.	- (5)	n.a.	n.a.

R=resistant; n.a.=not available; +=reactive for presence; -=non-reactive; * previously ASca; anti-ASc_1 does not react with amyloids of AA, Alzheimer's disease, lichen amyloidosis (11), pancreatic islets (10,11), Isolated Atrial Amyloid (3,5,11,13), or Congophilic angiopathy (3); ** various subtypes, see references; # aortic adventitial deposits defined by location, not antigenic reactivity.

Careful appraisal of these case histories has revealed no historical, clinical, or pathological feature which correlated with the presence or absence of evidence of plasma cell dyscrasia. Mean ages for myelomatous and primary groups were 51.6 and 56 years respectively, the difference of 4.4 years not significant by Student's "t" test (two tailed), and the variances were also closely similar. This apparent coincidence of age prevalence for these two classification groups has been recognized in general for amyloidosis as far back as 1946 (1) and has given rise to conjecture that many examples of systemic primary amyloidosis actually represent occult plasma cell dyscrasias. Another apparent coincidence is that approximately 75% of both of these groups of SAAIS were male. No other gender differences were evident.

A quarter of the examples of this syndrome have thus been myelomatous in origin, and it may be supposed that some designated "primary" in the older literature in reality were cases of myeloma with missed diagnosis. Nevertherless, the majority of the cases of this syndrome appear to represent primary disease. As yet, the numbers are too small for useful consideration of their relationship of increasing age to prevalence and extent, but most of the subjects were elderly, their condition worsened with increasing age, and the vascular involvement was either very predominant or almost exclusive of other tissues and in this sense restricted in distribution. Indeed, as noted above, not all have been systemic and in three reports of sixteen subjects (two myelomatous and fourteen primary) along with some dogs it was emphasized that the intracerebral vessels were not affected (28,38,43).

Thus, the features of the apparently primary form of SAAIS seem to satisfy most of the criteria of senile as opposed to other forms of amyloidosis, and so might be considered to qualify at least tentatively for inclusion in the category. The reservation here is that the only outstanding characteristic which clearly distinguishes the putative primary from the myelomatous cases is absence of evidence of myeloma; and absence of evidence is not, of course, evidence of absence. In spite of this suspicion, it is of couse eminently possible that a smaller or larger proportion of such putative cases were truly primary and represented the deposition of amyloid fibrils of some protein other than AA or immunoglobulin light chains.

11. Prospects and Conclusion

One outstanding feature of the senile amyloidoses in general is restriction of anatomical distribution, of which the peripheral angiopathies show two forms. First, they seem to be very largely confined to the arterial side of the blood vascular system and second, the different types appear to occur in circumscribed regions of the system. Anatomically the arterial system is divided into two main parts, the aorta and elastic arteries being clearly different and fairly sharply demarcated from the muscular arteries and arterioles. However, the diversity of senile vascular amyloid deposition referred to in this chapter suggests that each of these two major territories may be further subdivided by features presently unknown. These may reside in cell membrane components (4,7), or connective tissue fibrils or mucopolysaccharides - variations of which with age in different parts of the arterial tree have been recognized since at least 1959 (58,59). Such features may indicate the selective localization of the various forms of senile amyloid peripheral angiopathy, which in turn suggests the possibility of a different amyloid fibril protein in each. Apart from SSA there is as yet little evidence available on this point and such differences may be very subtle, as with the minor variations of primary structure, size, and molecular charge which distinguish the selectively vascular from the predominantly parenchymatous subvariants of AA fibril protein deposition in the kidney (60-64). As has so long been the case with many other areas of amyloidosis, exact identification of individual amyloid fibril proteins in each of the senile peripheral angiopathies will probably be required for final resolution of these puzzles. At the same time, it should be clearly understood that the limitation of distribution in the different types has up to the present been incompletely defined. Their presence in certain areas has been much more studied than their absence in others. What is now needed is a thorough survey of the whole of the arterial tree in a large enough number of. elderly subjects and with sufficient sampling sites to allow construction of an exact map of the extent and any correlations characterizing these apparently individual forms of senile amyloid peripheral angiopathy.

References

1.Eisen, H.N. Am. J. Med. 1, 144-160, 1946.
2.Westermark, P., Natvig, J.B. & Johansson, B. J. Exp. Med. 146, 631-636, 1977.
3.Pitkänen, P., Westermark, P. & Cornwell III, G.G. Am. J. Pathol. 117, 391-399, 1984.
4.Störkel, S., Schneider, H.M. & Thoenes, W. Virchows Arch. (A) 401, 185-201, 1983.
5.Cornwell III, G.G., Westermark, P., Murdoch, W.L., et al. Am. J. Pathol. 108, 135-139, 1982.
6.Ishii, T., Hosoda, Y., Ikegami, N., et al. J. Pathol. 139, 1-22, 1983.
7.Störkel, S., Bohl, J. & Schneider, H.M. Virchows Arch. (Cell. Pathol.) 44, 145-161, 1983.
8.Yamaguchi, A., Nasu, M., Esaki, Y. et al. J. Oral Pathol. 11, 237-244, 1982.
9.Ravid, M., Gafni, J., Sohar, E., et al. J. Clin. Pathol. 20, 15-20, 1967.
10.Cornwell III, G.G., Natvig, J.B., Westermark, P., et al. J. Immunol. 120, 1385-1388, 1978.
11.Cornwell III, G.G., Westermark, P., Natvig, J.B., et al. Immunology 44, 447-452, 1981.
12.Gorevic, P.D., Cleveland, A.B., Wright, J.R., et al. In Amyloid and Amyloidosis. Glenner, G.G., Costa, P.P., Freitas, A.F., Eds. Excerpta Medica, Amsterdam, 366-372, 1980.
13.Westermark, P., Johansson, B. & Natvig, J.B. Scand. J. Immunol. 10, 303-308, 1979.
14.Sletten, K., Westermark, P. & Natvig, J.B. Scand. J. Immunol. 12, 503-506, 1980.
15.Westermark, P., Pitkänen, P., Benson, L., et al, Lab. Invest. 52, 314-318, 1985.
16.Muckle, T.J., Hall, M. Symposium "The Milieu Interieur of Old Age", British Geriatric Society, Royal College of Physicians (London, U.K.).
17.Buerger, L. & Braunstein, H. Am. J. Med., 28, 357-367, 1960.
18.Puchtler, H., Waldrop, F.S. & Meloan, S.N. Histochemistry 77, 431-445, 1983.
19.Puchtler, H., Sweat, F. & Levine, M. J. Histochem. Cytochem. 10, 355-364, 1962.
20.Schwartz, Ph. Amyloidosis: Cause & Manifestation of Senile Deterioration. Charles C. Thomas, Springfield, Illinois, 80-110, 1970.
21.Brigger, D. & Muckle, T.J. J. Histochem. Cytochem. 23, 84-88, 1975.
22.Iwata, T., Kamei, T., Uchino, F., et al. Acta Pathol. Jpn. 28, 193-203, 1978.
23.Battaglia, S. & Trentini, G.P. Virchows Arch. (A) 378, 153-159, 1978.
24.Cornwell III, G.G., Murdoch, W.L., Kyle, R.A., et al. Am. J. Med. 75, 618-623, 1983.
25.Wright, J.R. & Calkins, E. Lab. Invest. 30, 767-773, 1974.
26.Wright, J.R., Calkins, E., Breen, W.J., et al. Medicine (Baltimore) 48, 39-60, 1969.
27.Muckle, T.J. Unpublished observations.
28.Schwartz, P. & Wolfe, K. J. Am. Geriatr. Soc. 15, 640-650, 1967.
29.Adams, C.W.M. J. Clin. Pathol. 10, 56-62, 1957.
30.Muckle, T.J. IInd International Meeting on Vascular Pathology, Coimbra, Portugal, May 26-29, 1980.
31.Linke, R.P. Personal communication, 1982.
32.Muckle, T.J. In XXth Colloquium Protides of the Biological Fluids, Peeters, H., Ed. Pergamon Press, Oxford, 141-144, 1973.
33.Schwartz, Ph. Deutsches Arzteblatt 8, 576 (photo 19.II), 1970.
34.Meretoja, J., Teppo, L. Acta Pathol. Microbiol. Scand. (A) 79, 432-440, 1971.
35.Meretoja, J. Ann. Clin. Res. 1, 314-324, 1969.
36.Meretoja, J. & Tarkkanen, A. Ophthalmologica (Basel) 170, 337-344, 1975.
37.Yamada, M., Hatakeyama, S. & Tsukagoshi, H. Acta Pathol. Jpn. 34, 1251-1266, 1984.
38.Barth, R.F., Willerson, J.T., Buja, L.M. et al. Arch. Intern. Med. 126, 627-630, 1970.
39.Breathnach, S.M. & Wells, G.C. Br. J. Dermatol. 102, 591-595, 1980.
40.Buja, L.M., Khoi, N.B. & Roberts, W.C. Am. J. Cardiol. 26, 394-405, 1970.
41.Case 23-1968, Case Records Massachusetts General Hospital. N. Engl. J. Med. 278, 1276-1286, 1968.
42.Jennette, J.C., Sheps, D.S. & McNeill, D.D. Arch. Pathol. Lab. Med. 106, 323-327, 1982.
43.Ng, L.L. & Gresham, G.A. J. Roy. Soc. Med. 79, 111-112, 1986.
44.Saffitz, J.E., Sazama, K. & Roberts, W.C. Am. J. Cardiol. 51, 1234-1235, 1983.
45.Saltissi, S., Kertes, P.J. & Julian, D.G. Br. Heart J. 52, 233-236, 1984.
46.Smith, R.R.L. & Hutchins, G.M. Am. J. Cardiol. 44, 413-417, 1979.
47.Zelis, R., Mason, D.T. & Barth, W. Ann. Intern. Med. 70, 1167-1172, 1969.
48.Barnard, W.G., Smith, F.B. & Woodhouse, J.L. J. Pathol. Bacteriol. 47, 311-315, 1938.
49.Bero, G.L. Ann. Intern. Med. 46, 931-955, 1957.
50.Brandt, K., Cathcart, E.S. & Cohen, A.S. Am. J. Med. 44, 955-969, 1968.
51.Brigden, W. Prog. Cardiovasc. Dis. 7, 142-150, 1964.
52.Bruni, J., Bilbao, J.M. & Pritzker, K.P.H. Can. J. Neurol.Sci. 4, 77-80, 1977.
53.Capone, R., Amsterdam, E.A., Mason, D.T., et al. Ann. Intern. Med. 76, 599-603, 1972.

54.Langsch, H.G. Beitr. Pathol. Anat. 125, 123-128, 1961.
55.Pomerance, A. In Pathology of the Heart. Pomerance, A. & Davies, M., Eds. Blackwell Scientific Publ., Oxford, 251-268, 1975.
56.Symmers, W.St.C. J. Clin. Pathol. 9, 212-228, 1956.
57.Weber, F.P., Cade, S., Stott, A.W. et al. Q. J. Med. 6, 181-193, 1937.
58.Zugibe, F.T. & Brown, K.D. Circulation 20, 971-972, 1959.
59.Zugibe, F.T. J. Histochem. Cytochem. 10, 448-461, 1962.
60.Westermark, P., Sletten, K. & Eriksson, M. Lab. Invest. 41, 427-431, 1979.
61.Falck, H.M., Törnroth, T. & Wegelius, O. Clin. Nephrol. 19, 137-142, 1983.
62.Westermark, P. & Nilsson, G.T. In Amyloidosis. Glenner, G.G., Osserman, E.F., Benditt, E.P., Calkins, E., Cohen, A.S., Zucker-Franklin, D., Eds. Plenum Press, New York, 19-26, 1986.
63.Skogen, B., Sletten, K., Lea, T. et al. In Amyloidosis. Glenner, G.G., Osserman, E.F., Benditt, E.P., Calkins, E., Cohen, A.S., Zucker-Franklin, D., Eds. Plenum Press, New York, 11-18, 1986.
64.Törnroth, T., Falck, H.M. & Wegelius, O. Scand. J. Urol. Nephrol. 19, Suppl.(90), 9-21, 1985.

VI.7 ANIMAL MODELS

Keiichi Higuchi and Toshio Takeda

Department of Pathology,
Chest Disease Research Institute,
Kyoto University, Sakyo-ku, Kyoto 606, Japan.

1. Introduction

Progress in medical science during the past 40 years has significantly increased average human life expectancy and, of course, the number of individuals who now reach old age. As life expectancy increases, the increase in age-associated disorders is one of the greatest problems facing most of the countries in the world at the present time. Senile amyloidosis is one of the most difficult pathological conditions affecting the aged.

In recent years, it has become increasingly evident that amyloidosis represents a family of diseases, each member of which may be characterized by a unique amyloid fibril protein in humans (1). It is now clear that amyloidosis associated with aging is very common, and the so-called senile amyloidoses are rather distinct members of this family (2-18). Although senile amyloidosis shares histochemical and morphological features with other forms of amyloidosis, it possesses unique biochemical and immunochemical characteristics. Moreover, there is evidence that amyloid deposits present in heart, brain, pancreas, and other tissues of the aged can be distinguished from one another on the basis of unique histochemical, biochemical and immunochemical properties (5,6,10-12,17,18). In spite of the huge accumulation of information in this field, the pathogenesis of amyloidosis, including senile amyloidosis, remains unexplained.

Advances in many fields of biomedical research depend to a considerable extent on the availability of relevant and appropriate experimental animals, preferably animals that have not previously been subjected to experimental manipulation (19-21). This is particularly true for studies in basic research to determine the mechanism of amyloid deposition or the pathogenesis of senile amyloidosis.

This report describes spontaneous or senile amyloidosis in animals with special reference to murine amyloidosis, in which biochemical and immunochemical as well as morphological studies have been performed. The characteristic biological features of SAM (Senescence Accelerated Mouse) established by Takeda and his colleagues at Kyoto University are presented (22). Finally, senile amyloidosis, one of the most characteristic pathological findings in SAM, is described in detail.

2.Spontaneous or senile amyloidosis in animals

Amyloid has been noted to occur spontaneously in a variety of animal species (Table I).

TABLE I: SPONTANEOUS NON-HUMAN AND NON-MURINE AMYLOIDOSIS

Animals	Reports (44,45)
Monkeys	Systemic in rhesus (Casey et al. 1972) and squirrel (Banks and Bullock, 1967), Islets of Langerhans (Sheldon and Gilbert, 1971)
Baboon	Gillman and Gilbert (1955)
Cattle	Primgaard (1930), Hjärre (1933), Murray et al. (1972)
Horse	Hjärre (1933), Sorenson et al. (1966), Trautwein (1965)
Goat	Sorenson et al. (1966)
Sheep	Sorenson et al. (1966)
Otter	Hjärre (1933), Sorenson et al. (1966)
Dog	Hjärre (1933), Braunmuhl (1956), Osborne (1968), Slauson (1970), Schwartz (1970), Wisniewski et al. (1970), Cheville et al. (1970)
Cat	Hjärre (1933), Clark and Seawright (1969), DiBartola et al. (1985)
Mink	Kenyon (1968), Nordstoga (1972), Lewis (1974)
Hamster	Sorenson et al. (1966), Gleiser et al. (1971)
Rabbit	Sorenson et al. (1966)
Guinea pig	Taylor et al. (1971)
Opossum	Sherwood et al. (1968)
Nutria	Karstad and Budd (1964)
Chicken	Sorenson et al. (1966)
Pekin ducks	Rigdon (1961), Dougherty and Rickard (1963)
Anatidae	Cowan (1968)
Turkey	Sorenson et al. (1966)
Turtle	Trautwein and Pruksaraj (1967)
Snake	Cowan (1968)

Although spontaneous amyloidosis is not always the same as senile amyloidosis, it is assumed that in most cases of spontaneous amyloidosis amyloid deposition increases in incidence and severity with advancing age without any apparent predisposing conditions, particularly infectious diseases; that is, it develops into senile amyloidosis.

In addition to the essential features described above, desirable criteria for an animal model of senile amyloidosis might be as follows: 1. Ease of obtaining the model in large numbers. 2. Ease of handling it in the laboratory. 3. Sufficient information on the biochemical, immunochemical as well as morphological characteristics of amyloidosis in the species selected. 4. Uniform genetic background. 5. Short life span. From this point of view, rodents, particularly mice, might be the most suitable model. In Table II murine spontaneous amyloidoses are listed; many reports on spontaneous or senile amyloidosis in mice have been published since the first description of renal glomerular lesions by Gorer in 1940 (23).

TABLE II: SPONTANEOUS AMYLOIDOSIS IN MICE

Reporters	Strains	Remarks	Ref
Gorer (1940)	A, C57BL	Cystic disease of the kidney age-associated	23
Dunn (1944)	A, ABC (hybrid)	Kidney (papilla), stomach, Brunner's gland	24
Thung (1957)	A, $O_{20}(O_{20}$x DBA$_f$)F$_1$, (C57BL x DBAf)F1, C57BL, CBA	Systemic, age-associated	25
West and Murphy (1965)	A/Sn	Systemic, age-associated	26
Ram et al. (1969)	A/HeN, AL/N, AALF$_1$		27
Glenner et al. (1971)	GP	Wounded in fighting activity	28
Zschiesche (1972)	AB/Jena, A/J Han Jena	Type I and Type II	29
Chai (1976)	LLC	Systemic, low leukocyte count	30
Eisenbud et al. (1981)	LLC	Not AA	31
Scheinberg et al. (1976)	SJL/J	Systemic, age-associated, not AA, 8000 dalton, blocked N-terminus	32
Westermark et al. (1979)	Obese-hyperglycemic mice	Protein AA	33
Takeda et al. (1981)	SAM	Accelerated senescence	22
Takeshita et al. (1981)	SAM	Systemic, age-associated	34
Matsumura et al. (1982)	SAM	Senile amyloid protein AS$_{SAM}$	35
Koeger et al. (1984)	PS	Not AA, light chain?	36

Biochemical information, however, on spontaneous amyloidosis of laboratory animals, including mice, is scant. Amyloid fibril proteins which have been demonstrated biochemically and immunochemically are AA protein in GP (28) and obese hyperglycemic mice (33), and AS$_{SAM}$ (35). In SJL/J mice with a high incidence of reticulum cell neoplasm, age-associated amyloidosis has been reported. The biochemical nature of the amyloid protein in this SJL/J amyloidosis has been partially established: molecular weight (8,000 dalton), amino acid composition and N-terminus (blocked) (32). In LLC mice, with characteristically low leucocyte counts, spontaneous amyloidosis was reported by Chai (30).

Preliminary reports revealed that the amyloid protein was not related to AA protein immunochemically (31). Koeger et al described spontaneous amyloidosis in the PS strain of mice (36). Biochemical, immunochemical and histochemical analysis suggested that the amyloid protein, 1,000-2,000 dalton in molecular weight, was related to immunoglobulin light chains. It might be reasonable to consider that deposition of AA protein in GP mice is secondary to wounds due to fighting. Amyloidosis with a definite close association with aging or senility was observed only in SJL/J and SAM. SAM amyloidosis (22,34) is the only murine senile amyloidosis in which the patho-biological, biochemical and immunochemical characteristics of its fibril protein (35) as well as its serum precursor (37), have been clarified to great extent (Table III).

TABLE III: BIOCHEMICAL AND IMMUNOCHEMICAL ASPECTS OF MURINE AMYLOID PROTEIN IN SPONTANEOUS AMYLOIDOSIS

Strain	M.W. dalton	Amino acid composition	Amino- terminus	Fibril protein	Precursor	Comments	Ref
GP	7,000- 7,200	AA	blocked	AA	n.d.	wounded in in fighting	28
SJL/J	8,000	not AA	blocked	n.d.	n.d.	reticulum cell neoplasm(75%)	32
Obese hyper- glycemic mice	8,600	AA	glycine	AA	SAA	obese hyper- glycemic	33
LLC	n.d.	n.d.	n.d.	not AA	n.d.	low leukocyte counts	30,31
PS	1,000- 2,000	not AA	n.d.	L-chain?	n.d.		36
SAM	5,200	not AA	blocked	AS_{SAM}	$HDL-$ SAS_{SAM}	accelerated senescence	35,37

[n.d. = not determined]

3.Development of the the SAM model; a historical review

Several pairs of the AKR strain of mice were donated by the Jackson Laboratory (Bar Harbor, Maine, U.S.A.) to the Department of Pathology, Chest Disease Reseach Institute, Kyoto University, in 1968. While continuing the sister-brother mating to maintain this inbred strain, we became aware of the presence of certain litters in which most of the mice showed a moderate to severe degree of loss of activity, alopecia and lack of glossiness of the fur, skin coarseness, periophthalmic lesions, increased lordokyphosis and a shortened life span, despite a relatively low incidence of thymic lymphoma. From these mice with severe exhaustion we selected five litters as the progenitors of the "senescence-prone" series (P series). Three litters in which the aging process was normal were selected as the progenitors of the "senescence-resistant" series (R series) in 1975. From the selected litters with severe exhaustion, five series, designated P-1, P-2, P-3, P-4 and P-5, were obtained. In the P-5 series, however, breeding was not succeful after six generations (22). Excluding P-5, these series have recently been named SAM-P/1, SAM-P/2, SAM-P/3 and SAM-P/4 (38). From the selected litters with normal aging, three different series designated R-1,R-2 and R-3 have been named SAM-R/1, SAM-R/2 and SAM-R/3, respectively (38).

The abnormal findings in the survivors, the Gompertz function and body weight curves suggest that the aging pattern in this model is accelerated senescence rather than premature aging or senescence. Therefore this model was named Senescence Accelerated Mouse (SAM). The characteristics of the aging phenomena in the P series are an earlier onset and irreversible advance of senescence manifested by several signs and gross lesions, such as the general deterioration of behaviour, various skin lesions, cataract (39), increased lordokyphosis, etc. after a period of normal development (22).

4. Spontaneous senile amyloidosis; one characteristic of SAM

4.1 Incidence

Morphological studies were conducted on 222 SAM-P and 150 SAM-R mice which had died naturally. Among the pathologic findings, amyloidosis showed the highest incidence in both SAM-P (79.7%) and SAM-R (32.7%). The incidence increased with age and reached over 80% in mice dying at 7 months of age. In the P-2 series, it was especially high: 100% after 6 months of age. In the R series, however, the incidence continued low up to 20 months of age and then increased gradually to reach high levels. Finally, the incidence of amyloidosis was comparable to that seen in the P series (Fig. 1). There was a statistically significant relationship between the incidence of amyloid deposition and age, as calculated by Spearman's rho test. Although a heavy deposition of amyloid was also evident in some aged mice in the R series, a more severe and higher incidence of amyloidosis occurred in the P series. There were no differences in organ distribution and mode of amyloid deposition. The autopsy findings in mice killed between 14 and 18 months of age showed that 60% of amyloid positive mice in the P series had no primary pathology such as abscess, pneumonia or neoplasm (34).

4.2 Morphology

The organs, except for bone and brain parenchyma, were systemically involved with amyloid deposition (Fig. 2). The morphological criteria for amyloid: congophilia, green birefringence of Congo red-stained sections under polarized microscopy and a non-branching felt-like fibril structure under electron microscopy, were completely in accord with the

287

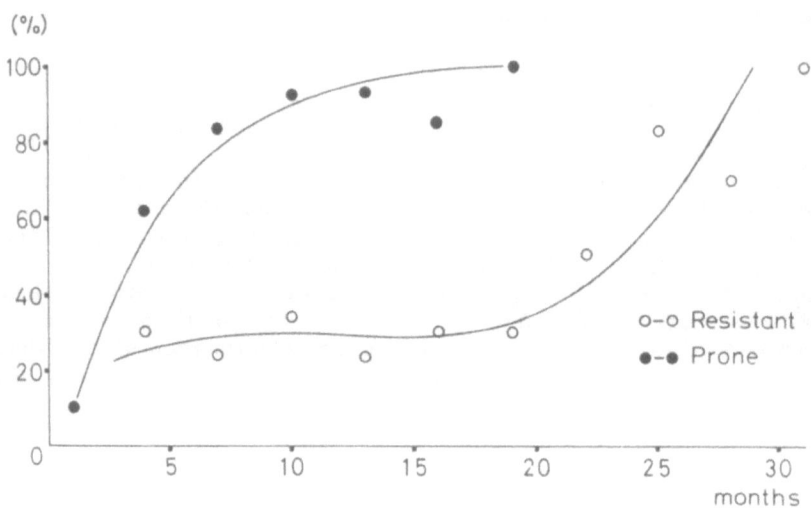

Figure 1: Incidence of amyloidosis in SAM-P (● — ●) and SAM-R (o — o) mice.

amyloid deposited in our model (20,34,40). Tissue sections of SAM-P and SAM-R were studied by the peroxidase-antiperoxidase (PAP) method with specific antisera against a unique amyloid fibril protein (AS$_{SAM}$) and against murine protein AA. Amyloid deposits in liver, kidney, spleen, gastro-intestinal tract, lung, heart, gonads, pancreas, salivary glands, adrenals, thyroid, skin, epineurium and blood vessels were positive for AS$_{SAM}$ in both the SAM-P and SAM-R groups. The amyloid deposited in gonads, papillary layer of the dermis and epineurium was exclusively AS$_{SAM}$ (41). The amyloid observed in most of the SAM-P/1 was AS$_{SAM}$. In the SAM-P/2 and SAM-R, however, protein AA frequently coexisted with AS$_{SAM}$ as demonstrated by a double staining method (41). Recent immunohistochemical studies with the PAP method have demonstrated AS$_{SAM}$-related antigenic substance

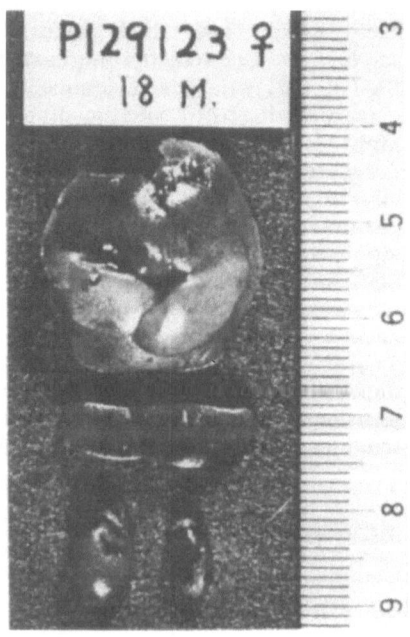

Figure 2: Liver, spleen and kidney of a 18 month-old SAM-P/1 mouse. Note the enlarged liver and spleen due to heavy amyloid deposition.

in the cytoplasm of hepatocytes and columnar epithelium of the small intestine suggesting that hepatocytes and intestinal mucosal epithelium are possible production sites of the precursor of AS_{SAM} (42).

4.3 Biochemistry

Characteristic biochemical features of AS_{SAM}, a novel amyloid fibril protein isolated from SAM-P/1 liver, and its serum precursor are described in detail in Section VII.

5. Usefulness of the SAM-P and SAM-R models

1. The demonstration in large quantities in the spontaneous deposition of a novel senile amyloid fibril protein (90-100% at 10 months of age) in SAM-P in contrast to a very slight deposition and low incidence in SAM-R (20-30% at 10 months of age) validate the usefulness of these models for studies on the pathogenesis of senile amyloidosis.

2. Since amyloid deposition is closely associated with aging or senescence, as mentioned previously, the model should contribute to the clarification of the relationship between amyloidosis and senescence which has long been one of the themes in the investigations of the aging process.

3. In addition to its contribution to clarify the pathogenesis of senile amyloidosis, this model might aid in the search for effective methods of preventing or inhibiting amyloidogenesis by environmental or nutritional changes, for example (43).

4. Molecular-genetic studies of this model will enable us to determine the complete gene structure related to amyloidogenesis and to diagnose senile amyloidosis by DNA analysis.

6. Relation of SAM to human senile amyloidosis

As far as the biochemical aspects of amyloid fibril protein and its serum precursor are concerned, there is no analogy between senile amyloidosis and SAM amyloidosis. In humans, senile systemic amyloidosis (SSA), which was previously called senile cardiac amyloidosis, has been described as a systemic disease with amyloid deposits in many organs (17).

The subunit protein of amyloid fibril in SSA, provisionally named ASc_1, has been partially characterized and shown to be closely related to human prealbumin. Biochemical and immunochemical analyses of AS_{SAM}, a novel amyloid fibril protein in SAM amyloidosis, however, showed no similarity to prealbumin (6). Moreover, prealbumin related to amyloid protein has not yet been reported in any kind of murine amyloidosis. Thus, there seems to be a species difference in the amyloidogenic protein in senile amyloidosis.

Pathologically, systemic involvement with amyloid deposition in many organs is common to both SAM amyloidosis and SSA. The degree of amyloid deposition in each involved organ, however, is somewhat different in the two species. In SSA, amyloid deposition is relatively severe in the cardiovascular and respiratory systems, but mild in the liver and spleen (17). On the other hand, amyloid deposition in SAM is fairly severe in each involved organ, and the spleen and liver are the most severely affected (34,41).

Acknowledgements

We thank Drs. E. Tsubura (Toneyama National Hospital), F.Uchino (Yamaguchi University) and S. Ohashi (Nagoya University) for pertinent advice and all our colleagues for their valuable contributions. We also thank Dr. A. Cary, Kyoto Baptist Hospital, for critical reading of the manuscript.

This work was supported by grants from the Ministry of Education, Culture and Science and the Ministry of Health and Welfare of Japan.

References

1.Cornwell III, G.G. & Westermark, P. J. Clin. Pathol. 33, 1146-1152, 1980.
2.Soyka, J. Prager Med. Wschr. 1, 165-171, 1876.
3.Husselmann, H. Virchows Arch. Pathol. Anat. 327, 607-628, 1955.
4.Wright, J.R., Calkins, E., Breen, W.J., et al. Medicine 48, 39-60, 1969.
5.Westermark, P., Johansson, B. & Natvig, J.B. Scand. J. Immunol. 10, 303-308, 1979.
6.Sletten, K., Westermark, P. & Natvig, J.B. Scand. J. Immunol. 12, 503-506, 1980.
7.Ehrlich, J.C. & Ratner, I.M. Am. J. Pathol. 38, 49-59, 1961.
8.Melato, M., Antonutto, G. & Falconieri, G. Path. Res. Pract. 170, 1-23, 1980.
9.Tomonaga, M. J. Am. Geriatr. Soc. 29, 151-157, 1981.
10.Shirahama, T., Skinner, M., Westermark, P., et al. Am. J. Pathol. 107, 41-50, 1982.
11.Cornwell III, G.G., Westermark, P., Murdoch, W., et al. Am. J. Pathol. 108, 135-139, 1982.
12.Pitkänen, P., Westermark, P., Cornwell III, G.G., et al. Am. J. Pathol. 110, 64-69, 1982.
13.Ravid, M., Gafni, J., Sohar, E., et al. J. Clin. Pathol. 20, 15-20, 1967.
14.Uchino, F., Nakamura, H., Kamei, T., et al. In Amyloid and Amyloidosis. Glenner, G.G., Costa, P.P., Freitas, A.F., Eds. Excerpta Medica, Amsterdam, 55-59, 1980.
15.Takeda, T., Sanada, H., Ishii, M., et al. Arthritis Rheum. 27, 1063-1065, 1984.
16.Ishii, T., Hosokawa, Y., Ikegami, N., et al. J. Pathol. 136, 1-22, 1983.
17.Pitkänen, F., Westermark, P. & Cornwell III, G.G. Am. J. Pathol. 117, 391-399, 1984.
18.Westermark, P., Natvig, J.B. & Johansson, B. J. Exp. Med. 146, 631-636, 1977.
19.Okamoto, K. & Aoki, K. Jpn. Circ. J. 27, 282-293, 1963.
20.Nakamura, M. & Yamada, K. Diabetologia 3, 212-221, 1967.
21.Watanabe, Y. Atherosclerosis 36, 261-268, 1980.
22.Takeda, T., Hosokawa, M., Takeshita, S., et al. Mech.Ageing Dev. 17, 183-194, 1981.
23.Gorer, P.A. J. Pathol. Bact. 50, 25-30, 1940.
24.Dunn, T.B. J. Natl. Cancer Inst. 5, 17-28, 1944.
25.Thung, P.J. Gerontologia 1, 259-279, 1957.
26.West, W.T. & Murphy, E.D. J. Natl. Cancer Inst. 35, 167-174, 1965.
27.Ram, J.S., DeLellis, R.A. & Glenner, G.G. Proc. Soc. Exp. Biol. Med. 130, 462-464, 1969.
28.Glenner, A.S., Page, D., Isersky, C., et al. J. Histochem. Cytochem. 19, 16-28, 1971.
29.Zschiesche, W. Acta Pathol. Microbiol. Scand. (A) 80, Suppl. 233, 135-140, 1972.
30.Chai, C.K. Am. J. Pathol. 85, 45-52, 1976.
31.Eisenbud, L.E., Lerner, C.P. & Chai, C.K. Proc. Soc. Exp.Biol. Med. 168, 172-174, 1981.
32.Scheinberg, M.A., Cathcart, E.S., Eastcott, J.W., et al. Lab. Invest. 35, 47-54, 1976.
33.Westermark, P., Sletten, K., Naeser, P., et al. Scand. J. Immunol. 9, 193-196, 1979.
34.Takeshita, S., Hosokawa, M., Irino, M., et al. Mech. Ageing Dev. 20, 13-23, 1982.

35.Matsumura, A., Higuchi, K., Shimizu, K., et al. Lab. Invest. 47, 270-275, 1982.
36.Koeger, A.C., Branellec, A., Hirbec, G., et al. Pathol. Biol. 32, 959-964, 1984.
37.Higuchi, K., Matsumura, A., Hashimoto, K., et al. J. Exp. Med. 158, 1600-1614, 1983.
38.Hosokawa, M., Kasai, R., Higuchi, K., et al. Mech. Ageing Dev. 26, 91-102, 1984.
39.Hosokawa, M., Takeshita, S., Higuchi, K. et al. Exp. Eye Res. 38, 105-114, 1984.
40.Shimizu, K., Ishii, M., Yamamuro, T., et al. Arthritis Rheum. 25, 710-712, 1982.
41.Higuchi, K., Matsumura, A., Honma, A., et al. Lab. Invest. 48, 231-240, 1983.
42.Takeshita, S., Higuchi, K., Hosokawa, M., et al. Am. J. Pathol. 121, 455-465, 1985.
43.Kohno, A., Yonezu, T., Matsushita, M. et al. J. Nutr. 115, 1259-1266, 1985.
44.Glenner, G.G. & Page, D.L. Int. Rev. Exp. Pathol. 15, 1-92, 1976.
45.Cohen, A.S. Int. Rev. Exp. Pathol. 4, 159-243, 1965.

SECTION VII

EXPERIMENTAL AMYLOIDOSIS

sub-editor: Keith P.W.J. McAdam

VII.1 PATHOLOGY OF EXPERIMENTAL AMYLOIDOSIS

Tsuranobu Shirahama and Alan S. Cohen

The Arthritis Center, Boston University School of Medicine,
and the Thorndike Memorial Laboratory and the Division of
Medicine,
Boston City Hospital,
Boston, MA 02118, U.S.A.

1. Introduction

The histopathology of amyloidosis is well established. In this brief review we shall focus on a few issues which may need some clarification; i.e. 1. tinctorial properties of amyloid, 2. two-phase theory of amyloidogenesis, and 3. immunohistochemistry of amyloid. We will discuss the first two "classic" issues in the light of current amyloid research, and evaluate the role of the third more recent issue.

2. Tinctorial properties of amyloid

Although recent achievements in amyloid research made it abundantly clear that amyloid is proteinaceous substance, amyloid was historically first defined as cellulose-like substance in animal tissues based on its tinctorial properties (1). Amyloid is still histologically characterized, for example, as positive for iodine reaction, metachromatic with crystal violet, violaceous with periodic acid-Schiff and positive for Congo red staining (2-9). While all these stains are known more commonly as stains for substances of carbohydrate nature such as cellulose and glycosaminoglycans (GAGs), they are historically accepted as the amyloid stains as well. At the present stage of amyloid research when the chemical nature of amyloid as fibrillar protein is so well established, however, we consider that each of these staining properties of amyloid should be carefully re-evaluated. This issue became a practical question for us when we became interested in the role of GAGs in amyloidogenesis and attempted to find a way to stain differentially amyloid and GAGs. For example, we have faced a question as to which the so-called amyloid stains indeed do stain the proteinaceous amyloid fibrils, or the carbohydrate elements (associated with but not essential part of the amyloid) of the amyloid deposits, or even both. Thus far, we have not been able to find a definitive answer to this question.

It appears certain though that one of the amyloid stains, i.e Congo red, indeed binds with the amyloid fibril protein (Figs. 1 and 2). This conclusion is derived from published findings and our own experience with amyloid fibrils that were synthesized in vitro from Bence-Jones proteins (10-13) and β_2-microglobulin (14).

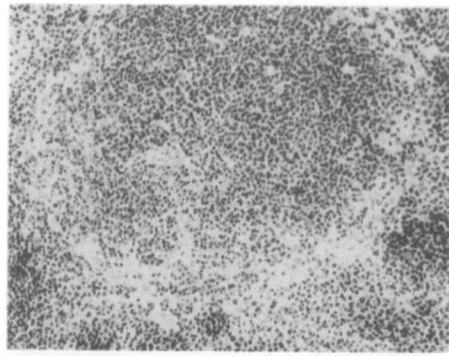

Figure 1: Spleen of a mouse in a very early stage of casein-induced amyloidosis, stained with Congo red and hematoxylin. Congophilic substance in the widened intercellular spaces of the perifollicular zone represents amyloid. [magnification x 120]

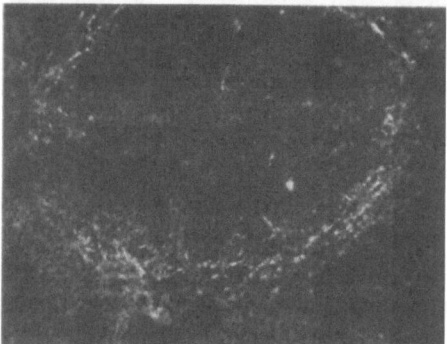

Figure 2: Same area as figure 1, photographed through polarized light. The Congo red positive deposits demonstrate (green) birefringence that is considered characteristic of amyloid. [magnification x 120]

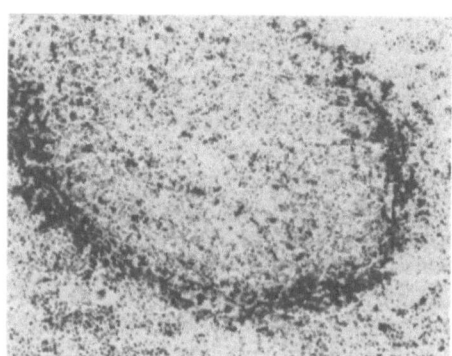

Figure 3: A section from the same mouse spleen as the one shown in figures 1 and 2, immunohistochemically (using an avidin-biotin-peroxidase method) reacted with anti-mouse AA. The amyloid deposits that are primarily localized in the perifollicular zone demonstrate positive reaction. [magnification x 120]

The amyloid fibrils thus constituted indeed stain well with Congo red and demonstrate characteristic green birefringence under polarized light, while they are not associated with GAGs. Thus, Congo red binds with the proteinaceous amyloid fibril proper, while a question still remains as to whether or not this dye binds with GAGs (which may be closely associated with the amyloid) as well.

Many of the amyloid stains differ from Congo red in their basic nature as stains. For example, Alcian blue has long been used as an amyloid stain, but it is a cationic dye differing from anionic Congo red (15,16). Indeed, in a recent study that dealt with the role of GAGs in amyloidogenesis, this dye was used as specific stain for GAGs that differentiates GAGs from Congo red positive amyloid (17). Although the latter use of Alcian blue seems not unreasonable when the nature of this dye is considered, it still leaves open the questions as we set forth above.

The point we are trying to make here is that the specificity of amyloid stains is not well defined. Probably with sole exception of Congo red, although they indeed stain amyloid deposits, it is not clear as to which dyes bind with which component(s) of amyloid deposits. This issue need to be clarified, and until then one must be very cautious in use of these stains and interpretation of the results.

3. Two-phase theory of amyloidogenesis

The two-phase theory of amyloidogenesis that was first postulated by Teilum nearly two decades ago (18,19) stands well in principle today after a period where such rapid developments occurred in amyloid research. Orginally, Teilum developed this theory through his histologic observation of the sequence of changes that took place in tissues, especially spleens, during experimental amyloid induction in mice. The first phase was a preamyloidotic period where a series of cellular proliferations were observed but not yet amyloid deposition. The second phase was the amyloid deposition phase. This theory fitted well the fact that in any experimental amyloidosis model a certain lag time existed between the start of the regimen and the onset of amyloid deposition, and therefore the theory received strong popularity (2-9).

This theory with some modification fits well the contemporary concepts of amyloidogenesis (20,21). For example, in AA amyloidogenesis, the phase of active SAA biosynthesis (by the hepatocytes and probably some other cell types as well) can be considered as the first, and the transformation of SAA to AA and subsequent fibril formation (presumably with the role of the reticulendothelial cells) can be considered the second stage. Nonetheless, some areas of the original two-phase theory need to be re-evaluated in the light of contemporary data. One area deals with whether the sequence of changes observed in the tissues, especially the spleens, during the preamyloidotic phase are indeed directly or indirectly related to amyloidogenesis or simply are coincidental changes. It is now well known that the major site of SAA biosynthesis is liver, and SAA synthesis in lymphoid tissues, e.g. spleen, is at best low (22-31). Furthermore, active SAA synthesis does not appear to require drastical morphologic changes in the tissues and cells that are actively synthetic (22,25,28-30). In this context, the preamyloidotic changes in tissues and cells do not fit too well contemporary modifications of the two-phase theory. If the preamyloidotic histologic changes are indeed related to amyloidogenesis, they could relate to something other than SAA synthesis; for example, to the development of amyloid enhancing factor. In any case, these histopathologic events need to be re-evaluated in the light of current knowledge of amyloid research.

4. Immunohistochemistry of amyloid

Advances in immunohistochemical methodology and the development of antisera to a variety of amyloid-related proteins have made the application of immunohistochemistry to amyloid studies very practical (8,32,33). With this approach it has become possible to localize amyloid proteins and to identify amyloid types in tissue sections (Figs. 1-3). In experimental amyloidosis, this technique was used for localization of amyloid deposits, for identification of extracellular nonfibrillar deposits such as AA-related substance, for localization of newly synthesized SAA in tissues and cells, e.g. hepatocytes, and for the differentiation of deposited amyloid in respect to species specificity (8,22,25,28-30, 34-36). Applicability of this technique will surely increase as more antibodies are developed against increasingly specific amyloid related proteins. Clearly, this method is one of most useful histopathologic techniques of the present era.

From the information available in literature and our own experience with human and animal amyloid (8,22,25,28-30,34-40), it is clear that certain precautions should be applied in using this method. One of such areas concerns with selection of antisera or antibodies. Due to the extremely high sensitivity of modern immunohistochemical methods, antisera with low specificity create many problems, i.e. false negatives due to high background staining caused by the contaminating antibodies or false positives created by nonspecific antibodies (8,32,33). On the other hand, highly specific antibodies can cause or highlight other problems. For example, with monoclonal antibodies against AA, Linke observed some degrees of variation in staining intensity among the AA-amyloid deposits from different patients (39). In our experience (Shirahama, T. & Ju, S.T. unpublished observation), a line of monoclonal antibodies to AA demonstrated highly specific and intense reaction with AA-amyloid deposits from some patients, specific but weaker reaction with some others, and virtually no reaction with some. Another line of the antibodies showed similarly varying reaction but with different population of tissues. These results were not completely unexpected, but we were rather surprised with the wide range of degrees of variation in reaction and high frequency of the occurrence of negative reaction. It is not yet known whether such antigenic heterogeneity exists among AA proteins within an animal species, but it is a realistic possibility that these immunohistochemical observations with human specimens have suggested.

Another uncertainty with amyloid immunohistochemistry concerns interpretation of positive reaction, i.e. whether the reaction is indeed produced by the target element (e.g. amyloid protein) or by a substance simply nearby (for example, proteins simply trapped in amyloid deposits). The latter kind of reaction has indeed been reported and we have often experienced such problem.

5. Final remarks

We discussed the current status, the achievements, the problems and the future possibilities concerning classic histopathologic approaches to amyloid research, using three subjects as examples. While most of the histopathologic studies on amyloidosis are now considered to be well established as classic textbook subjects, there are many areas that need to be improved and re-evaluated. With these improved methodologies and concepts, the histopathologic approach will certainly continue to be one of vital tools in amyloid research.

Acknowledgements

Supported by grants from the United States Public Health Service, National Institute of Arthritis, Diabetes, Digestive and Kidney Disease (AM-04599 and AM-07014), National Institutes of Health, Multipurpose Arthritis Center (AM-20613), the General Clinical Research Centers Branch of the Division of Research Resources, National Institutes of Health (RR-533) and the Arthritis Foundation.

References

1. Virchow, R. Virchows Arch. 6, 416-426, 1854.
2. Cohen, A.S. Int. Rev. Exp. Pathol. 4, 159-243, 1965.
3. Cohen, A.S. New Engl. J. Med. 277, 522-530, 574-583, 628-638, 1967.
4. Franklin, E.C. & Zucker-Franklin, D. Adv. Immunol. 15, 249-304, 1972.
5. Glenner, G.G. New Engl. J. Med. 302, 1283-1292, 1333-1343, 1980.
6. Eds. Glenner, G.G. Costa, P.P. & Freitas, A.F., Amyloid and Amyloidosis, Excerpta Medica, Amsterdam, 1980.
7. Eds. Mandema, E., Ruinen, L., Scholten, J.H. & Cohen, A.S., Amyloidosis, Excerpta Medica, Amsterdam, 1968.
8. Shirahama, T., Cohen, A.S. & Skinner, M. In Advances in Immunohistochemistry. DeLellis, R.A., Ed. Masson Publishing, New York, 277-302, 1984.
9. Amyloidosis. Wegelius, O., Pasternack, A., Eds. Academic Press, London, 1976.
10. Epstein, W.V., Tan, M. & Wood, I.S. J. Lab. Clin. Med. 84, 107-110, 1974.
11. Glenner, G.G., Ein, D., Eanes, E.D. et al. Science 174, 712-714, 1971.
12. Linke, R.P., Zucker-Franklin, D. & Franklin, E.C. J. Immunol. 111, 10-23, 1973.
13. Shirahama, T., Benson, M.D., Cohen, A.S. & Tanaka, A. J. Immunol. 110, 21-30, 1973.
14. Connors, L.H., Shirahama, T., Skinner, M. et al. Biochem. Biophys. Res. Commun. 131, 1063-1068, 1985.
15. Mowry, R.W. & Scott, J.E. Histochemie 10, 8-32, 1967.
16. Puchtler, H., Sweat, F. & Levine, M. J. Histochem. Cytochem. 10, 355-364, 1962.
17. Snow, A.D. & Kisilevsky, R. Lab. Invest. 53, 37-44, 1985.

18.Teilum, G. Acta Pathol. Microbiol. Scand. 61, 21-45, 1964.
19.Teilum, G. In Amyloidosis. Mandema, E., Ruinen, L., Scholten, J.H., Cohen, A.S., Eds. Excerpta Medica, Amsterdam, 37-41, 1968.
20.Cohen, A.S., Shirahama, T., Sipe, J.D. & Skinner, M. Lab. Invest. 48, 1-4, 1983.
21.Kisilevsky, R. Lab. Invest. 49, 381-390, 1983.
22.Benson, M.D. & Kleiner, E. J. Immunol. 124, 495-499, 1980.
23.Hoffman, J.S. & Benditt, E.P. J. Biol. Chem. 257, 10518-10522, 1982.
24.McAdam, K.P.W.J., Li, J., Knowles, J. et al. Ann. N.Y. Acad. Sci. 389, 126-136, 1982.
25.Miura, K., Takahashi, Y. & Shirasawa, H. Lab. Invest. 53, 453-463, 1985.
26.Morrow, J.F., Stearman, R.S., Peltzman, C.G. & Potter, D.A. Proc. Natl. Acad. Sci. USA 78, 4718-4722, 1981.
27.Ramadori, G., Sipe, J.D. & Colten, H.R. J. Immunol. 135, 3645-3647, 1985.
28.Shirahama, T. & Cohen, A.S. Am. J. Pathol. 118, 108-115, 1985.
29.Shirahama, T., Skinner, M. & Cohen, A.S. Cell Biol. Int. Reports 8, 849-856, 1984.
30.Takahashi, M., Yokota, T., Yamashita, Y. et al. Lab. Invest. 52, 220-223, 1985.
31.Tatsuta, E., Sipe, J.D., Shirahama, T. et al. J. Biol. Chem. 258, 5414-5418, 1983.
32.Hus, S.M. & Raine, L. In Advances in Immunohistochemistry. DeLellis, R.A., Ed. Masson Publishing, New York, 31-42, 1984.
33.Sternberger, L.A. Immunocytochemistry, 2nd edition. John Wiley and Sons, New York, 1979.
34.Shirahama, T., Skinner, M. & Cohen, A.S. In Amyloid and Amyloidosis. Glenner, G.G., Costa, P.P., Freitas, A.F., Eds. Excerpta Medica, Amsterdam, 278-282, 1980.
35.Van de Kaa, C.A., Hol, P.R., Huber, J. et al. Virchows Arch. A. (Pathol. Anat.) 408, 649-664, 1986.
36.Varga, J., Flinn, M.S.M., Shirahama, T. et al. Virchows Arch. B (Cell Pathol.) 51, 177-185, 1986.
37.Fujihara, S. & Glenner, G.G. Lab. Invest. 44, 55-60, 1981.
38.Fujihara, S., Balow, J.E., Costa, J.C., et al. Lab. Invest. 43, 358-365, 1980.
39.Linke, R.P. J. Histochem. Cytochem. 32, 322-328, 1984.
40.Shirahama, T., Skinner, M. & Cohen, A.S. Histochemistry, 72, 161-171, 1981.

VII.2 WHAT FACTORS ARE NECESSARY FOR THE INDUCTION OF AA
AMYLOIDOSIS?
(AA amyloid, glycosaminoglycans, amyloid enhancing factor,
apo-SAA)

R. Kisilevsky, A.D. Snow, L. Subrahmanyan, L. Boudreau,
and R. Tan

Department of Pathology,
Queen's University and Kingston General Hospital,
Kingston, Ontario, Canada K7L 3N6.

1.Introduction

The essential elements involved in the pathogenesis of AA amyloidosis
have, over the last 10-15 years, been shown to be events associated
with acute inflammation (1). As part of the process of inflammation
cytokines (the effect of interleukin-1 being the best characterized) are
released from inflammatory cells and stimulate the synthesis of acute
phase proteins by the liver. Among the various acute phase proteins
is the putative precursor of the AA deposit, apo-SAA, an apoprotein of
HDL but one seen associated with HDL primarily during inflammation.

Persistent inflammation also results in the appearance of a second factor, amyloid enhancing factor (AEF), which has now been identified in
several experimental models (2-4), human tissue (5), and which alters
the metabolism of apo-SAA (6). As shown in mice (2), the purified denatured AA protein does not possess AEF activity but isolated AA
fibrils may possess such AEF activity (7). Experimentally AEF always
appears before AA deposits can be demonstrated by light microscopy
and amyloid is never seen in the absence of AEF (2).

These observations suggest that at a minimum two coincidental factors
are necessary for AA deposition - an elevated plasma level of apo-SAA
and the presence of AEF.

In the experiments described below elevated levels of apo-SAA were
induced in vivo by administering supernatants from macrophages cultured in the presence of lipopolysaccharide (LPS). The presence of a
full blown inflammatory reaction for apo-SAA stimulation was therefore
not necessary. Such animals could be treated with AEF and examined
for AA deposition. The presence or absence of amyloid would indicate
whether high plasma apo-SAA levels and AEF are sufficient, or whether
additional factors stemming from a full blown inflammatory reaction are
necessary for AA deposition. Some potential additional factors are identified.

301

2.Materials and methods

2.1.Preparation of macrophage supernatants

Cytokine rich and cytokine poor supernatants were prepared as described by Tatsuta et al (8). CBA/J mice were given 1 ml of sterile thioglycolate medium (BDH Chemicals) by IP injection and the cells harvested 6 days later by rinsing the peritoneum with 5 ml of cold RPMI 1640 (Gibco) medium. The cells were washed three times in the same medium and pelleted at 300 x g for 7 min. at 4°C. Cells were plated in 25 ml tissue culture dishes at a concentration of 10^6 cells/ml. After incubation at 37°C for 2 hours the medium and non-adherent cells were removed and replaced with fresh medium $\pm$ 10 μg/ml of LPS from E. coli (BDH Chemicals). After incubation at 37°C for 72 hours in a 5% CO_2 humid atmosphere the supernatants were harvested, centrifuged, filter sterilized, and stored in small aliquots at -20°C.

2.2.AEF preparation and fractionation

AEF was prepared as described previously (2) using animals that received daily subcutaneous injections of 7% azocasein 0.5 ml, for 3 weeks. Four molar (4M) glycerol extracts were prepared from their spleens as described previously (2), and aliquots dialysed against phosphate buffered saline. Protein concentrations were determined by the technique of Lowry et al (9) and the samples then diluted to 1 mg/ml. Animals received 500 μg i.v. administered by tail vein.

In anticipation of fractionating AEF extracts by chromatofocusing spleens were also extracted with 8 volumes of 0.025 M ethanolamine-HCl pH 9.4. Undialysed samples of the ethanolamine extract were subjected to Sephacryl - 200 separation. The peaks were tested for AEF activity and those which were positive were subjected to DEAE separation using a linear (0.0 - 0.5M) KCl gradient, or step elution at 0.3M and 1M KCl. All peaks were tested for activity at a dose of 100 and 500 μg. An ultraviolet spectrum was determined for the active material recovered from the DEAE chromatography steps.

Spleens were also prepared in the manner of Pras et al (10) for the preparation of amyloid fibrils. Amyloidotic spleens were washed extensively in 0.15M NaCl followed by successive washes in distilled water. The first water wash was discarded. The subsequent two water washes were pooled and tested for AEF activity as described above.

Azocasein was prepared according to Janigan and Druet (11).

2.3.AgNO$_3$ as an inflammatory stimulus

AgNO$_3$ was dissolved in pyrogen free water as a 2% solution and 0.5 ml/animal was injected subcutaneously.

2.4. Effect of macrophage cytokines and AEF on splenic AA deposition

The experiments with macrophage supernatants were performed in C3H/HeJ mice to obviate the possibility that the LPS in the supernatant was serving as a source of apo-SAA stimulation. The mice were divided into several groups:
1. Untreated controls
2. Positive controls
   [given AEF (4M glycerol extracts from CBA animals) + $AgNO_3$]
3. AEF alone
4. Supernatant from LPS-stimulated macrophages
5. Supernatant from LPS-stimulated macrophages + AEF
6. Supernatant from non-stimulated macrophages
7. Supernatant from non-stimulated macrophages + AEF

Forty-eight hours later the animals were anesthetized with Metofane (Pitman-Moore Ltd) exsanguinated from the retro-orbital sinus, and killed by cervical dislocation. Plasma was saved for apo-SAA determination. Spleens were harvested for AA quantitation.

2.5. RIA determination of apo-SAA or AA

Plasma, 50-100 μl was diluted with 500-1,000 μl of 10% formic acid and incubated for 1 hour at $60^{\circ}C$. Following incubation 2-3 vol of distilled water were added and the samples lyophilized. Spleens were homogenized in 0.1 vol PBS to which was added an equal volume of 20% formic acid. The homogenates were incubated at $60^{\circ}C$ for 1 hour, the particulates removed by centrifugation, and the supernatant diluted with 2-3 vol of distilled water and lyophilized.

The quantity of apo-SAA and AA were measured by solid phase radioimmunoassay as described by Sipe et al (12) using purified AA protein as standards. The results are therefore expressed as AA equivalents.

2.6. Glycosaminoglycan (GAG) quantitation and characterization during amyloid induction

CBA/J mice were divided into four groups:
1. untreated
2. AEF treated (4M glycerol extracts)
3. $AgNO_3$ treated
4. AEF + $AgNO_3$ treatment

Animals in each group were sacrificed at varying intervals from 0-9 days, following their injections.

Spleens were harvested and following delipidation by acetone extraction, GAGs were isolated and quantitated using the technique of Niebes and Schifflers (13). Recovery was monitored by adding radioactive

GAGs during the initial homogenization and counting an aliquot of the final GAG extract. Recoveries ranged between 50-70%. Quantitation of total GAGs was measured as μg hexuronate isolated /mg dry defatted tissue. Subsequent characterization of GAGs and their proportions were carried out by high voltage electrophoresis, using a modification of the technique of Cappelletti et al (14).

3. Results

3.1. Partial purification of AEF

As demonstrated previously 4M glycerol extracts of amyloidotic spleens when fractionated by Sepharose 4B chromatography provides 3 peaks with AEF activity (2). Similar peaks are seen in the ethanolamine extracts. To coalesce these peaks the ethanolamine extracts were chromatographed on various grades of Sephacryl. Sephacryl-200 proved best, as demonstrated in Figure 1.

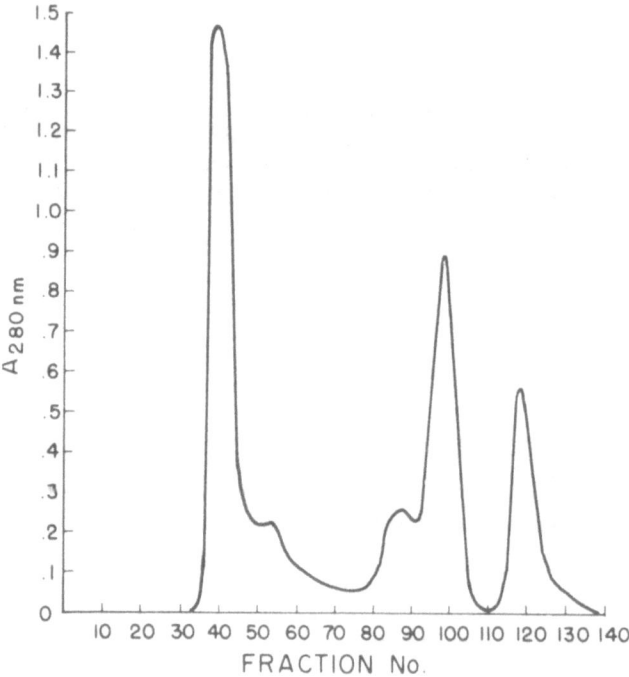

Figure 1: AEF fractionation on Sephacryl-200. Five ml of 0.025 M ethanolamine, pH 9.4 extract of amyloidotic spleen was chromatographed on a 2.5 x 85 cm Sephacryl-200 column at a flow rate of 20 ml/hr. Five ml fractions were collected. The AEF activity was present in the void volume (fractions 35-50). Fractions 92-105 represent hemoglobin at a molecular weight of 68,000 dalton.

All activity emerged in the void volume. This peak was then loaded onto a DEAE Sephacel column and the chromatographic pattern developed with a 0 - 0.5M KCl gradient. A final 1M KCl step was also included (Fig. 2).

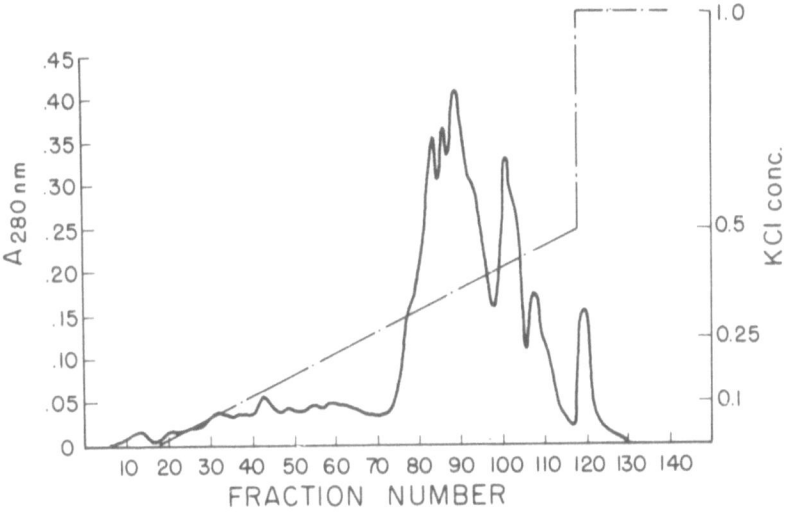

<u>Figure 2</u>: AEF fractionation on DEAE Sephacel. The void volume peak obtained from Sephacryl-200 fractionation, which contained the AEF activity, was applied to a 1 x 15 cm DEAE Sephacel column and the chromatographic pattern developed with a 0-0.5 M KCl gradient in 0.025 M ethanolamine, pH 9.4. This was followed by a 1.0 M KCl step. AEF activity emerged in fractions 75-115 and 117-125. [Fraction size = 5 ml].

The active material emerged at a KCl concentration greater than 0.3M. AEF activity could also be eluted at 1M KCl. Stepwise elution of DEAE Sephacel bound material (Fig. 3) with 0.3M and 1M KCl provided two fractions which both had activity but with different U.V. spectra. Material eluting at 0.3M KCl had a spectrum typical of protein with peaks at 278 and 216 nm. Material eluting at 1M KCl had peaks at 254 and 212 nm, more typical of nucleic acids (Fig. 4).

Homogenization and extensive washing of amyloidotic spleen in 0.15M saline followed by distilled water extractions, as one would prepare amyloid fibrils, provided material which had more potent AEF activity than any previous extraction procedure. Although the data is not shown, a comparison of amyloidotic and non-amyloidotic water washes showed activity only in extracts of amyloidotic spleen. The latter had five times as much glycosaminoglycan content (as hexuronic acid) as the controls. It also contained abundant amyloid fibrils.

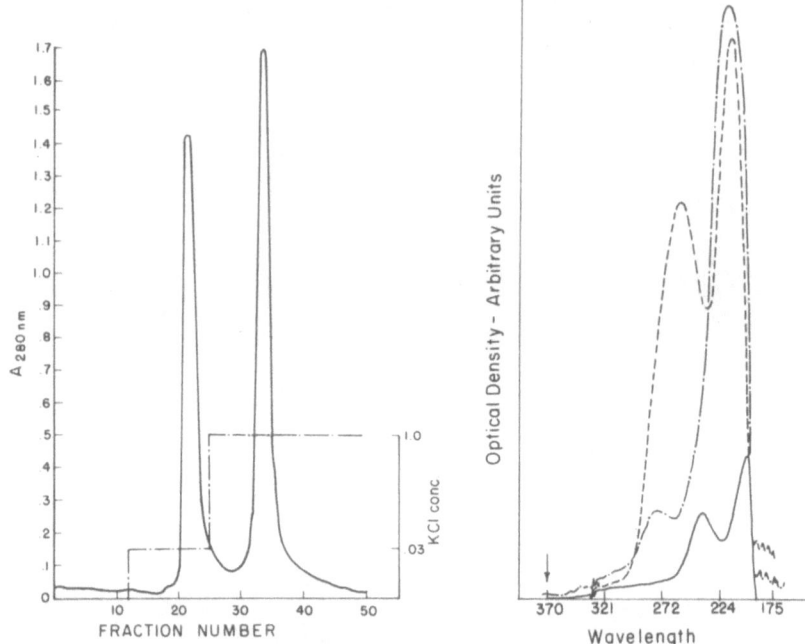

Figure 3: AEF fractionation on DEAE Sephacel using 0.3 M and 1 M KCl. The void volume from Sephacryl-200 fractionation of AEF was applied to DEAE-Sephacel as in Figure 2. Two steps, 0-0.3 M and 0.3-1 M KCl were used to elute the samples. AEF activity was present in both samples. The U.V. spectrum of each fraction was determined (see Figure 4). SDS polyacrylamide gel electrophoresis of the 1.0 M KCl fraction failed to reveal any protein bands.

Figure 4: The U.V. spectrum of .03 M and 1.0 M samples from DEAE Sephacel. The —·— line represents the spectrum of the 0.3 M KCl sample. Note the peaks at 278 and 216 nm. The --- line represents the spectrum of the 1.0 M KCl sample. Note the peaks at 254 and 212 nm. The ——— line represents the spectrum of the 0.025 M ethanolamine buffer. Note the peaks at 240 and 200 nm.

3.2. Effect of cytokines and AEF on AA and apo-SAA induction

The effect of various animal treatments on the production of apo-SAA and AA _in vivo_ is demonstrated in Figure 5. Neither the administration of AEF alone (15), nor supernatants from non-stimulated macrophages, with or without AEF, resulted in an increase in apo-SAA 48 hours after their administration. Supernatants obtained from macrophages stimulated with LPS however caused a marked and significant rise in circulating apo-SAA levels when examined 48 hours later. This was true whether or not these animals received AEF. The results compare favourably with an inflammatory stimulus produced by $AgNO_3$ + AEF which was used as our positive control. The absolute level of apo-SAA induced by culture cytokines though lower than that seen in AgNO$_3$ treated animals, is at a level sufficient to support continued AA deposition (16).

As can be seen in Figure 5, no group other than the AgNO$_3$ + AEF group deposited substantial amyloid. All other groups had AA determinations at control levels. Elevated levels of apo-SAA even in the presence of AEF are insufficient to lead to amyloid deposition. An additional

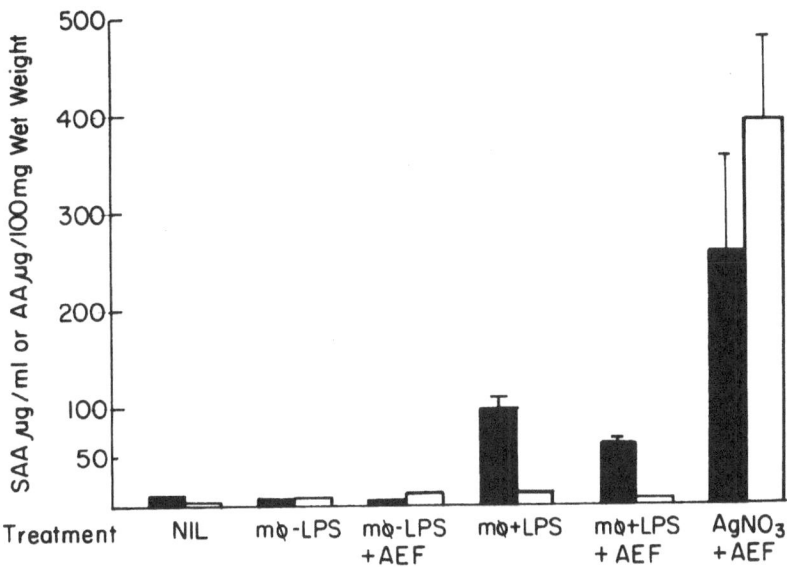

Figure 5: Effects of various *in vivo* treatments on SAA induction and splenic AA deposition. Solid bars represent SAA as µg/ml determined as AA equivalents. Open bars represent AA as µg/100 mg splenic wet weight. The results are the means ± S.E.M. of at least 7 animals per group. Error bars were too small to be shown on values less than 25 µg. Note that of the two groups of mice with elevated SAA levels that also received AEF, only the AgNO$_3$ + AEF group deposits amyloid.

process, or factor(s) set in motion from the acute inflammatory reaction is necessary. One of these potential processes is the synthesis of GAGs which, as demonstrated previously (17), are deposited in a temporally related manner with the amyloid protein.

Tables I and II show the time course of GAG accumulation during AA induction. The increase in total GAGs commences at 48 hours but only in the group depositing AA amyloid. During the 9 day period under observation the increase progressed unabated. An apparent increase, statistically significant at $p \leq 0.01$, was also seen in the AgNO$_3$ treated group late in the course of induction (6-9 days).

Following electrophoretic separation of the GAG samples and densitometry (data not shown), we were able to determine which GAGs were responsible for this increase.

Table II shows that the entire increase in GAG content can be accounted for by heparin and heparan sulphate. This was also true in the group treated with $AgNO_3$ at nine days when these animals also start depositing the AA protein.

TABLE I: CHANGES IN GLYCOSAMINOGLYCAN CONTENT OF SPLEEN DURING AA AMYLOID INDUCTION
[measured as hexuronate]

Treatment	Hexuronate µg/mg dry defatted tissue days following treatment					
	0	1	2	3	6	9
None	0.39 ± 0.04					
AEF		0.31 ± 0.03	0.45 ± 0.06	0.28 ± 0.05	0.54 ± 0.04	0.38 ± 0.02
$AgNO_3$		0.45 ± 0.05	0.45 ± 0.02	0.34 ± 0.02	0.56 ± 0.02	0.56 ± 0.05
AEF + $AgNO_3$		0.33 ± 0.02	0.55 ± 0.04	$0.67 \pm 0.03^*$	$1.05 \pm 0.09^*$	1.18 ± 0.09

Glycosaminoglycans were measured at varying intervals during amyloid induction. The data represent the mean $\pm$ S.E.M. of four animals. * represents a significant difference at a p value ≤ 0.01.

TABLE II: HEPARIN/HEPARAN SULPHATE CHANGES IN SPLEEN DURING AA AMYLOID INDUCTION

Treatment	Hexuronate µg/mg dry defatted tissue days following treatment					
	0	1	2	3	6	9
None	0.05 ± 0.01					
AEF			0.06 ± 0.01	0.02 ± 0.01	0.06 ± 0.01	$0.03 + 0.01$
$AgNO_3$			0.06 ± 0.01	0.04 ± 0.01	0.05 ± 0.01	$0.38 \pm 0.04^*$
AEF + $AgNO_3$			$0.14 \pm 0.02^*$	$0.13 \pm 0.05^*$	$0.61 \pm 0.01^*$	$0.82 \pm 0.04^*$

Heparin and heparan sulphate content were calculated by determining the relative % of each GAG in the isolated GAG samples. The relative % was determined using high voltage electrophoresis, Alcian blue staining, densitometry, and the relative affinities of various GAGs for Alcian blue. The results represent the mean $\pm$ S.E.M. of at least 3 determinations per time point. * represents a significant difference at the $p \leq 0.01$ level. Heparin and heparan sulphate were the only GAGs undergoing increases in spleen during AA amyloid induction.

4.Discussion

While the skeleton of the mechanism involved in AA amyloid deposition is now reasonably well established, the details have yet to be elucidated (1). The present work shows that at least three coincident processes are necessary. Firstly any one of a number of inflammatory stimuli can activate inflammatory cells to produce cytokines among which is inter-leukin-1. The latter serves as a stimulus for the hepatic production of apo-SAA, which upon entering the circulation associates with high density lipoproteins to complete the SAA-complex (18). The elevation of serum SAA levels during inflammation is insufficient to lead to AA depo-sition as this is a relatively uncommon complication of inflammatory dis-orders. Precisely where SAA or apo-SAA are normally metabolized or how this metabolism is altered to lead to AA deposition remains to be determined.

Secondly, the demonstration in a variety of mouse strains that AEF is not only a constant companion of amyloid deposition but appears in tis-sues 24-48 hours prior to AA deposition suggests that AEF is not sim-ply an enhancing factor but is essential for this process (2). AEF ap-pears in tissues only with longstanding inflammation, and when it does it sets the stage for an alteration in apo-SAA metabolism (6).

The present work demonstrates that elevated levels of apo-SAA even in the presence of AEF are not sufficient for amyloid deposition. Ani-mals with apo-SAA levels of 60-100 µg/ml (Fig. 1), which are sufficient to maintain continued amyloid deposition in animals with a complete inflammatory reaction (16), even in the presence of AEF, do not deposit the AA protein. Further factors or processes stemming from a full blown inflammatory reaction are necessary. The precise nature of the additional factor(s) is not clear. Nevertheless the present work shows that glycosaminoglycan (GAG) deposition occurs virtually coincidentally with AA deposition, and that the GAGs involved are heparin and/or heparan sulphate.

The origin of this GAG is apparently not from the serum, as the plasma GAG showing the major alterations during both inflammation and amyloidogenesis is chondroitin-4-sulphate (19). If AA associated splenic heparin/heparan sulphate is being derived from the plasma, the plasma pool would of necessity be turning over at a markedly increased rate. The most likely source of tissue GAGs is therefore local synthesis. Endothelial and presumably reticulo-endothelial cells do possess the ca-pacity to synthesize GAGs of the appropriate class (20). Precisely how inflammation influences these cells to alter their capacity to synthesize GAGs remains to be investigated.

Notwithstanding recently published work characterizing AEF (3) the question of the nature of AEF and how it operates remains unanswered. The chromatographic separation and purification of AEF continues to pose significant problems, though some headway is being made. As extracted in 4M glycerol, or 0.025M ethanolamine pH 9.4, AEF activity is part of a large complex which elutes close to the void volume, and void volume itself, on Sepharose 4B and Sephacryl-200 respectively. The requirement of high (0.3M - 1M KCl) salt concentrations to elute AEF activity from DEAE Sephacel indicates a substantial negative charge associated with this complex. SDS polyacrylamide gel electrophoretic separation of the step eluted samples from the DEAE columns showed a few minor protein bands of low molecular weight (10-25,000 dalton) in the 0.3M KCl peak, but not demonstrable Coomassie blue staining material in the 1M KCl peak (data not shown). The latter finding coupled with the U.V. spectral analysis of these peaks (Fig. 4) would suggest that the active material may be a nucleoprotein, as has been suggested by others (3). An alternative suggestion is that the active material is not protein but one which co-elutes with nucleic acid from DEAE columns, and which of necessity would also have large numbers of negative charges. Highly sulphated glycosaminoglycans or proteoglycans do elute from DEAE columns at such salt concentrations and higher, and may represent such a class of compounds.

The ability to show large quantities of AEF activity in fibril preparations suggests a further possibility. AEF, though not the AA protein per se (2), may represent early fibrils, too early to detect histologically, but which once formed, in some way catalyze extensive and further fibril formation.

One last concept deserves consideration. The literature both in the past (2,3) and present (4) shows AEF activity in diverse preparations with seemingly no consistent molecular relationship. One should consider that AEF may not be a specific molecular entity but rather a specific cell response to a variety of stimuli.

Acknowledgements

This work was supported by Grant MT-3153 from the Medical Research Council of Canada. The authors gratefully thank Mrs. M. Jones and Mrs. B. Latimer for their able secretarial assistance.

References

1. Kisilevsky, R. Lab. Invest. 49, 381-390, 1983.
2. Axelrad, M.A., Kisilevsky, R., Willmer, J., et al. Lab. Invest. 47, 139-146, 1982.
3. Hardt, F., & Ranløv, P. Int. Rev. Exp. Path. 16, 273-334, 1976.
4. Hol, P.R., van Andel, A.C.J., van Ederen, A.M., et al. Br. J. Exp. Pathol. 66, 689-697, 1985.
5. Varga, J., Shirahama, T. & Cohen, A.S. Fed. Proc. 44, 747, 1985.
6. Deal, C.L., Sipe, J.D., Tatsuta, E., et al. Ann. N.Y. Acad. Sci. 389, 439-441, 1982.
7. Baltz, M.L., Caspi, D., Hind, C.R.K., et al. In Amyloidosis. Glenner, G.G., Osserman E.F., Benditt, E.P., Calkins, E., Cohen, A.S., Zucker-Franklin, D., Eds. Plenum Press, New York, 115-121, 1986.
8. Tatsuta, E., Sipe, J.D., Shirahama, T., et al. J. Biol. Chem. 258, 5414-5418, 1983.
9. Lowry, O.H., Rosebrough, N.H., Farr, A.L. & Randall, R.J. J. Biol. Chem. 193, 265-275, 1951.
10. Pras, M., Schubert, M., Zucker-Franklin, D., et al. J. Clin. Invest. 47, 924-933, 1968.
11. Janigan, D.T. & Druet, R.L. Am. J. Pathol. 48, 1013-1026, 1966.
12. Sipe, J.D. Ignaczak, T.F., Pollock, P.S. & Glenner, G.G. J. Immunol. 16, 1151-1156, 1976.
13. Niebes, P. & Schifflers, M.H. Clin. Chim. Acta 62, 195-202, 1975.
14. Capelletti, R., Rosso, M.D. & Chiaruvi, V.P. Anal. Biochem. 99, 311-315, 1979.
15. Kisilevsky, R., Benson, M.D., Axelrad, M.A. & Boudreau, L. Lab. Invest. 41, 206-210, 1979.
16. Kisilevsky, R., Boudreau, L. & Foster, D. Lab. Invest. 48, 60-67, 1983.
17. Snow, A.D. & Kisilevsky, R. Lab. Invest. 53, 37-44, 1985.
18. Hoffman, J.S. & Benditt E.P. J. Biol. Chem. 257, 10518-10522, 1982.
19. Snow, A.D. & Kisilevsky, R. Fed. Proc. 45, 465, 1986.
20. Atkins, F.M., Friedman, M.M. & Metcalfe, D.O. Lab. Invest. 52, 278-286, 1985.

Keiichi Higuchi and Toshio Takeda

Department of Pathology, Chest Disease
Research Institute, Kyoto University,
Sakyo-ku, Kyoto 606, Japan.

1. Introduction

Amyloidosis can be induced in mice by casein, endotoxin, or other substances. Results of biochemical studies on the amyloid protein in experimentally induced amyloidosis (1-2) are similar to the findings of secondary amyloidosis in humans. There have also been numerous reports on spontaneous amyloidosis in mice (3-6). However, information about the biochemical features of amyloid proteins in spontaneous amyloidosis has been sparse until recently.

The first report of biochemical characterization of murine spontaneous amyloidosis by Glenner et al (7) described protein AA deposits in GP mice. Subsequently, protein AA deposits were noted in several strains of mice (8,9) without any obvious association with chronic infections or inflammatory conditions similar to the spontaneous protein AA deposits in the cat, dog and duck (10-12).

Spontaneous age-associated and systemic deposits of amyloid proteins which are distinctly different from protein AA have been reported in SJL/J mice (13), and recently in LLC (14) and SAM-P mice (15). In another interesting amyloidogenic protein in mice, the amino acid sequence of prion protein in amyloid plaques in the brains of mice inoculated with human Creutzfeldt-Jakob or scrapie brain homogenates have been partially determined (16,17).

Since protein AA is described in detail in other chapters, we will describe in this chapter the amyloid proteins in SAM-P and SJL/J mice.

2. AS_{SAM}: Senile Amyloid Fibril Protein in the Senescence Accelerated Mouse(SAM)

A murine model of accelerated senescence, Senescence Accelerated Mouse (SAM), comprising the SAM-P/1 SAM-P/4 series and the control SAM-R/1 SAM-R/3 series with normal aging characteristics, was recently developed in our laboratory (18). Aging in SAM is marked by the early onset and irreversible progress of aging phenomena after a period of normal development (19,20).

Spontaneous age-associated amyloidosis is one of the most characteristic findings in SAM. The incidence of amyloidosis increases with age, and about 90% of SAM-P mice have amyloid deposits after 8 months of age (21). Amyloidosis is systemic in SAM-P, and amyloid fibril deposits are observed in all organs except the bone marrow and the brain (21-23). A unique amyloid fibril protein: AS_{SAM} has been isolated from the livers of SAM-P/1 mice by Matsumura et al (15).

Amyloid fibrils were isolated as the water soluble fraction from the livers of SAM-P/1 mice by the method of Pras et al (23). Electron micrographs of the extracted proteins showed a nonbranched filament structure 50 to 100 Å in width, characteristic of amyloid fibrils (Fig.1). Amyloid protein was purified from the fibril fraction by gel chromatography under denaturing conditions (Fig. 2).

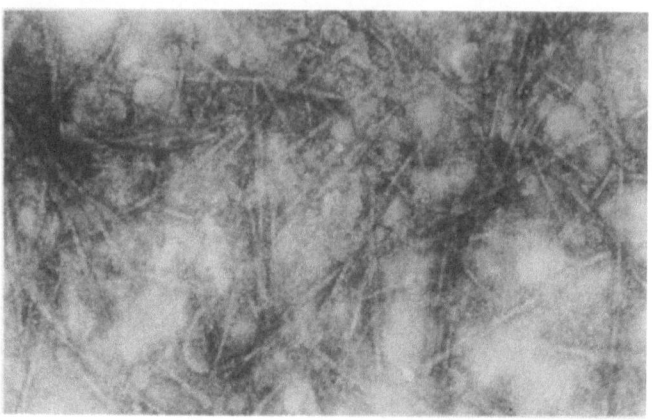

Figure 1: Electron micrograph of amyloid fibrils isolated from liver of SAM-P/1, negatively stained with 2% phosphotungstic acid. Magnification: x 162,300. Reproduced from Lab. Invest. 47, 271, 1982, by copyright permission of US-Canadian Div. of the IAP.

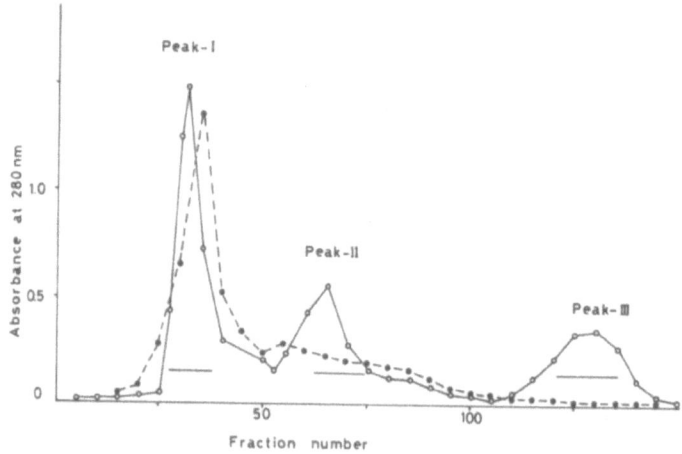

Figure 2: Gel chromatography of amyloid fibril protein from SAM-P/1 through Sephadex G-100 (90x2.5 cm) eluted with 5M guanidine-HCl, 1N acetic acid (o—o). Elution of proteins from liver (●—●) did not show a second peak corresponding to peak II in SAM-P/1. Protein was not contained in peak III. Reproduced from Lab. Invest. 47, 272, 1982, by copyright permission of US-Canadian Div. of the IAP.

Three major protein peaks were observed in chromatography; the second peak contained a protein which could not be found in normal liver or in liver laden with protein AA on 8M urea sodium dodecyl sulfate (SDS) polyacrylamide gel electrophoresis. This protein showed a single band, and its molecular weight was calculated to be about 5,200 dalton in SDS polyacrylamide gel electrophoresis.

The amino acid composition of the purified amyloid protein is shown in Table I. The amino acid composition of murine protein AA is listed for comparison. The protein had relatively large amounts of glutamic and aspartic acid, alanine and leucine, no tryptophan and half-cystine. The profile of the amino acid composition of the protein was clearly different from that of murine protein AA. Automatic sequence analysis revealed a blocked N-terminus, unlike murine protein AA (1,2).

TABLE I: AMINO ACID COMPOSITIONS OF MURINE AMYLOIDOGENIC PROTEINS AND APO-SAS$_{SAM}$
[residues per 100 residues]

Amino acid	Murine protein AA (1)	AS$_{SAM}$	SJL/J (13)	Apo SAS$_{SAM}$	Rat apo A-II (34)
Lys	6.3	6.8	8.1	7.2	5
His	2.6	1.5	2.3	1.2	0
Arg	5.6	3.0	5.4	1.2	4
Asp	10.4	7.0	8.5	6.7	9
Thr	3.1	6.6	5.2	7.1	7
Ser	6.1	8.2	6.5	11.1	6
Glu	12.7	17.0	11.6	17.7	21
Pro	2.1	4.2	5.3	5.5	6
Gly	14.3	7.0	8.5	6.8	3
Ala	12.7	9.9	8.3	9.5	12
Cys	0	0	3.0	0	0
Val	2.3	5.1	5.7	3.6	3
Met	2.9	2.8	2.0	3.6	3
Ile	2.8	3.5	4.0	1.5	1
Leu	1.8	9.0	8.0	8.2	11
Tyr	3.8	3.0	3.1	3.1	4
Phe	7.7	4.9	4.6	5.7	5
Trp	2.9	0	n.d.	0	0

[n.d. not determined]

Specific antiserum was prepared in rabbits by immunizing with guanidine-denatured unfractionated amyloid fibril protein. Double immunodiffusion analysis demonstrated that the specific antibody did not react with murine protein AA, mouse IgG, mouse immunoglobulins or water-extracted proteins from normal liver. Thus, we have characterized a novel amyloid fibril protein that is distinguishable from protein AA and is not related to immunoglobulin. We designated this amyloid protein "AS$_{SAM}$": Senile Amyloid protein (AS) in SAM. Immunohistochemical investigation using anti-AS$_{SAM}$ anti-serum showed AS$_{SAM}$ deposits in all tissues of every SAM-P series and aged SAM-R series (24).

3. SAS$_{SAM}$: Serum AS$_{SAM}$ Related Antigenic Substance

Using specific antiserum against AS$_{SAM}$, we observed that normal mouse serum contains a substance that reacts with anti-AS$_{SAM}$. We termed this substance "SAS$_{SAM}$": Serum AS$_{SAM}$ related antigenic substance and we thought it was probably a precursor of AS$_{SAM}$ (25).

Fig. 3 shows the detection of SAS$_{SAM}$ by double immunodiffusion. All sera obtained from mice of several strains (SAM-P/1, SAM-R/1, A/J, CBA/St, CBA/HeN, C57BL/6J, SJL/J, B10A, Slc:ICR and DDD) showed a single precipitation line with anti-AS$_{SAM}$ antiserum. However, rat and human sera showed no precipitation line. SAS$_{SAM}$ migrated to the albumin/prealbumin region in immuno-electrophoresis, and the precipitation line formed with anti-AS$_{SAM}$ antiserum was stained positively with dyes for both protein and lipid. SAS$_{SAM}$ was eluted as a high molecular weight form of approximately 200,000 dalton in gel chromatography. These data suggested that SAS$_{SAM}$ might be high density (α) lipoprotein: HDL.

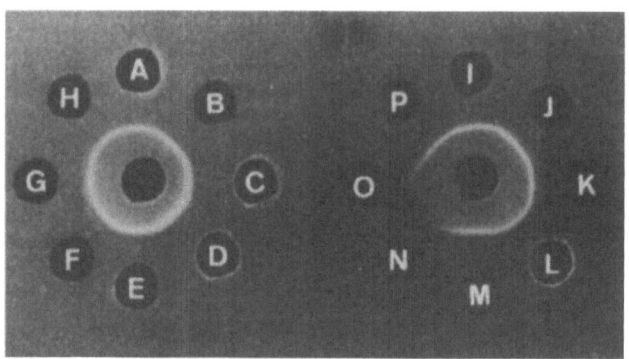

Figure 3: Detection of SAS$_{SAM}$ by immunodiffusion. Anti-AS$_{SAM}$ antiserum in central wells was tested against purified AS$_{SAM}$ (H, D, and P), SAM-P/1 (A and B), SAM-R/1 (C), DDD (D), Slc:ICR (F), CBA/St (G), C3H/HeN (I), C57BL6J (J), A/J (L), B10A (M), rat (N), and human (O) serum. Reproduced from J. Exp. Med. 158, 1600-1614, 1983, by copyright permission of the Rockefeller University Press.

To confirm this suggestion, the amount of SAS$_{SAM}$ in each lipoprotein fraction of normal mouse serum was determined with antiserum against AS$_{SAM}$. SAS$_{SAM}$ was found mainly in HDL (the density is between 1.063 and 1.21 g/ml) and the largest amount of SAS$_{SAM}$ was contained in the HDL$_2$ fraction (1.063 <d< 1.125 g/ml). After the delipidation of HDL, the protein components (apo-HDL) were chromatographed with Sephadex G-200 and DEAE-Cellulose, and an apoprotein which cross-reacted with anti-AS$_{SAM}$ antiserum was purified (26). The apoprotein, designated "apo-SAS$_{SAM}$", had the same molecular weight as tissue amyloid fibril protein AS$_{SAM}$ (Fig. 4). The amino acid composition of apo-SAS$_{SAM}$ closely resembled that of AS$_{SAM}$ (Table I). Furthermore, antiserum against apo-SAS$_{SAM}$ reacted with AS$_{SAM}$. These data indicate that AS_{SAM} originates from apo-SAS_{SAM}. Its lower molecular weight amino acid composition and concentration in serum (0.6-1.5 mg/ml) (27) indicate that apo-SAS_{SAM} is an apoliprotein corresponding to human and rat apoA-II, a major apolipoprotein in HDL (murine apo-A-II) (Table I).

4. Amyloid Protein in SJL/J Mice

A high incidence of spontaneous amyloidosis has been described in SJL/J mice, a model for human Hodgkin's disease, and reticulum cell neoplasms are frequently seen in aging SJL/J mice (13). Amyloid deposition is systemic in SJL/J mice, and amyloid fibril protein has been isolated from spleens and livers. The molecular weight was calculated to be about 8,000 dalton by gel filtration. The amino acid composition of SJL/J amyloid is very different from that of murine protein AA and somewhat different from AS_{SAM} in the content of cystine and glutamic acid (Table I). The N-terminus of SJL/J amyloid protein is blocked, similar to that of AS_{SAM}. Immunologic characterization of SJL/J amyloid protein failed to show any relation between SJL/J amyloid protein and anti-murine protein AA. The serum precursor of SJL/J amyloid protein has not yet been demonstrated.

Nearly 100% development of amyloid was observed in LLC (Low Leucocyte Count) mice (3). The tissue amyloid protein of LLC mice has not been determined, but neither antiserum against murine protein AA nor immunoglobulin light chain (AL) reacted with amyloid deposits in LLC mice (14).

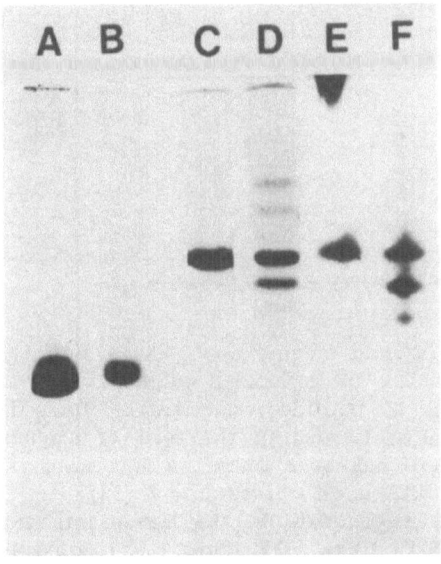

Figure 4: Comparison of apo-SAS_{SAM} with AS_{SAM} in electrophoresis. 8 M-urea-SDS--polyacrylamide gel electrophoresis of (A) apo-SAS_{SAM}, (B) AS_{SAM}, urea-polyacrylamide gel electrophoresis (pH 9.4) of (C) apo-SAS_{SAM} and (D) AS_{SAM}. Antibody labelling of (E) apo-SAS_{SAM} and (F) AS_{SAM}. Protein bands separated by urea--acrylamide gel electrophoresis were labelled with anti-apo-SAS_{SAM} antiserum and detected by immunoperoxidase method on the nitrocellulose paper. Reproduced from Amyloidosis, 1986 (Ref. 26) by copyright permission of Plenum Publishing Corporation, New York.

5.Discussion

In humans more than ten kinds of amyloid fibril proteins from several types of systemic and localized amyloidosis have been isolated and characterized. In mice only three kinds of amyloid fibril protein have been confirmed biochemically in systemic amyloidosis: Protein AA, AS_{SAM} and SJL/J amyloid protein. Physicochemical information about these proteins in mice is sparse, but electron micrographs of their amyloid fibrils show nonbranched filament structures, similar to the amyloid fibrils in humans. Thus, the β-fibril conformation is a common structure. AS_{SAM} isolated from SAM, a mouse model for accelerated senescence, was shown by us to originate from apoA-II, a major apoprotein of HDL (26). AS_{SAM} is synthesized in the liver and small intestine (28) and contains HDL particles with other apoproteins and lipid components (triglyceride, cholesterol, phospholipid) in the serum. In tissues in which amyloidosis is developing, apo-SAS_{SAM} (apoA-II) may change its conformation to β-fibrils after separation from other HDL components (Fig. 5). The relationship of aging and nutrition with the pathogenesis of amyloidosis is now being investigated in our laboratory (25,29).

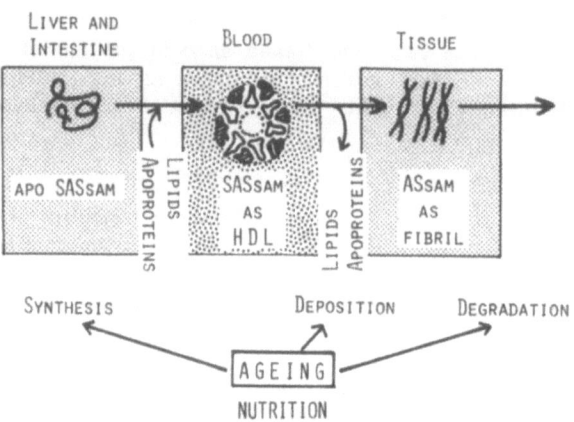

Figure 5: Schematic diagram demonstrating the pathologic pathway of apo-SAS_{SAM}.

It is noteworthy that apo SAS_{SAM} and murine apo-SAA, a putative precursor of protein AA, have a similar low molecular weight to that of apoprotein in HDL (30). This class of peptides, carriers of lipids in serum, may be prone to deposition in tissues in the form of amyloid fibrils. A gene coding murine apoA-II has been found on chromosome 1 (31) and a gene coding murine apo-SAA is on chromosome 7 (32).

Zschiesche classified spontaneous amyloidosis in the mouse into two types according to the morphological findings (33). Type I is frequently associated with malignant or inflammatory lesions and is considered to be a protein AA deposition. In type II, no underlying disease could be found, and the morphological features seem to resemble these in SAM, SJL/J and LLC mice. Although there is some difference between the amino acid compositions of AS_{SAM} and SJL/J amyloid protein, it is tempting to postulate that AS_{SAM} is a common fibril protein in murine spontaneous amyloidosis. Although amyloid deposition of AL, prealbumin (in human FAP and senile systemic amyloidosis), and amyloid proteins of endocrine origin have not been found in mice, as far as we know, the availability of numerous mutant strains of mice and their usefulness in all sorts of experiments make it the most appropriate animal for the investigation of the mechanism of deposition of amyloidogenic proteins.

Acknowledgments

We thank Drs E. Tsubura (Toneyama National Hospital) and F. Uchino (Yamaguchi University) for pertinent advice and all our colleagues for their valuable contributions. We also thank Dr A. Cary, Kyoto Baptist Hospital, for critical reading of the manuscript.

This work was supported by grants from the Ministry of Education, Culture and Science and the Ministry of Health and Welfare of Japan.

References

1. Ericksen, N., Ericsson, L.H., Pearsall, N., et al. Proc. Natl. Acad. Sci. USA. 73, 964-967, 1976.
2. Skinner, M., Shirahama, T. & Benson, M.D. Lab. Invest. 36, 420-427, 1977.
3. Chai, C.K. Am. J. Pathol. 85, 5-52, 1976.
4. Dunn, T.B. J. Natl. Cancer Inst. 5, 17-28, 1944.
5. Ram, J.S., DeLellis, R.A. & Glenner, G.G. Proc. Soc. Exp. Biol. Med. 130, 462-464, 1969.
6. Thung, P.J. Gerontologia 1, 259-279, 1957.
7. Glenner, G.G., Page, D.L., Isersky, C., et al. J. Histochem. Cytochem. 19, 16-28, 1971.
8. Page, D.L., Glenner, G.G. Am. J. Pathol. 67, 555-570, 1972.
9. Westermark, P., Sletten, K., Naeser, P., et al. Scand. J. Immunol. 9, 193-196, 1979.
10. DiBartola, S.P., Benson, M.D., Dwulet, F.E. et al. Lab. Invest. 52, 485-489, 1985.
11. Benson, M.D., Dwulet, F.E. & DiBartola, S.P. Lab. Invest. 52, 448-452, 1985.
12. Gorevic, P.D., Greenwald, M., Frangione, B., et al. J. Immunol. 118, 1113-1118, 1977.
13. Scheinberg, M.A., Cathcart, E.S., Eastcott, J.W., et al. Lab. Invest. 35, 47-54, 1976.
14. Chai, C.K. & Lerner, C. Exp. Cell. Biol. 52, 339-346, 1984.
15. Matsumura, A., Higuchi, K., Shimizu, K., et al. Lab. Invest. 47, 270-275, 1982.
16. Chesebro, B., Race, R., Wehrly, K., et al. Nature 315, 331-333, 1985.
17. Hikita, H., Tateishi, J. & Nagara, H. Acta Neuropathol. (Berl) 68, 138-144, 1985.
18. Takeda, T., Hosokawa, M., Takeshita, S. et al. Mech. Ageing Dev. 17, 183-194, 1981.
19. Hosokawa, M., Kasai, R., Higuchi, K., et al. Mech. Ageing Dev. 26, 91-102, 1984.
20. Hosokawa, M., Takeshita, S., Higuchi, K., et al. Exp. Eye Res. 38, 105-114, 1984.
21. Takeshita, S., Hosokawa, M., Irino, M., et al. Mech. Ageing Dev. 20, 13-23, 1982.
22. Shimizu, K., Ishii, M., Yamamuro, T., et al. Arthritis Rheum. 25, 710-712, 1982.
23. Pras, M., Zucker-Franklin, D., Rimon, A., et al. J. Exp. Med. 130, 777-795, 1969.
24. Higuchi, K., Matsumura, A., Honma, A., et al. Lab. Invest. 48, 231-240, 1983.
25. Higuchi, K., Matsumura, A., Hashimoto, K., et al. J. Exp. Med. 158, 1600-1614, 1983.
26. Higuchi, K., Matsumura, A., Takeshita, S., et al. In Amyloidosis, Glenner, G.G., Osserman, E.F., Benditt, E.P., Calkins, E., Cohen, A.S., Zucker-Franklin, D. Eds. Plenum Press, New York, 669-677, 1986.
27. Higuchi, K., Matsumura, A., Honma, A., et al. Mech. Ageing Dev. 26, 311-326, 1984.
28. Takeshita, S., Higuchi, K., Hosokawa, M., et al. Am. J. Pathol. 121, 455-465, 1985.
29. Kohno, A., Yonezu, T., Matsushita, M., et al. J. Nutr. 115, 1259-1266, 1985.

30. Benditt, E.P., Ericksen, N. & Hanson, R.H. Proc. Natl. Acad. Sci. USA 76, 4092-4096, 1979.
31. Lusis, A.J., Taylor, B.A., Wangenstein, R.W., et al. J. Biol. Chem. 25, 5071-5078, 1983.
32. Taylor, B.A. & Rowe, L. Mol. Gen. Genet. 195, 491-499, 1984.
33. Zschiesche, W. Acta Pathol. Microbiol. Scand. A (80), Suppl. 233, 135-140, 1972.
34. Herberd, P.N., Windmueller, H.G., Bersot, T.P., et al. J. Biol. Chem. 249, 5718-5724, 1974.

VII.4 SITES OF SAA/AA SYNTHESIS

Jean D. Sipe[1] and Giuliano Ramadori[2]

Arthritis Center
Boston University School of Medicine, Boston, U.S.A.[1]

First Department of Internal Medicine,
Mainz, F.R.G.[2]

1. Introduction

In the early 1970's, a new protein, serum amyloid A (SAA), was detected in serum by its cross-reactivity with antibodies raised to the
amyloid A (AA) fibril protein of amyloid deposits (1,2). Subsequently,
SAA was shown to consist of the entire polypeptide sequence of AA
together with an extension of 20 to 50 amino acids at the carboxyl portion of the molecule (3-6). Three immunochemically distinct forms of
AA-related proteins have been identified (7), varying in size, charge
and antigenic presentation. They are SAA's associated with HDL (8),
the isolated 12.5 Kdalton SAA (called SAAL), and the amyloid fibril
protein AA. Although SAA is primarily contained in serum and AA in
amyloidotic tissues, SAA(L) has been identified in amyloid depositis and
AA in SAA-containing human plasma (7,9). SAA is thought to be degraded to AA by enzymes on the surface of monocytes (10,11). Both
human and mouse SAA have been characterized as polymorphic apoproteins of serum high density lipoprotein (12,13) and as major induc-
ible acute phase proteins (14,15).

The pathogenesis of amyloidosis has been investigated since Virchow
first used the term amyloid to define a pathologic substance deposited
extracellularly in tissues, a substance subsequently shown to be
proteinaceous and fibrillar in nature (reviewed in reference 16). The
experimental mouse model has been frequently employed for nearly one
hundred years (17-23), and with only a rare exception (24), the
amyloid protein has been shown to be of the AA type. Both histologic
(25) and biochemical (22) studies have shown experimental amyloidosis
to be a biphasic process, consisting of a primary or preamyloid phase
which varies from one or two weeks to a few months depending upon
the induction method employed, followed by the amyloidotic phase which
is defined by the appearance of insoluble fibrils in the extracellular
spaces of tissues. The preamyloid phase is characterized by markedly
elevated, but steadily decreasing SAA concentrations (22,26). In the
face of persistent inflammation, the second stage (amyloid formation) is
marked by the appearance of fibrils in numerous organs and tissues.

2. Serum amyloid A precursor

After its detection, SAA was readily accepted as the circulating precursor of the AA fibril protein. Thus, the inflammation-associated AA amyloidosis was considered to be analogous to the immunoglobulin form of the disease in which there are identical light chains both in the circulation and, intact and partially digested, in tissue deposits of amyloid fibrils (27). However, as the acute phase nature of SAA became clear a puzzling question about the pathogenesis of amyloidosis became apparent: if SAA levels are highest 24 hours after the onset of inflammation, then why is there a lag period before amyloid fibrils are deposited in tissues? Using a quantitative immunoassay for the AA fibril protein (28), the fluctuations in concentrations of amyloid A proteins during the development of amyloidosis in C3H/HeN mice were monitored relative to the A/J strain of mice in which the onset of amyloidosis was delayed and diminished (22). The SAA profiles in C3H and A/J mice after a single injection of mycobacterium butyricum in Freund's adjuvant were similar (Fig. 1a), but the concentration of AA proteins in the spleens were different (Fig. 1b).

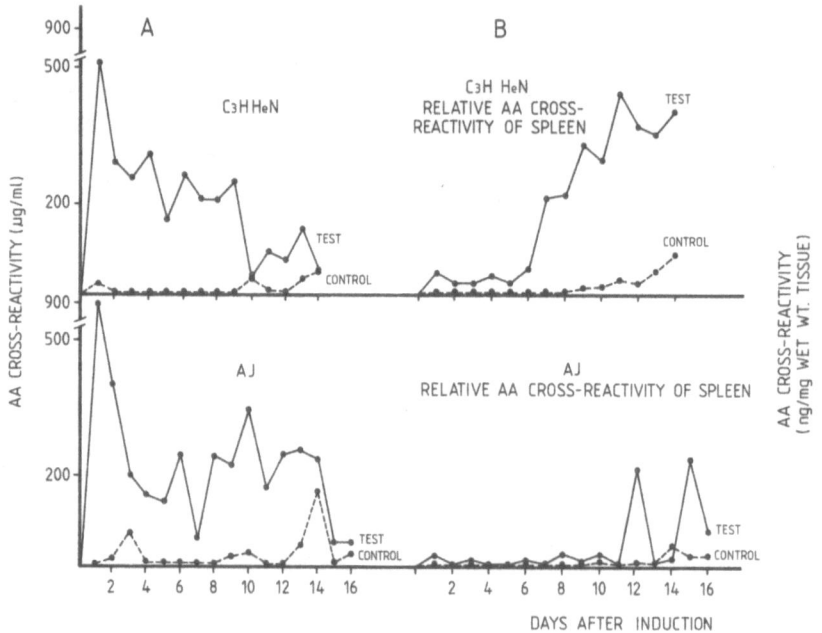

Figure 1: a. SAA profiles in C3H/HeN and A/J mice during the induction of amyloidosis by a single intraperitoneal injection of mycobacterium butyricum in complete Freund's adjuvant. b. AA-related protein profiles in spleens of above C3H/HeN and A/J mice. Reprinted with permission from Lab. Invest. 38, 110-114, 1978.

320

In C3H mice, the amyloidotic phase was marked by a 1000-fold in-crease in the concentration of AA-related proteins in the spleen approx-imately 7 days after the injection of the amyloidogenic stimulus (Fig. 1b), whereas in A/J mice lesser amounts of AA proteins were found in spleen much later and only in amyloidotic tissues. This study estab-lished that there is no correlation between circulating SAA concentration and AA fibril deposition in tissues. These biochemical observations are consistent with the earlier concept of Teilum (25) that amyloid fibrils may arise from local cellular secretion.

3. Induction of SAA synthesis

Since 1970, the mechanism by which the SAA genes are regulated has been studied with inbred strains of mice differing in sensitivity to the lipid A portion of LPS (29-31). Acute phase SAA biosynthesis proceeds by two steps, the first of which is macrophage production of interleukin 1 (IL-1) (Fig.2), which is maximal 90 minutes after LPS injection (30); the second is a dose-dependent exponential increase in SAA con-centration which is detectable 3 hours after LPS administration and reaches a maximum 16 to 24 hours later (15).

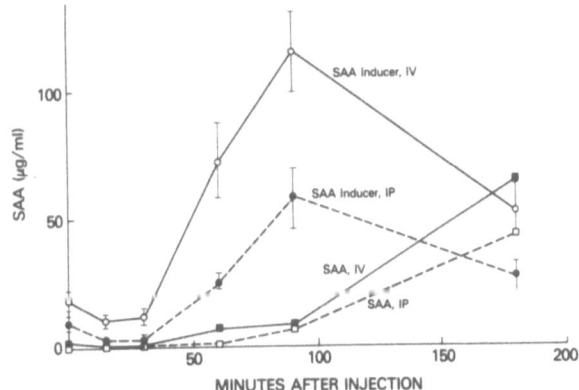

Figure 2: Time course of appearance of SAA mediator in serum of C3H/HeN mice after either i.p. or i.v. injection of LPS. Reprinted with permission from J. Exp. Med. 150, 597-606, 1979.

A comparison of the kinetics of appearance of total SAA mRNA in liver and the serum SAA profile following injection with LPS is shown in Figure 3. SAA mRNA was not detected in livers from control mice and is barely detectable in animals 1 hour after injection of LPS. A sub-stantial amount of SAA mRNA is detected at 2 hours and is quite abundant from 4 to 15 hours after injection of LPS, after which it begins to decrease and is no longer detectable by 54 hours. There is still a substantial amount of SAA mRNA present in liver when the SAA concentration in serum abruptly begins to decline.

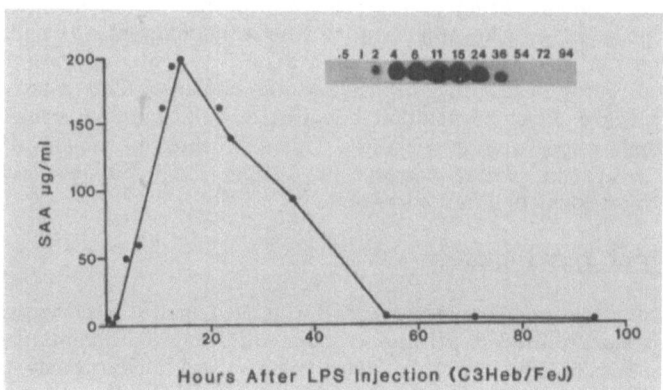

Figure 3: Serum concentration of SAA in responder C3Heb/FeJ mice after intraperitoneal injection of 20 μg of protein-free LPS. SAA concentrations at intervals after injection were measured by radioimmunoassay (28). SAA mRNA was determined by Northern blot hybridization with pAla (5).
Reprinted in part with permission from Dtsch. Med. Wochenschr. (Ramadori et al. 1986).

It has been definitively established that IL-1 acts upon liver to effect SAA synthesis. The SAA inducing substance appearing in vivo prior to the acute phase elevation of SAA (Fig. 2) had previously been documented to be IL-1 (32,33). When recombinant generated murine IL-1 was injected intravenously into C3H/HeJ (LPS non-responder) mice, we observed a dose-dependent increase in hepatic SAA total mRNA and a corresponding increase in plasma SAA concentration (Fig. 4) (34). A more detailed time course of SAA mRNA and protein response to recombinant IL-1 using LPS responder C3Heb/FeJ mice is shown in Figure 5. SAA mRNA was detectable in liver by two hours, was maximal between 4 and 15 hours and was virtually undetectable by 32 hours. It was demonstrated that IL-1 acts directly upon the hepatocyte (34), both upon resting cells and hepatocytes which are synthesizing SAA (Figs. 6a, 6b).

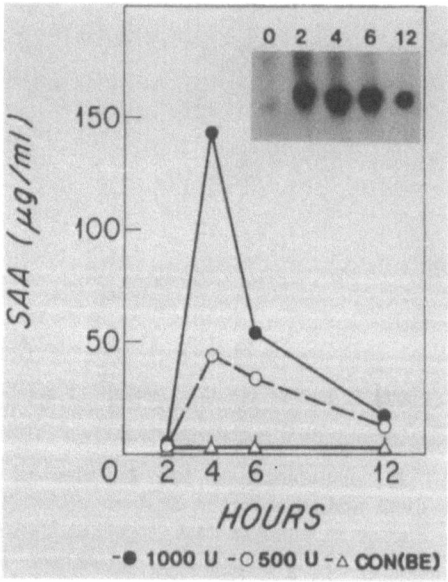

Figure 4: Kinetics of induction of SAA gene expression in C3H/HeJ mice by recombinant IL-1. Insert is Northern blot analysis of SAA mRNA in liver by 500 units of IL-1. Reprinted with permission from J. Exp. Med. 162, 930-942, 1985.

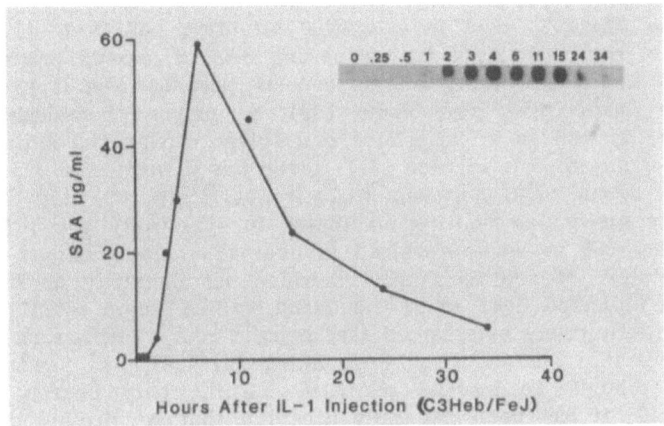

Figure 5: Serum concentration of SAA in responder C3Heb/FeJ mice after intraperitoneal injection of 2500 units of recombinant murine IL-1 as above. SAA was measured by radio-immunoassay (28) and SAA mRNA was determined by Northern blot hybridization with pAla (5).

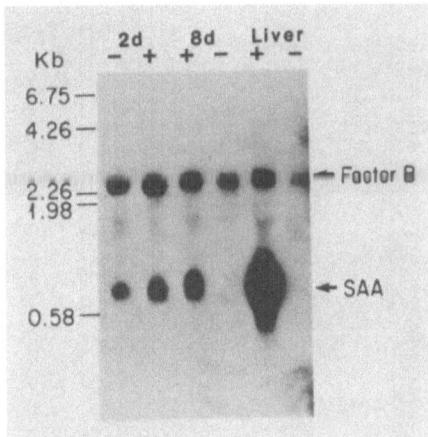

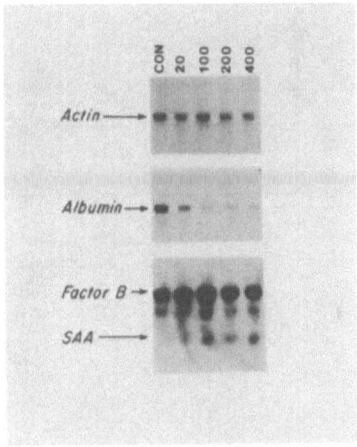

Figure 6: a. Northern blot analysis of RNA extracted from hepatocytes isolated from a C3H/HeJ mouse and kept in culture for 2 or 8 days. Cultures were incubated for 20 hours as indicated with medium containing either 200 units/ml of IL-1 or with medium containing non-transformed bacterial extract. As controls liver RNA from a C3HeB/FeJ mouse 16 hours after intraperitoneal injection of 10 μg LPS or saline was included. Radiolabelled factor B and SAA cDNA were used as probes. [Reprinted with permission from J. Exp. Med. 162, 930-942, 1985]. b. Northern blot analysis of actin, albumin, factor B, and SAA mRNA in hepatocytes cultured with increasing doses of recombinant murine IL-1. Radiolabelled actin, albumin, factor B, and SAA cDNA probes were used for hybridization.

4.Sites of SAA synthesis

Until the present, most investigative attention has been devoted to definition of the role played by circulating SAA of hepatic origin in the genesis of the AA protein, despite reports that SAA/AA is present in connective tissue (35), fibroblasts (36), in polymorphonuclear leukocytes (37), as well as in both liver and spleen during the experimental induction of amyloidosis in mice (22). Liver was identified as the probable site of serum SAA synthesis when it was found (38) that SAA is a major acute phase protein that fluctuates in synchrony with CRP, determined in 1966 to be synthesized in liver (39). In addition, a study using inhibitors of protein synthesis which act primarily on liver but not spleen indicated liver to be the tissue of SAA origin (40,41). Finally, it was definitively established that hepatic SAA synthesis is regulated by increased production of SAA mRNA (5,34,42-44). Because liver has been thought to be the main, if not the only source of SAA (40,42,45,46) it has been generally accepted that AA protein deposited in tissues has been derived by proteolysis of a circulating precursor of hepatic origin (9,46,47). Our recent studies, however, have demonstrated extrahepatic SAA gene expression in resident peritoneal macrophages of control mice and at numerous peripheral sites in mice following administration of LPS (Fig. 7) and recombinant generated IL-1 (49), and raise the possibility that amyloid deposits may be derived from local protein synthesis.

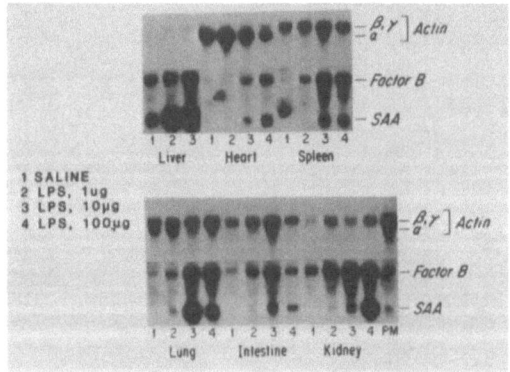

Figure 7: In vivo modulation of SAA, factor B, and actin gene expression in tissues of mice treated with endotoxin. Tissues were taken 16 hours after injection with saline or LPS as indicated. [Reprinted with permission from J. Immunol. 135, 3645-3647, 1985].

If so the situation would be one in which not only the enzymes (50,51) involved in conversion of SAA to AA but also the substrate is produced by cells in the organs in which amyloid is deposited. In addition to predominant hepatocyte production, SAA synthesis has been demonstrated in macrophages at both the message and protein level and SAA mRNA has been demonstrated in many organs, one of which, heart, does not have a recognizable macrophage population (52). Recently, synthesis and secretion of SAA has been demonstrated in peritoneal macrophages and Kupffer cells of the mouse (53). There are differences in the size patterns of immunoprecipitable SAA proteins synthesized by hepatocytes and Kupffer cells. Antiserum which precipitates a single population of preSAA of 14.3 Kdalton molecular weight from cell-free translation of RNA from acute phase liver, but not normal mice, identifies the 12.5 Kdalton mature SAA secreted by hepatocytes, but in addition a higher molecular weight 14.5 Kdalton is coprecipitated. However, from peritoneal macrophages or Kupffer cells, the 14.5 Kdalton species is predominant although the 12.5 Kdalton species is produced in significant quantity. Other workers, using poly A+ acute phase liver RNA, have separated cell-free translation species as SAA1 and SAA2 by SDS-PAGE either directly (54,55), or after immunoprecipitation (56). It is known that the human SAA primary translation product has a signal peptide of 18 amino acids and thus is converted from a species of 14 to 12.5 Kdalton, upon removal of the signal peptide sequence (5).

5. SAA gene expression

Recent studies have addressed the site of synthesis of the AA protein using the mouse model of accelerated amyloidogenesis (23). In the initial survey (53) of extrahepatic SAA gene expression in C3Heb/FeJ mice, there was a significant amount of SAA mRNA in spleens of mice 24 hours after injection of LPS. This observation is in contrast to the report from Benditt's laboratory that injection of casein only, does not stimulate demonstrable SAA gene expression in spleens of CBA/J mice. When we compared (23) total SAA gene expression in tissues of mice given three distinct types of inflammatory stimulation; casein in Freund's adjuvant and Amyloid Enhancing Factor (AEF), casein-adjuvant alone, and intraperitoneal LPS; the splenic SAA mRNA concentration in CBA/J mice following treatment with LPS was markedly elevated at 24 hours and diminished but detectable 48 and 72 hours later, similar to the earlier observation (53) with C3H mice. Furthermore LPS was a more potent stimulus for SAA gene expression in spleen than casein-adjuvant, although the latter elicited a greater SAA concentration in serum at 24 hours. The amount of SAA total mRNA in the spleens of mice after 24 hours of treatment with casein adjuvant only was reduced by 50% from that seen in the LPS treated mice. In the case of amyloidotic mice which had received both casein-adjuvant and AEF the amount of total SAA mRNA was reduced by 75% from that seen in the LPS treated mice. The concentration of total SAA mRNA is lower in liver of amyloidotic mice than in the control group of mice given the casein-adjuvant inflammatory stimulus alone (90% at 24 hours and 60% at 48 and 72 hours) and the concentration of SAA in serum was lower in amyloidotic mice than in those treated with casein-adjuvant only (23). Experiments are in progress to determine whether the decreased SAA gene expression associated with amyloidosis is part of a generally reduced protein synthesis, and how reduced SAA gene expression may be related to impaired Kupffer cell function demonstrated in C57BL/6J mice made amyloidotic by repeated injections of casein. Future investigations will be required to determine whether other cell types such as endothelial cells or fibroblasts are able to express the SAA gene.

Acknowledgements

This work was supported by USPHS grants AM04599, AM20193 and AM35337 and by grant Ra 362/1-4 of the Deutsche Forschungsgemeinschaft. We wish to thank Drs. A.S. Cohen, K.H. Meyer zum Buschenfelde and H.R. Colten for encouragement and support.

References

1. Isersky, C., Page, D.L., Cuatrecasas, P. et al. J. Immunol. 107, 1690-1698, 1971.
2. Levin, M., Pras, M. & Franklin, E.C. J. Exp. Med. 138, 373-380, 1973.
3. Gorevic, P.D., Levo, Y., Frangione, B. & Franklin, E.C. J. Immunol. 121, 131-140, 1978.
4. Parmalee, D.C., Titani, K., Ericsson, L.H. et al. Biochemistry 21, 3298-3303, 1982.
5. Sipe, J.D., Colten, H.R., Goldberger, G. et al. Biochemistry 24, 2931-2936, 1985.
6. Yamamoto, K.I. & Migita, S. Proc. Natl. Acad. Sci. USA 82, 2915-2919, 1985.
7. Linke, R.P. In Amyloid and Amyloidosis. Glenner, G.G., Costa, P.P., Freitas, A.F., Eds. Excerpta Medica, Amsterdam, 313-319, 1979.
8. Benditt, E.P. & Eriksen, N. Proc. Natl. Acad. Sci. USA 74, 4025-4028, 1977.
9. Husebekk, A., Skogen, B., Husby, G. & Marhaugh, G. Scand. J. Immunol. 21, 283-287, 1985.
10. Lavie, G., Zucker-Franklin, D. & Franklin, E.C. J. Exp. Med. 148, 1020-1031, 1978.
11. Fuks, A. & Zucker-Franklin, D. J. Exp. Med. 161, 1013-1028, 1985.
12. Bausserman, L.L., Herbert, P.N. & McAdam, K.P.W.J. J. Exp. Med. 152, 641-656, 1980.
13. Benditt, E.P., Hoffman, J.S., Eriksen, N. & Walsh, K.A. Ann. N.Y. Acad. Sci. 389, 183-189, 1982.
14. McAdam, K.P.W.J., Anders, R.F., Smith, S.R. et al. Lancet ii, 572-576, 1975.
15. McAdam, K.P.W.J. & Sipe, J.D. J. Exp. Med. 144, 1121-1127, 1976.
16. Glenner, G.G. In Amyloid and Amyloidosis. Glenner, G.G., Costa, P.P. & Freitas, A.F. Eds. Excerpta Medica, Amsterdam, 3-13, 1979.
17. Davidsohn, D. Virchows Arch. Pathol. Anat. 150, 16-32, 1897.
18. Kuczynski, M.H. Virchows Arch. Pathol. Anat. 239, 185-302, 1922.
19. Dunn, T.B. In Pathology of Laboratory Rats and Mice. Cotchin, E., Roe, F.J., Eds. F.A. Davis Co., Philadelphia, 181,1967.
20. DeLellis, R.A., Ram, J.S. & Glenner, G.G. Int. Arch. Allergy Appl. Immunol. 37, 175-183, 1970.
21. Cohen, A.S. & Cathcart, E.S. Methods Achiev. Exp. Pathol. 6, 207-242, 1972.
22. Sipe, J.D., McAdam, K.P.W.J. & Uchino, F. Lab. Invest. 38, 110-114, 1978.
23. Sipe, J., Rokita, H., Shirahama, T. et al. In XXXIVth Colloquium Protides of the Biological Fluids, 1986 (In press).
24. Higuchi, K., Matsumura, A., Honma, A. et al. Lab. Invest. 48, 231-240, 1983.
25. Teilum, G. Acta Pathol. Microbiol. Scand. 61, 21-45, 1964.
26. Brandwein, S.R., Sipe, J.D., Skinner, M. et al. J. Rheumatol. 12, 418-426, 1985.
27. Glenner, G.G. & Page, D.L. Int. Rev. Exp. Pathol. 15, 1-81, 1976.
28. Sipe, J.D., Ignaczak, T.F., Pollock, P.S. & Glenner, G.G. J. Immunol. 116, 1151-1156, 1976.
29. Rosenstreich, D.L. & McAdam, K.P.W.J. Infect. Immun. 23, 181-183, 1979.
30. Sipe, J.D., Vogel, S.N., Ryan, J.L. et al. J. Exp. Med. 150, 597-606, 1979.
31. Sipe, J.D. Lymphokines 12, 87-106, 1985.
32. McAdam, K.P.W.J. & Dinarello, C.A. In Bacterial Endotoxins and Host Response. Agarwal, M.K. Ed., 167-178, 1980.
33. Sztein, M.B., Vogel, S.N., Sipe, J.D. et al. Cell. Immunol. 63, 164-176, 1981.

34.Ramadori, G., Sipe, J.D., Dinarello, C.A. et al. J. Exp. Med. 162, 930-942, 1985.
35.Linder, E., Anders, R.F. & Natvig, J.B. J. Exp. Med. 144, 1336-1346, 1976.
36.Linder, E., Lehto, V.P., Virtanen, I. et al. J. Exp. Med. 146, 1158-1163, 1977.
37.Rosenthal, C.J. & Sullivan, L. J. Clin. Invest. 62, 1181-1186, 1978.
38.McAdam, K.P.W.J., Elin, R.J., Sipe, J.D. & Wolff, S.M. J. Clin. Invest. 61, 390-394, 1978.
39.Hurliman, J., Thorbecke, G.J. & Hochwald, J.M. J. Exp. Med. 123, 365-378, 1966.
40.Sipe, J.D. Br. J. Exp. Pathol. 59, 305-310, 1978.
41.Kisilevsky, R., Benson, M.D., Axelrad, M.A. & Boudreau, L. Lab. Invest. 41, 206-210, 1979.
42.Moorow, J.F., Stearman, R.S., Peltzman, C.G. & Potter, D.A. Proc. Natl. Acad. Sci. USA 78, 4718-4722, 1981.
43.Stearman, R.S. Lowell, C.A., Pearson, W.R. & Morrow, J.F. Ann. N.Y. Acad. Sci. 389, 106-115, 1982.
44.Lowell, C.A., Stearman, R.S. & Morrow, J.F. J. Biol. Chem., 1986 (In press).
45.Selinger, M.J., McAdam, K.P.W.J., Kaplan, M.M. et al. Nature 285, 498-500, 1980.
46.Tatsuta, E., Sipe, J.D., Shirahama, T. et al. J. Biol. Chem. 258, 5414-5418, 1983.
47.Glenner, G.G. New Engl. J. Med. 302, 1333-1343, 1980.
48.Kisilevsky, R. Lab. Invest. 49, 381-390, 1983.
49.Ramadori, G., Sipe, J.D. & Colten, H.R. J. Immunol. 135, 3645-3647, 1985.
50.Fuks, A. & Zucker-Franklin, D. J. Exp. Med. 161, 1013-1028, 1985.
51.Lavie, G., Zucker-Franklin, D. & Franklin, E.C. J. Exp. Med. 148, 1020-1031, 1978.
52.Lee, S.H., Starkey, P.M. & Gordon, S. J. Exp. Med. 161, 475-489, 1985.
53.Ramadori, G., Rieder, H., Mitch, A. et al. In XXXIVth Colloquium Protides of the Biological Fluids, 1986 (In press).
54.Yamamoto, K.I. & Migita, S. Proc. Natl. Acad. Sci. USA 82, 2915-2919, 1985.
55.Yamamoto, K.I., Shiroo, M. & Migita, S. Science 232, 227-229, 1986.
56.Meek, R.L., Hoffman, J.S. & Benditt, E.P. J. Exp. Med. 163, 499-510, 1986.

VII.5 THE ROLE OF THE MACROPHAGE PHAGOCYTIC SYSTEM (MPS) IN THE DEVELOPMENT OF SECONDARY AMYLOIDOSIS

Dorothea Zucker-Franklin and Alejandro Fuks

Department of Medicine
New York University Medical Center
550 First Avenue
New York, New York 10016, U.S.A.

1.Introduction

That the acute phase reactant, serum amyloid A (SAA) is synthesized in the liver is beyond dispute (1). The derivation of the peptide amyloid A (AA) from SAA is also no longer questioned (2-4). In order to elucidate the pathogenesis of secondary amyloidosis, attention must now be focused on the structural variants of SAA (5,6), its behaviour in diverse disease conditions, and on the mechanism whereby the soluble degradation product of SAA becomes polymerized into insoluble fibrils. As described elsewhere in this volume (sections 3 and 7), several investigators are addressing the first aspect of amyloidogenesis, i.e., whether the development of amyloidosis is contingent on a structural variation of the SAA molecule, whereas in our laboratory, studies have concerned mostly the second aspect. We have postulated that the deposition of the AA protein may be attributable, in part, to faulty processing of its precursor peptide, SAA. This hypothesis is based on the observation that in vitro SAA is degraded to completion by surface enzymes of normal monocyte/macrophages, but that peripheral blood monocytes of patients with amyloidosis degrade the peptide incompletely (7-9). While the intermediate degradation product was found to have electrophoretic mobility and virtually complete immunologic cross-reactivity with AA, it was not known whether incomplete processing could be attributed to faulty macrophage function per se. Thus, it seemed possible that, in patients with conditions prone to develop amyloidosis, e.g. patients subject to chronic inflammatory stimuli, the cells belonging to the monocyte/macrophage system (MPS) became impaired. In order to investigate this possibility systematically, an animal model had to be chosen in which amyloidosis could be induced in a more or less predictable fashion. Casein-induced amyloidosis in mice fulfilled this requirement (10). The studies were initiated with Kupffer cells because these cells are quantitatively the most important macrophages involved in clearance of plasma components, and because they are strategically located in an organ whose involvement is the sine qua non of experimental amyloidosis. This brief report summarizes our observations.

2. Materials and methods

Kupffer cells (KC) were isolated from the livers of normal C57BL/6J mice and of mice sacrificed at various time intervals, i.e., 0, 8, 13, 18 and > 30 days, during the induction of amyloidosis with daily injections of casein. Details of the methods used have been published (11). The isolated KC were cultured for 48 hours on 35 mm Petri dishes at a concentration of 7×10^6 per ml, after which the serum containing supernate was replaced with serum-free medium containing 200 µg SAA. The supernates of such cultures were collected at 0, 4, 8 and 18 hrs after appropriate preparation (11) and further analyzed on 10% to 20% SDS polyacrylamide slab gels. The density of the protein bands obtained was quantified and expressed as percentage of residual SAA of AA after incubation with KC. In addition, freshly isolated as well as cultured KC were subjected to electron microscopy and a variety of histochemical and immunochemical analyses as discussed below.

3. Results and discussion

The results were clear cut. The Kupffer cells of all animals which had received more than 20 injections of casein and had developed frank amyloidosis detected by Congo red staining of their organs, could no longer degrade SAA to completion (Figs. 1 and 2).

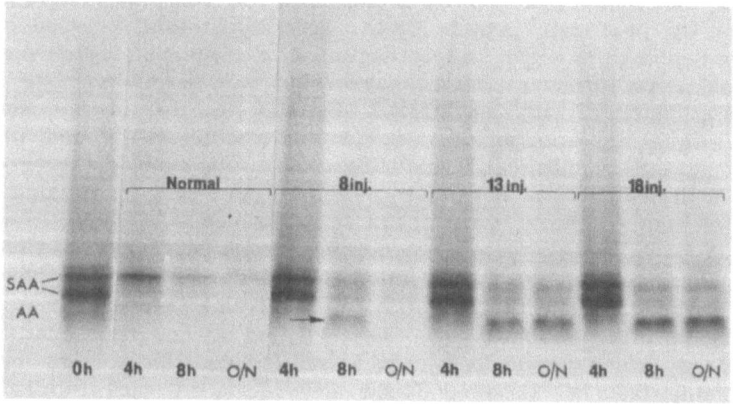

Figure 1: SDS polyacrylamide gel patterns obtained with the supernatants of Kupffer cell cultures. The KC were isolated from livers of mice which had received 0, 8, 13, or 18 injections of casein. Subsequently, the cells were incubated with SAA for 4 h, 8 h and overnight (O/N). The control lane shows the 2 SAA isotypes characteristic for mice. The arrow indicates the AA band.

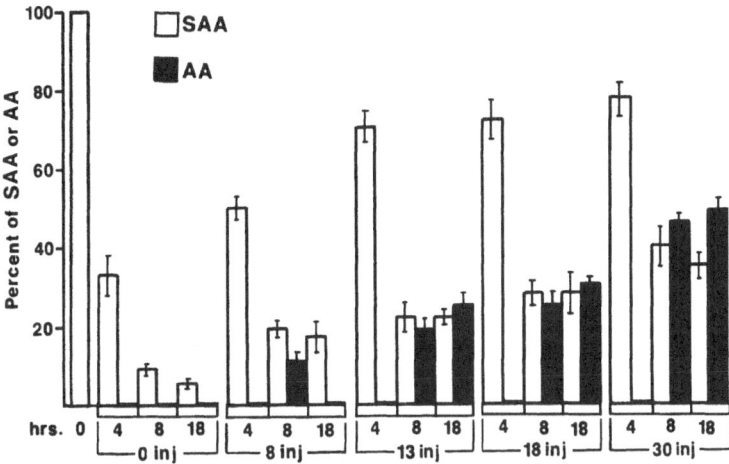

Figure 2: Spectrophotometric quantitation of residual SAA and AA in the supernatants of Kupffer cell cultures. The cells were obtained from mice which had received 0, 8, 13, or 30 injections of casein and were incubated for 4, 8, or 18 h with SAA. Larger amounts of residual SAA and increasing quantities of AA appeared during the amyloid induction period. Note that when the animals had been given more than 18 injections of the stimulant, their KC were no longer able to eliminate the AA intermediate product.

An additional band appeared on the gels which had the same electro- phoretic mobility as AA and was seen in the supernates of all KC cul- tures prepared from amyloidotic animals. More interesting, however, was the observation that during the course of casein injections, a decrease in the ability of KC to process SAA was manifested before any evidence of amyloidosis could be detected in the relevant organs of the animals, even on electron microscopy. Since the AA product was found in KC cultures very early during stimulation of the animals, the possibility was considered that casein stimulation had caused the synthesis of an aberrant molecule which could not be hydrolyzed by normal Kupffer cells. Therefore, KC isolated from unstimulated, healthy animals were added to supernates containing the intermediate cleavage product.

As illustrated in Fig. 3, such cells were able to digest the AA peptide to completion. Therefore, it must be concluded that the KC of amyloidotic mice were defective as regards the enzyme(s) necessary for the hydrolysis of AA. On the basis of previous studies (7) we assumed that the KC of casein-stimulated mice had lost some of their elastase- -like surface enzymes known to be involved in SAA degradation. Yet, the isolated Kupffer cells from animals which had received as few as 8 injections of casein showed ample evidence of normal stimulation. The cells exhibited increased spreading, adhesiveness, inclusions and vacuoles. Histochemical analysis also showed a marked increase in α-napthyl acetate esterase and tartrate inhibitable acid phosphatase typical of stimulated macrophages. Therefore, the reduction in the ability of the cells to degrade SAA could not be interpreted to reflect an overall suppression of cell function.

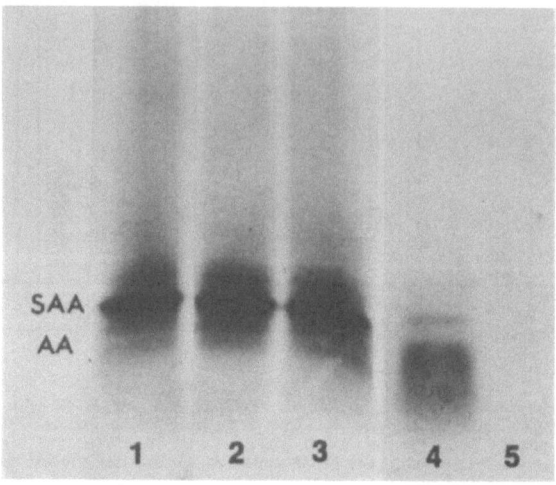

Figure 3: SDS polyacrylamide gel patterns showing that normal Kupffer cells can degrade the intermediate AA product elaborated by Kupffer cells from casein-injected animals. Lane 1 - SAA; Lane 2 - SAA incubated with supernates of normal KC culture showing that the cells do not secrete the enzymes responsible for SAA degradation into the medium; Lane 3 - SAA incubated with supernate of Kupffer cell culture prepared from an amyloidotic liver; Lane 4 - pattern obtained when SAA was incubated with intact Kupffer cells isolated from a mouse which had received 18 injections of casein, showing the AA intermediate product; Lane 5 - result obtained when normal KC were added to the supernate shown in Lane 4. The SAA as well as the intermediate AA fragment were eliminated.

Recently, we have shown that stimulation of mouse peritoneal macrophages with LPS or interferon, stimuli known to increase the bactericidal and tumoricidal capacities of these cells, will at the same time, markedly decrease their production of lysozyme (12). Other examples showing that increased synthesis of some enzymes is accompanied by down-regulation of others could be cited (13-16). However, even if the appearance of the AA cleavage product were attributable to down-regulation of the enzyme(s) required to degrade SAA to completion, the process by which soluble AA detected by SDS-PAGE polymerizes into fibrils, still needs to be explained. Two possibilities may be considered. The abnormal SAA cleavage product may polymerize spontaneously, as appears to be the case in primary amyloidosis, where one or another amino acid substitution in the L-chain of the immunoglobulin molecule seems to be sufficient to cause polymerization (17). The second possi-

bility is that enzymatic cross-linking of the cleavage peptides is responsible for the formation of insoluble deposits. In this regard, we have
speculated that Kupffer cells/macrophages could play yet another role in
amyloidogenesis by virtue of the observation that these cells elaborate
transglutaminase, when stimulated. This enzyme cross-links peptide-
-bound glutamine to primary amines, such as the ε-NH_2 groups of
lysine. Glutaminase-catalyzed reactions are exemplified by factor XIII,
which stabilizes the fibrin clot (18), and they probably mediate the
formation of keratin (19) and the development of cataracts (20).

With the help of an antiserum to transglutaminase kindly provided to
us by Dr. L. Lorand, we were not able to detect this enzyme in freshly
isolated Kupffer cells of healthy animals or in the peripheral blood
monocytes prepared from normal volunteers. However, in Kupffer cells
isolated from mice which had received more than 8 injections of casein
or human monocytes which had been cultured for ten days, the enzyme
could be demonstrated by indirect immunofluorescence (Figure 4).

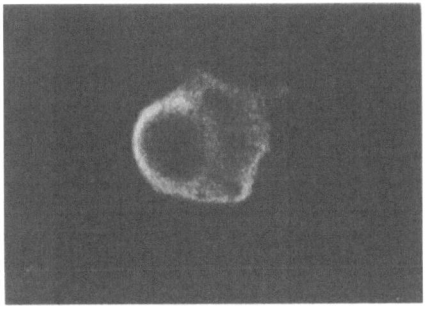

Figure 4: Kupffer cell isolated from the liver of a mouse sacrificed after 8 injections of
casein. The cell was incubated with anti-transglutaminase and then prepared for indirect
immunofluorescence. Note that the peripheral cytoplasm and membrane areas appear to be
more reactive than the remainder of the cell suggesting preferential localization of the
enzyme (see text).

An additional observation suggesting that Kupffer cells or other tissue macrophages may play more than a "bystander" role in amyloid
fibrillogenesis is the intimate relationship between fibrils and such cells.
This phenomenon has been commented on by numerous investigators
(21,22). As illustrated in Fig. 5, the fibrils often occupy deep invaginations of the plasma membrane into the cytoplasm of the cells.
These may be in continuity with the "worm-like" structures (Fig. 6)
believed to be characteristic of Kupffer cells as well as other cells constituting the MPS (23, 24).

Although it is now generally accepted that the SAA polypeptide is
degraded by surface-associated elastase-like enzymes of macrophages,
the involvement of the cell in polymerization of the intermediate AA
product is completely speculative at this time. The concept is offered on

the occasion of this Symposium as a current working hypothesis, meant to help design experiments which will further our understanding of amyloidogenesis in the future.

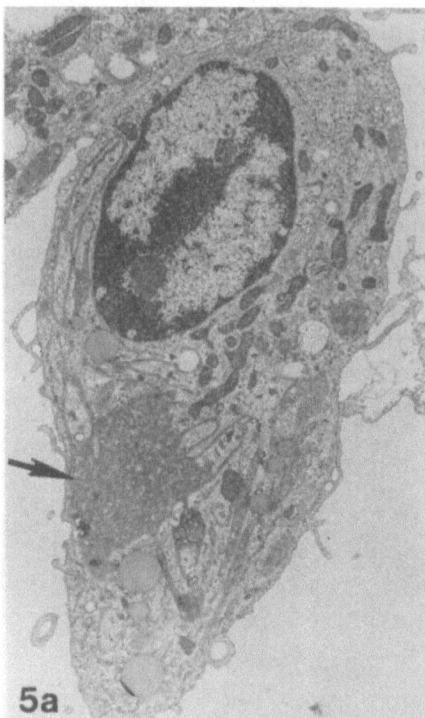

Figure 5a: A Kupffer cell isolated from the liver of a mouse after 30 injections of casein. The fibril-containing inclusion has an irregular circumference and appears to be in continuity with narrow channels and the cell's surface. These membrane-bound spaces do not resemble phagocytic vacuoles. It is suggested that the fibrils form in association with the "worm-like" processes which are in continuity with the extracellular space (see Fig. 6). Magnification x 8000. A detail of the inclusion is seen at higher magnification in Fig. 5b.

Figure 5b: Higher magnification of the area indicated by the arrow in Fig. 5A showing the amyloid fibrils and narrow membrane-bound channels (arrows) to better advantage. Magnification x 34,000.

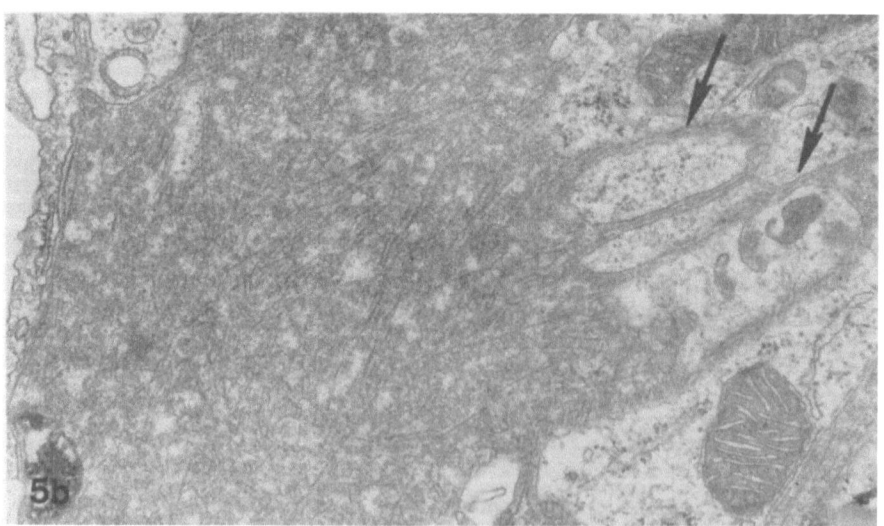

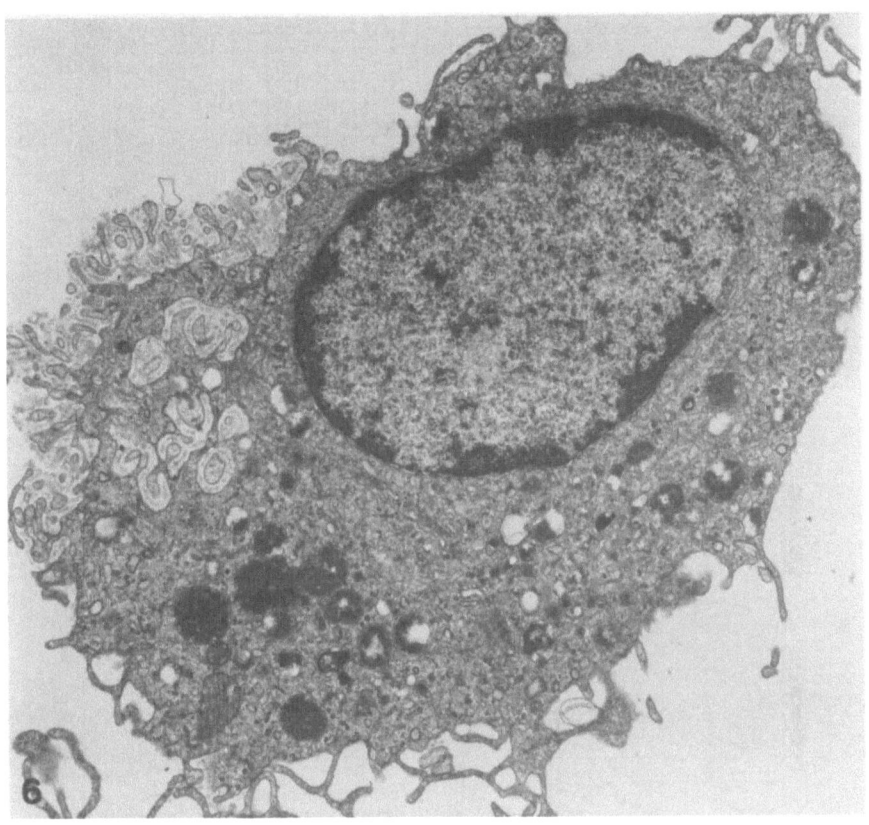

Figure 6: Kupffer cells isolated from a normal animal to illustrate the "worm-like" processes. These structures are usually located at the vascular pole of the cell. They consist of parallel membranes filled with material which resembles the "coat" of the plasma membrane. Magnification x 13,000.

Acknowledgement

This work was supported by the National Institutes of Health Grants #AM 012274 and AM 01431.

References

1. Selinger, M.J., McAdam, K.P.W.J., Kaplan, M.M. et al. Nature 285, 498-500, 1980.
2. Levin, M., Franklin, E.C., Frangione, B. & Pras, M. J. Clin. Invest. 51, 2773-2776, 1972.
3. Levin, M., Pras, M. & Franklin, E.C. J. Exp. Med. 138, 373-380, 1973.
4. Eriksen, N., Ericsson, L.H., Pearsall, N. et al. Proc. Natl. Acad. Sci. USA 73, 964-967, 1976.
5. Bausserman, L.L., Herbert, P.N. & McAdam, K.P.W.J. J. Exp. Med. 152, 641-656, 1980.

6. Hoffman, J.S., Ericsson, L.H., Eriksen, N. et al. J. Exp. Med. 159, 641-646, 1984.
7. Lavie, G., Zucker-Franklin, D. & Franklin, E.C. J. Exp. Med. 148, 1020-1031, 1978.
8. Lavie, G., Zucker-Franklin, D. & Franklin, E.C. J. Immunol. 125, 175-180, 1980.
9. Zucker-Franklin, D., Lavie, G. & Franklin E.C. J. Histochem. Cytochem. 29, 451-456, 1981.
10. McAdam, K.P.W.J. & Sipe, J.D. J. Exp. Med. 144, 1121-1127, 1976.
11. Fuks, A., & Zucker-Franklin, D. J. Exp. Med. 161, 1013-1028, 1985.
12. Warfel, A.H. & Zucker-Franklin, D. J. Immunol. (In press).
13. Edelson, P.J. & Cohen, Z.A. J. Exp. Med. 144, 1581-1595, 1976.
14. Werb, Z. & Chin, J.R. J. Exp. Med. 158, 1272-1293, 1983.
15. Varesio, L. J. Immunol. 134, 1262-1267, 1985.
16. Varesio, L., Issaq, H.J. & Taramelli, D. Eur. J. Immunol. 13, 959-964, 1983.
17. Solomon, A., Frangione, B. & Franklin, E.C. J. Clin. Invest. 70, 453-460, 1982.
18. Lorand, L & Stenberg, P. C.R.C. Handbook Biochem. Mol. Biol. 2, 669-685, 1976.
19. Rice, R.H. & Green, H. Cell 11, 417-422, 1977.
20. Lorand, L., Hsu, L.K.M., Siefring, G.E., Jr. & Rafferty, N.S. Proc. Natl. Acad. Sci. USA 78, 1356-1360, 1981.
21. Ranløv, P. & Wanstrup, J. Acta Pathol. Microbiol. Scand. 71, 575-591, 1967.
22. Franklin, E.C. & Zucker-Franklin, D. Adv. Immunol. 15, 249-304, 1972.
23. Emeis, J.J. J. Reticuloendothelial. Soc. 20, 31-50, 1976.
24. Brederoo, P. & Daems, W.Th. Z. Zellforsch. 126, 135-156, 1972.

VII.6 SAA KINETICS IN ANIMALS

Linda L. Bausserman

Division of Nutrition and Metabolism,
The Miriam Hospital, Brown University,
Providence, Rhode Island 02906, U.S.A.

1. Introduction

Kinetic models have been established for the study of plasma proteins in which tracer quantities of radiolabelled proteins are administered intravascularly to animals and disappearance of radioactivity from the plasma compartment is monitored. Two conditions must be met. First, it is essential that the tracer be distributed and metabolized identically to the tracee. Secondly, the system must be in dynamic equilibrium, i.e., plasma concentrations must not fluctuate during the course of the study. If these criteria are met, one can plot a disappearance curve of radioactivity remaining in the plasma versus time on a log-linear scale. Slopes and intercepts extrapolated from the curve are then used to calculate half-life and fractional catabolic rate. If one also knows the plasma concentration of the protein of interest, it is possible to calculate synthesis rate. The total plasma mass of the protein can be determined from the initial specific activity (usually measured 5-10 minutes after infusion of tracer) and the dose of tracer (1).

The study of SAA kinetics is complicated by the fact that SAA is transported in association with the high density lipoproteins (HDL) (2-4). Therefore, one must consider not only the metabolic rate of SAA but also its interaction with a complex system of lipids and other lipid-bound proteins. It is not known if SAA clearance is affected by either its ability to compete for lipid binding sites on HDL or by the normal cycle of HDL metabolism.

Technically, the fact that SAA is associated with HDL makes preparation of a valid tracer difficult. If one labels intact SAA-rich HDL, all of the HDL proteins are labelled. It then becomes necessary to separate the proteins in each assay sample to quantitate SAA. This procedure is not only very laborious but may also introduce errors. Alternatively, one can isolate the SAA, label it, and reincorporate the tracer into HDL. Analysis is simplified but the SAA may no longer be native after isolation and radiolabelling. Shepherd et al (5) have investigated the effect of labelling methods on the clearance rates of apo A-I and apo A-II, the major HDL apoproteins. They found that purified apo A-I, that had been radiolabelled and reincorporated into HDL, was cleared faster than apo A-I labelled in situ. Such differences were not observed with apo A-II.

Hoffman and Benditt (6) have addressed this issue in studies of SAA kinetics in mice (see below). In our studies in rodents we have used SAA intercalated in HDL and biologically screened before use. Recoveries after screening are only 10-15% but results using screened preparations are identical to those obtained with native SAA-rich HDL (unpublished observation).

A second major obstacle in studying SAA kinetics is that it is virtually impossible to obtain steady-state conditions. During an acute phase response there are wide fluctuations in SAA plasma concentrations (7). Most studies have been performed in normal animals. However, concentrations are very low in normal animals and turnover rates may be different from those obtained when high levels of SAA are present. Three patterns of the relationship between plasma concentration and catabolic rate have been described. Catabolic rate may be independent of pool size (e.g., IgA, IgM, fibrinogen), inversely related (e.g., IgD, haptoglobin, transferrin), or directly related to pool size (e.g., IgG) (8). It is not known into which class SAA falls. Moreover, SAA production may be induced by the conditions of the experiment (4,9) so that SAA concentrations may not be constant even in normal animals. In general, laboratories have not tried to develop rigorous kinetic models of SAA kinetics but have compared SAA clearance rates to those of the major HDL apoproteins in an attempt to determine whether SAA catabolism is related to that of HDL.

2. SAA kinetics in mice

Hoffman and Benditt (6) have compared turnover of radioiodinated normal and SAA-rich HDL in normal mice. The SAA-rich HDL was cleared faster. When the individual proteins were analyzed by polyacrylamide gel electrophoresis, SAA had a $T\frac{1}{2}$ of 85 minutes and apo A-I a $T\frac{1}{2}$ of 11 hours. Unlabelled SAA in SAA-rich plasma, injected into normal animals and monitored by radioimmunoassay, had a $T\frac{1}{2}$ of 72 minutes. This value was very close to that obtained with tracer despite possible plasma volume expansion and elevation (> 20 fold) of SAA concentration in these animals. Rapid clearance of SAA was not due to urinary excretion and did not appear to result from rapid uptake by a specific organ.

Different results were obtained with SAA that had been isolated, radiolabelled and reincorporated into HDL. In this case, SAA disappeared at the same rate as apo A-I. These results contrast with those of Shepherd et al (5) who found that exogenously labelled protein was cleared more rapidly than in situ labelled apo A-I and with our studies (10) in cynomolgus monkeys in which exogenously labelled SAA was cleared faster than apo A-I. The reason for the discrepancy is unclear.

3.SAA kinetics in subhuman primates

Our laboratory, in collaboration with the New England Regional Primate Center, has studied SAA clearance in cynomolgus monkeys (10). We used human proteins incorporated into monkey HDL and compared clearance of human SAA with human apo A-I, human apo C-III and monkey HDL. Human apo A-I disappeared from the plasma at the same rate as monkey HDL; SAA clearance was much faster than apo A-I, and apo C-III clearance was intermediate between apo A-I and SAA. Analysis of tracer distribution by ultracentrifugation indicated that 74-84% of the tracer remained HDL-bound during the first six hours of the study when more than 50% of the radioactivity was cleared.

In contrast to the rapid clearance of SAA observed in cynomolgus monkeys, Parks and Rudel (11) have reported a $T\frac{1}{2}$ of 2.5 days for HDL-associated SAA in African green monkeys. This is longer than would be expected on the basis of studies in other species. For comparison, the $T\frac{1}{2}$ of SAA in humans has been estimated as approximately 24 hours (12,13) whereas the A apoproteins have half-lives of 4-6 days (14). The half-life of apo A-I in cynomolgus monkeys is approximately 3 days (15). It is possible that the faster clearance of SAA in cynomolgus monkeys was due to the use of human protein. Alternatively, differences may be due to the way in which the data were expressed. SAA was labelled in situ and analyzed by isoelectric focusing. The results were calculated as percent of the SAA specific activity at 1 minute. If SAA concentrations were decreasing during the study, the $T\frac{1}{2}$ would appear to be longer.

Parks and Rudel (4) have reported that SAA production is induced by chair restraint; therefore, it is likely that there were fluctuations in SAA plasma concentrations.

4.Conclusion

It is clear from these studies that results of SAA kinetics studies are very dependent on the methods of tracer preparation and analysis of plasma samples. Interpretation of results is facilitated by including an HDL apoprotein for comparison. Experiments in mice using in situ labelled SAA and in cynomolgus monkeys using exogenously labelled SAA gave comparable results, i.e., SAA was cleared more rapidly than apo A-I. This conclusion was substantiated in mice using SAA-rich plasma in which the SAA underwent no modifications. These results are also analogous to those reported in humans. The mechanism of SAA clearance is not known. The data suggest that either a subset of HDL particles on which SAA is carried may be more rapidly cleared or that SAA is dissociated from HDL before clearance (6,8).

Acknowledgements

Research described was supported by NIH grant HL26156 and The Miriam Foundation.

References

1. Shipley, R.A. & Clark, R.E. Tracer Methods for in Vivo Kinetics. Academic Press, New York, 1-20, 1972.
2. Benditt, E.P. & Eriksen, N. Proc. Natl. Acad. Sci. USA 74, 4025-4028, 1977.
3. Benditt, E.P., Eriksen, N. & Hanson, R.H. Proc. Natl. Acad. Sci. USA 76, 4092-4096, 1979.
4. Parks, J.S. & Rudel, L.L. J. Lipid Res. 26, 82-91, 1985.
5. Shepherd, J., Packard, C.J., Gotto, A.M. & Taunton, O.D. J. Lipid. Res. 19, 656-661, 1978.
6. Hoffman, J.S. & Benditt, E.P. J. Clin. Invest. 71, 926-934, 1983.
7. McAdam, K.P.W.J., Elin, R.J., Sipe, J.D. & Wolff, S.M. J. Clin. Invest. 61, 390-394, 1978.
8. Waldmann, T.A. & Strober, W. In Progr. Allergy. Karger, Basel/New York. Vol. 13, 1-110, 1969.
9. Moon, E.A., MacKinnon, A.M. & Barter, P.J. Biochim. Biophys. Acta 796, 354-358, 1984.
10. Bausserman, L.L., Herbert, P.N., Rodger, R. & Nicolosi, R.J. Biochim. Biophys. Acta 792, 186-191, 1984.
11. Parks, J.S. & Rudel, L.L. Am. J. Pathol. 112, 243-249, 1983.
12. Raynes, J.G. & Cooper, E.H. J. Clin. Pathol. 36, 798-803, 1983.
13. Bausserman, L.L., Bernier, D.N., McAdam, K.P.W.J. & Herbert, P.N. Clin. Res. 33, 504A, 1985.
14. Herbert, P.N., Bernier, D.N., Cullinane, E.M. et al. JAMA 252, 1034-1037, 1984.
15. Chong, K.S., Nicolosi, R.J., Roger, R.F. et al. J. Clin. Invest. (In press).

VII.7 AMYLOID AND FEMALE PROTEIN: SEX-RELATED OCCURRENCE
IN THE SYRIAN HAMSTER

John E. Coe

U.S. Department of Health and Human Services, National
Institutes of Health, National Institute of Allergy and Infectious
Diseases, Laboratory of Persistent Viral Diseases,
Rocky Mountain Laboratories, Hamilton, Montana 59840, U.S.A.

1. Introduction

The prevalence of amyloidosis in Syrian hamsters has been reported
in a variety of reports (1-3). Our interest in hamster amyloid was related to previous studies on an unusual protein, female protein (FP),
found in the serum of these animals (4). Female protein was shown to
be a homologue of serum amyloid P component (SAP) and C-reactive
protein (CRP) (5). However, FP synthesis was regulated by sex
steroids so that normal males had serum levels about 100- to 200-fold
less than females. Actually, FP was present at extraordinarily high levels in female hamster serum (1-3 mg/ml) when compared to the usual
CRP-SAP homologues in other mammals. Functionally, FP shared a very
characteristic function with CRP, i.e., a Ca^{++} dependent phosphoryl-
choline (PC) binding capacity (5) with attendant complement activation
(6). However, at the amino terminus, FP was structurally more similar
to SAP (5). The question arose whether FP also could have a "SAP-
-like" role as an amyloid constituent. The results of this study indicated that FP was indeed an amyloid constituent. Furthermore, amyloid
deposition was correlated directly with serum FP levels, suggesting
more than a passive role of FP in pathogenesis of this disease. In addition, the metabolism of injected ^{125}I-FP was found to be characteristically altered in presence of amyloid (7).

2. Materials and methods

2.1. Amyloid studies

Normal and experimental Syrian hamsters (Mesocricetus auratus) were
tested for presence of amyloid by examination of histological sections
(liver, spleen, kidney) for Congo red birefringence. For experimental
induction of amyloid, treatments were routinely initiated at 3 months of
age so induced amyloid could be related to expected incidence of
amyloid in normal hamsters. Treatments were: (i) A subcutaneous implantation of one 12 mg pellet of diethylstilbestrol (DES - Pfizer, Inc.,
New York) every 3-4 months, (ii) 1 ml Na-caseinate (Difco Laboratories, Detroit, Michigan, 12.5% sterile) subcutaneous injection three times

341

per week. FP was detected in amyloid by fluorescence microscopy using a fluorescein isothiocyanate-labeled antibody to FP. In addition, the amount of FP extractable from normal and amyloid livers was determined according to reference (8).

2.2. Metabolic studies

Purified FP (5) and DEAE-purified rabbit gamma globulin (RGG) were labeled with ^{125}I and intravenously injected to determine plasma disappearance and/or tissue localization as previously described (9). ^{125}I--FP in organs was quantified by weighing organ and determining CPM per gram of tissue; to normalize for plasma CPM contribution in the organ, the individual animal's organ/plasma ratio was calculated. For autoradiography, histological sections were coated with NTB-2 emulsion (Eastman Kodak Co., Rochester, New York) and after suitable incubation, were developed and stained with Congo red.

3. Results

3.1. Incidence of amyloid in normal and experimental hamsters

Examination of normal hamsters at various ages revealed more amyloid in aging female hamsters than in aging male hamsters. That is, amyloid was detectable at an earlier age in females (8 months) and the deposits were consistently more extensive in female hamsters. In animals 1.5 years old, amyloid was a uniform finding in females (vs. 25% in males) and became progressively more severe with age. Indeed, females rarely lived longer than 24-30 months, whereas many males lived over 3 years and did not develop the consistent and extensive amyloidosis seen in females.

Amyloid induced by Na-caseinate was detected earlier and the deposits were much more extensive in females than in males. Repeated injections of Na-caseinate for 5 months resulted in amyloid deposits in 80% of females and in only 7% of males. After 7-9 months of Na-caseinate injections, minimal amyloid was present in about half of the males, whereas extensive deposits with a lethal result were characteristic for females. Implantation of a DES pellet (12 mg) was the most effective way of inducing deposits of amyloid in males; after 3 months, 55% of males were affected (and 82% of females).

3.2. Presence of FP in amyloid

By fluorescence microscopy, FP deposits were detected in circumscribed areas of histological sections of liver, spleen and kidney; these same areas were shown to contain amyloid when similar sections were examined for Congo red birefringence (Figs. 1A, 1B). Furthermore, amyloidotic tissue was greatly enriched for extractable FP content; for

example, female amyloid liver contained approximately 20-fold more extractable FP than that found in normal liver.

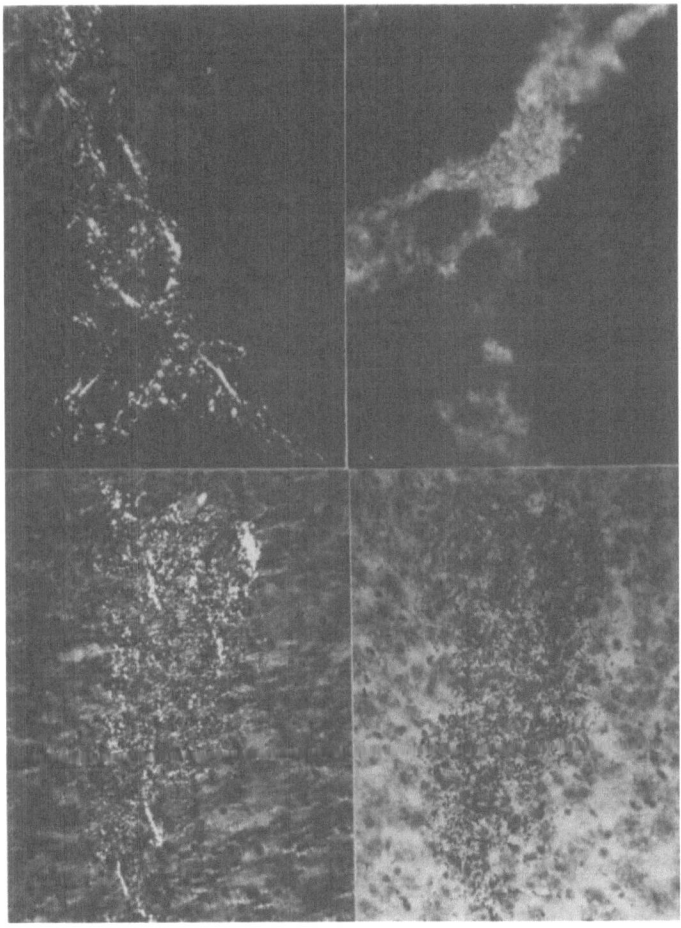

Figure 1: Photomicrograph of liver sections from amyloidotic hamsters. A (left top):
typical appearance of Congo red birefringent amyloid in periportal area during
illumination by polarized light. B (right top): similar periportal amyloid deposit with
green fluorescence after reaction with fluorescein-isothiocyanate-labelled anti-FP and
examination by fluorescent microscopy. C and D (bottom left and right): same histological
section from amyloid hamster injected intravenously with ^{125}I-FP seven days earlier; the
section was overlayed with photographic emulsion which after incubation was developed and
slide stained with Congo red. When examined by polarized light (C), the Congo red
birefringence of amyloid infiltrate was defined. When viewed with transmitted light (D),
the grains in the developed emulsion indicated the presence of ^{125}I-FP only within the
amyloid area.

3.3. Metabolism of ^{125}I-FP in amyloidotic hamsters

The plasma metabolism of ^{125}I-FP was determined in normal and amyloidotic Syrian hamsters. The disappearance of plasma ^{125}I-FP was relatively rapid in normal females (T½ approximately 15 hrs) and even faster in normal males because of their low FP serum level (Fig. 2). However, in either sex, the presence of amyloidosis resulted in a distinctly different metabolism, which was characterized by an initial rapid intravascular loss, followed by a very prolonged slower disappearance (T½ from terminal slope b approximately 30 hr) (Fig. 2).

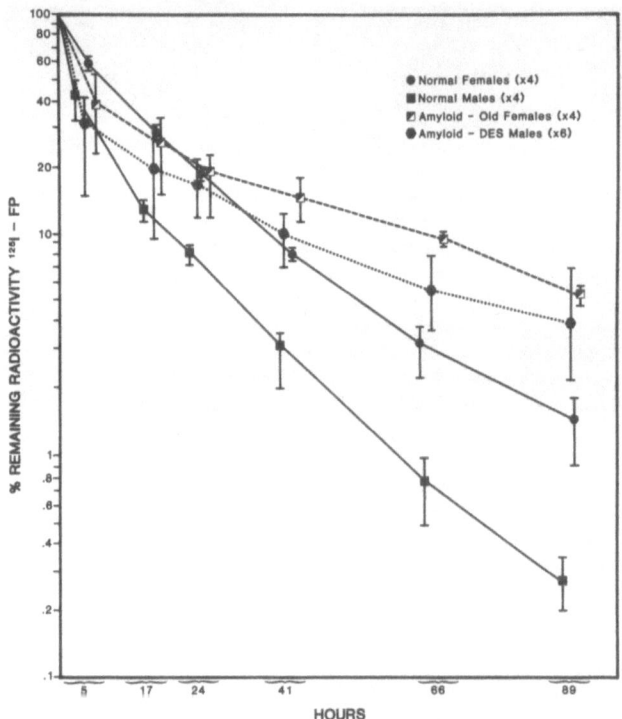

Figure 2: ^{125}I-FP plasma disappearance in four normal male (■) and four normal female (●) hamsters; plasma disappearance in males with increased serum FP levels (e.g. after DES treatment but before amyloid deposition, ref. 7) was similar to females (not shown). However, plasma metabolism was changed by the presence of amyloid within males (x6 from DES treatment ●) and females (x4 from old age ▨); ^{125}I-FP disappearance was characteristically altered with an initial rapid i.v. loss and a prolonged linear slope.
Bracket = range of group.
Reproduced from the Journal of Clinical Investigation 76:66-74, 1985 by copyright permission.

This pattern of plasma disappearance was seen only in amyloidotic hamsters and was similar regardless of the etiology of the amyloidosis (that is, amyloid associated with normal aging, DES or Na-caseinate treatment or sterile abscess formation after turpentine injection). The plasma disappearance of other ^{125}I-labeled proteins (hamster serum albumin, rabbit gamma globulin, bovine serum albumin) was evaluated in amyloidotic hamsters and found to be similar to that of the normal hamster. Thus, amyloid deposits had a specific effect on plasma ^{125}I-FP metabolism and the disappearance curve was suggestive of a dynamic extravascular deposition. To determine if the ^{125}I-FP was sequestered in amyloidotic tissues, the animals were sacrificed 7 days after ^{125}I-FP injection and various organs were assayed for content of ^{125}I-FP. Comparison of amyloid and non-amyloid organs showed a selective accumulation of ^{125}I-FP only within amyloidotic tissues. This localization of ^{125}I-FP in amyloid organs was specific, as a similar analysis of hamsters injected with ^{125}I-RGG did not show any preferential localization in amyloidotic organs (7).

In order to determine if the ^{125}I-FP was actually located within the amyloid deposits of the organ, histologic sections were examined by autoradiography for coincidence of Congo red birefringence and radio-activity. A positive correlation was evident, in that high silver grain counts (^{125}I-FP) were invariably associated with amyloid deposits (Figs. 1C, 1D).

4. Discussion

Female Syrian hamsters have a remarkable proclivity to develop systemic amyloidosis. Indeed, the extensive amyloid deposits in aging females probably explain their relatively early mortality when compared to male hamsters (2,3,10); Syrian hamsters are unusual mammals because the male actually outlives the female of the species (10).

Induction of amyloid also was accomplished more easily in females than in males; deposits were detected earlier and were more extensive in females after a variety of amyloid producing treatments. The capacity of DES to induce amyloid appears to be a unique event not described in any other species (1,11). Of special interest was the fact that DES injection also resulted in marked elevation of serum FP levels in male hamsters (4). The other amyloid inducing treatments (Na-caseinate, sterile abscess formation) also produced increases of serum FP levels as FP has an acute phase reaction (9). Thus, amyloid formation was associated with high serum FP levels either naturally present or experimentally induced. Studies in progress will determine if amyloid can be reduced (or even resorbed) by decreasing serum FP levels.

It is clear that ^{125}I-FP rapidly enters into and persists within amyloid deposits and that this is a specific process. The etiologic significance of this dynamic FP equilibrium between serum and amyloid is unknown. However, this altered metabolism of ^{125}I-FP does provide for hamsters a specific technique for noninvasive diagnosis of amyloidosis and also demonstrates the dynamic exchange ongoing between the intravascular compartment and extravascular amyloid deposits.

The presence of FP in amyloid was not unexpected as the sequence at the amino terminus indicated a close relationship to SAP (5); the complete sequence comparison of FP with SAP showed a 69% identity, whereas FP and CRP were 50% identical (12). FP has been shown to bind to preparations of human amyloid fibrils in a Ca^{++} dependent fashion (unpublished) similar to SAP (13). Like CRP, however, FP also contains a PC binding site, which is apparently contiguous with the area specific for fibrils, as free PC will interfere with the FP-fibril association.

The Syrian hamster is an intriguing amyloid model. Is the bizarre sex limited expression of amyloid in this species etiologically related to the unique sex-limited expression of its SAP homologue, i.e. FP? Are the extraordinary high serum levels of this homologue in females a primary cause for amyloid deposition? If FP is so deleterious to female hamsters, why has this system been maintained during Syrian hamster evolution? FP may play an especially important role in the physiology of the female Syrian hamster. Determination of this special function could elucidate the purpose of SAP and CRP homologues within other species.

Acknowledgements

Human amyloid fibrils were kindly provided by Dr. J. Sipe and Dr. K.P.W.J. McAdam.

References

1. Dontenwill, W., Ranz, H. & Mohr, U. Beitr. Pathol. Anat. 122, 390-405, 1960.
2. McMartin, D.N. J. Gerontol. 34, 502-511, 1979.
3. Schmidt, R.E., Eason, R.L., Hubbard, G.B., et al. Pathology of Aging Syrian Hamsters. CRC Press, Inc., Boca Raton, Florida, 219-242, 1983.
4. Coe, J.E. Proc. Natl. Acad. Sci. USA 74, 730-733, 1977.
5. Coe, J.E., Margossian, S.S., Slayter, H.S., et al. J. Exp. Med. 153, 977-991, 1981.
6. Etlinger, H.M. & Coe, J.E. Int. Arch. Allergy Appl. Immunol. (In press).
7. Coe, J.E. & Ross, M.J. J. Clin. Invest. 76, 66-74, 1985.
8. Skinner, M., Sipe, J.D., Yood, R.A., et al. Ann. N.Y. Acad. Sci. 389, 190-198, 1982.
9. Coe, J.E., & Ross, M.J. J. Exp. Med. 157, 1421-1433, 1983.
10. Kirkman, H. & Yau, P.K.S. Am. J. Anat. 135, 205-220, 1972.
11. Russfield, A.B. & Green, M.N. Am. J. Pathol. 46, 59-67, 1965.
12. Dowton, S.B., Woods, D.E., Mantzouranis, E.C., et al. Science 228, 1206-1208, 1985.
13. Pepys, M.B., Dyck, R.F., De Beer, F.C., et al. Clin. Exp. Immunol. 38, 284-293, 1979.

VII.8   ENDOCRINE AMYLOID IN ANIMALS

Per Westermark

Department of Pathology,
University Hospital,
S-751 85 Uppsala, Sweden.

1. Introduction

Amyloid, selectively deposited in peptide hormone producing tissues, is commonly associated with aging but occurs also in some endocrine tumours. The amyloid in the islets of Langerhans has especially attracted some interest due to its connection with type II (non insulin-dependent) diabetes mellitus (see Section VI, Chapter 3). In human medullary carcinoma of the thyroid gland, it has been shown that the amyloid fibrils are of hormonal nature (1) and it can be presumed that studies of the nature and of the pathogenesis of the amyloid in all endocrine tissues can give us valuable information in hormone physiology and pathophysiology.

No experimentally induced endocrine amyloid in animals has yet been established. If an animal model is desirable, a spontaneously developing endocrine amyloid has to be used. Unfortunately such spontaneously appearing endocrine amyloids are comparatively rare and have mainly been described in the islets of Langerhans in a few animals, as well in some endocrine tumours.

2. Amyloid in the islets of Langerhans in animals with spontaneous diabetes mellitus

Diabetes mellitus associated with amyloid of the islets of Langerhans has been reported to occur in several monkey species (2-4), cats (5), ocelots (6) and raccoons (7). It is easy to understand that animal islet amyloid has been studied most extensively in monkeys and cats.

Monkey islet amyloid has especially been studied by Howard and co-workers in Oregon. In their model, they use black Celebes apes (Macaca nigra) which quite frequently develop diabetes mellitus, resembling the human type II (non-insulin-dependent) form. These apes present abnormal glucose tolerance tests, hyperglycemia, impaired insulin response, reduced insulin secretion and occurrence of islet amyloid (3,8,9). As in humans, islet amyloid to a lesser extent is present also in non-diabetic individuals (9). Other monkey species may also get diabetes mellitus with islet amyloid (2,4). The islet amyloid of apes has not yet been characterized.

The cat model has been extensively studied by Johnson and coworkers in Minnesota. They investigate old domestic cats with spontaneous diabetes mellitus. The sampling procedure is laborious since the incidence of diabetes, although increasing with age, is only 1:100 for cats over 7 years old (10). The feline diabetes resembles human type II diabetes, and islet amyloid is quite common and can be as extensive as in human diabetics (7). Islet amyloid occurs less frequently and to a slighter degree in non-diabetic cats and, as in humans, the frequency increases with age (7,10,11). The feline islet amyloid closely resembles the human type. It does not contain tryptophan (10) and is permanganate-resistant (12). Furthermore, like the human islet amyloid, it does not react with antibodies to insulin but shows a distinctive reaction with an antiserum obtained by immunization with a B-chain rich insulin fraction (13). The cat islet amyloid has recently been purified and a fibril protein been isolated. A partial N-terminal amino acid sequence analysis of this protein (Westermark, Johnson and coworkers, result to be published) shows that it is homologous to the human insulinoma amyloid peptide (IAP) (see Section 6). This result further emphasizes that the feline spontaneous diabetes mellitus is a valid model for the human maturity onset diabetes.

3. Experimental model for amyloid of medullary carcinoma of the thyroid gland

As a good model for this amyloid, medullary carcinoma, spontaneously appearing in old bulls has been proposed (14,15). More than 10 years old bulls often get this form of tumour which may contain amyloid. To my knowledge, no studies of this amyloid have been performed, but bulls are kept only with some difficulty in the ordinary laboratory.

4. Conclusions

No easily available animal models of endocrine amyloid exist. Both the monkey and the cat forms of islet amyloid resemble the human, but in both species, mainly old animals get deposits. This means that it is difficult to obtain animals in sufficient number. Amyloid does, however, occur in animals without diabetes mellitus, but in smaller amount. Lastly, for a human pathologist the bull model of medullary carcinoma amyloid is a remote possibility. For this disease one can conclude that a human model of animal disease is more easy to study than the opposite.

Acknowledgements

Some of the studies, reviewed in this paper, have been supported by the Swedish Medical Research Council and The Research Fund of King Gustaf V.

References

1. Sletten, K., Westermark, P. & Natvig, J.B. J. Exp. Med. 143, 993-998, 1976.
2. Sheldon, W.G. & Gleiser, C.A. Vet. Pathol. 8, 16-18, 1971.
3. Howard, C.F. Diabetes 21, 1077-1090, 1972.
4. Howard, C.F. & Palotay, J.L. Lab. Anim. Sci. 25, 191-196, 1975.
5. Johnson, K.H. & Stevens, J.B. Diabetes 22, 81-90, 1973.
6. Frye, F.L., Detrick, J.F., Clement, E.D., et al. Vet. Med. Small Anim. Clin. 70, 860-862, 1975.
7. Yano, B.L., Hayden, D.W. & Johnson, K.H. Vet. Pathol. 18, 621-627, 1981.
8. Howard, C.F. Diabetologia 10, 671-677, 1974.
9. Howard, C.F. Diabetes 27, 357-364, 1978.
10. Johnson, K.H., Hayden, D.W., O'Brien, T. & Westermark, P. Am. J. Pathol. (In press).
11. Yano, B.L., Hayden, D.W. & Johnson, K.H. Vet. Pathol. 18, 310-315, 1981.
12. Yano, B.L., Johnson, K.H. & Hayden, D.W. Vet. Pathol. 18, 181-187, 1981.
13. Johnson, K.H., Westermark, P., Nilsson, G., et al. Vet. Pathol. 22, 463-468, 1985.
14. Black, H.E., Capen, C.C. & Young, D.M. Cancer 32, 865-878, 1973.
15. Capen, C.C. & Black, H.E. Am. J. Pathol. 74, 377-380, 1974.

VII.9   DIETARY TREATMENT DURING THE INDUCTION AND
        RESORPTION PHASES OF EXPERIMENTAL AMYLOIDOSIS

Edgar S. Cathcart, Crystal A. Leslie, Simin M. Meydani,
K.C. Hayes and Devayani Lathi

Geriatric Research, Educational and Clinical Center,
E.N. Rogers Memorial Veterans Administration Hospital,
Bedford, MA 01730 and
Boston University School of Medicine,
Boston, MA 02118, U.S.A.

1. Introduction

We have postulated that the administration of azocasein to amyloid
susceptible mice overwhelms the proteolytic capacity of the mononuclear
phagocytic system (MPS), either by inhibition of specific cell membrane
associated enzymes or by activation of serine esterase inhibitors, one of
which may be SAP or serum amyloid P component. The influence of
strain, age and gender of the mouse on the incidence and severity of
amyloid is presumably reflected in reduced MPS activity which in turn
can be modified by altering dietary factors, particularly the content of
milk protein (casein) and the level of antioxidants (vitamin E and
santoquin).

In this report we have examined the incidence and severity of type
AA amyloid (AA) produced experimentally in mice fed a diet in which
the only source of fat was either 1. low in polyunsaturated fatty acids
(PUFA's), 2. high in omega-6 PUFA's or 3. high in omega-3 PUFA's.
The design of out studies permitted comparison of cocoanut versus corn
versus fish oil diets during both the induction and resorption phases of
secondary amyloidosis.

Polyunsaturation of the fat per se did not affect the course of the
disease. However, a diet rich in eicosapentaenoic acid (EPA) had a significantly beneficial effect on AA induction while also altering the
prostaglandin (PG) profile of the macrophage (M).

2. Methods

Diet: the level of dietary fat was 5% of dry weight supplied as either
corn oil (Mazola corn oil, Best Foods, Union, NJ), fish oil (Maxepa,
R.P. Scherer, N.A. Troy, MI) or edible cocoanut oil (Capitol City
Product, Columbus, OH). Diets were made fresh every 2 to 3 weeks
and stored refrigerated. After 3 weeks of storage the fatty acid composition of the diet was not altered. The diet was fed fresh daily and the
left over diet discarded. Prior to being fed special diets, the mice were
given fresh rodent laboratory Chow (No. 5000, Purina, St. Louis, MO).

Mice: Six week old CBA/J mice were divided randomly into 3 dietary groups and fed either the corn oil, fish oil, or cocoanut oil diet, respectively. Mice were housed 4 or 5 to a cage and allowed access to food and water ad libitum.

Induction of amyloid: Azocasein was prepared from casein as previously described (1). After 2 weeks on the experimental diet, 25 mice in each dietary group received injections of azocasein subcutaneously (0,3 ml of 10% w/v 5 days per week). The remaining 25 mice were left untreated and served as controls. After 1 week of injections spleens from 5 mice in each treatment group and 3 control mice were screened for the presence of amyloid. After 2 weeks all the remaining mice were killed and their spleens, livers and kidneys removed for AA quantification (0 - 4+) (as per Janigan and Druet (1)).

Resorption of amyloid: Seventy three CBA/J mice were fed a corn oil diet for 9 weeks, given 14 azocasein injections and randomly distributed between the 3 dietary fatty acid regimens after AA induction. Mice were killed at random at regular intervals and the degree of AA assessed histologically after Congo red staining of formalin fixed sections.

Statistics: The Mann Whitney U non-parametric test was used to assess whether differences existed in the amount of amyloid under 3 different dietary conditions.

3. Results

In the first experiment, most spleens, few livers and none of the kidneys had developed AA after 10 injections of azocasein. Both the incidence and severity of AA was less in the livers of mice fed a fish oil diet (data not shown). The mean AA severity score of spleens from mice fed the fish oil diet was 1.80 ± 0.21 (S.E.) compared to 3.00 ± 0.28 for the corn oil fed mice and 3.53 ± 0.17 on the cocoanut oil fed mice. A similar pattern of amyloid distribution was found by 2 other observers.

When these scores were ranked and their distribution compared, fewer spleens of mice on the fish oil diet had high amyloid scores compared to the spleens from mice maintained on either of the other two diets $(p<0.02)$. Although there was a trend for the mice fed cocoanut oil to have more severe AA relative to mice on corn oil, the difference was not significant $(p>0.01)$. No amyloid was detected in any organs from mice not injected with azocasein.

In the second experiment, the mean AA spleen score prior to dietary manipulation was 2.6 ± 1.3 with only trace amounts noted in the liver. The amount of AA present in the spleens of each dietary group decreased over time (Table I). The results indicated that there was AA regression (resorption) which reached significance $(p<0.05)$ 15 weeks after stopping azocasein; this process was not affected by a change in diet from corn oil to fish oil or cocoanut oil.

TABLE I: REGRESSION OF AA IN CBA/J MICE FED FISH vs. CORN vs. COCOANUT OIL ENRICHED DIETS

	0-week	10-week	15-week
Fish oil		2.3 ± 0.8	1.2 ± 0.6
Corn oil	2.6 ± 1.3	2.5 ± 1.1	1.4 ± 1.3
Cocoanut oil		1.8 ± 1.2	1.4 ± 0.5

4. Discussion

These experiments demonstrate that a fish oil diet compared to a corn oil diet ameliorated the severity of secondary amyloidosis in CBA/J mice. The effect does not appear to be related to the higher percentage of saturated fat present in the fish oil (approximately 30% compared to less than 10% present in the corn oil diet) since the more highly saturated cocoanut oil diet did not offer any protection. In fact it is possible that an augmenting effect of the cocoanut oil diet relative to the corn oil diet might have been demonstrated if an earlier time point had been chosen. Interestingly, in view of the classic two-phase theory of amyloidogenesis, a switch from a corn oil diet to fish oil or cocoanut oil did not affect the late or resorption phase of amyloidosis.

We have recently shown that within one week of feeding a fish oil diet, EPA and its metabolites, docosapentaenoic acid and docosahexaenoic acid appear in the macrophage phospholipid pool (2). Concurrently, there is depletion, compared to corn oil fed mice, in the percentage of omega 6 fatty acids present in the phospholipid pool and a decrease in arachidonate metabolism. Since mice fed the cocoanut oil as well as those fed the fish oil tended to produce less archidonate metabolites from the macrophages compared to those fed corn oil, the implication is that the protective effect of the fish oil during AA induction may be related to EPA incorporation rather than arachidonate depletion.

Our finding that omega-3 fatty acids in the diet markedly altered the eicosanoid profile of the macrophage again hints at a PG-mediated control of AA deposition, possibly through modified MPS protease activity (3). On the other hand, the PG alterations could also be acting at other levels including modulation of interleukin-1 release to decrease the formation of serum amyloid precursor protein SAA. Several non PG-mediated mechanisms such as altered saturated/unsaturated fat ratios in the cell membrane or changes in vitamin E or cholesterol uptake might also affect the level of SAA or protease activity. Macrophages, especially those which are immunologically activated, can generate via a membrane bound NADPH oxidase, large amounts of highly oxidized molecules (4) that cause direct protein damage. Peroxide, by increasing available cellular hydroperoxide, will further stimulate PG synthesis (5). Thus changing the available fatty acid precursors by a fish oil diet could modulate the activity of NADPH oxidase to reduce free oxygen radical formation as well as producing different eicosanoids.

Many unanswered questions remain with respect to fat ingestion and the genesis of experimental and human amyloid disease. The role of saturated fats needs to be studied in more detail since the risk of developing AA in lepromatous leprosy rises sharply in populations where animal fats have replaced diets rich in vegetable fats (6). Finally, and most important, it remains to be shown if amyloid disease, once established and still progressing, can subsequently be altered by dietary manipulation. To date, true regression of type AA deposits in human tissues has only rarely been documented in the literature (7).

Acknowledgements

This work was supported in part by the United States Public Health Service grant #AM-32588 and by the Veterans Administration.

References

1. Janigan, D.T. & Druet, R.L. Am. J. Pathol. 48, 1013-1025, 1966.
2. Leslie, C.A., Gonnerman, W.A., Ullman, M.D. et al. J. Exp. Med. 162, 1336-1349, 1985.
3. Leslie, C.A., Lazzari, A.A. & Cathcart, E.S. In Amyloidosis. Glenner, G.G., Osserman, E.F., Benditt, E.P., Calkins, E., Cohen, A.S., Zucker-Franklin, D., Eds. Plenum Press, New York, 175-185, 1986.
4. Pick, E. & Bromberg, Y. Transplantation Proc. 14, 570-576, 1982.
5. Lands, W.E.M. Prostaglandins, Leukotrienes and Med. 13, 35-41, 1984.
6. Williams, R.C. Jr., Cathcart, E.S., Calkins, E. et al. Ann. Intern. Med. 62, 1000-1007, 1966.
7. Cathcart, E.S. & Ignaczak, T.F. In Textbook of Rheumatology, 2nd Ed. Kelley, W.N., Harris Jr., E.D., Ruddy, S, Sledge, C.B., Eds. W.B. Saunders, Philadelphia, 1469-1487, 1985.

SECTION VIII

VIII.1 FUTURE DIRECTIONS IN AMYLOID RESEARCH

George G. Glenner

Department of Pathology (M-012)
University of California, San Diego,
La Jolla, California 92093, U.S.A.

1. Introduction

Since its recognition, the subject of amyloid and amyloidosis has been fraught with misconceptions and errant pathways. Although Virchow applied to it a misnomer over 130 years ago, he correctly realized that the systemic disease was caused by a substance from the blood (1). Although it was authoritatively promulgated that amyloid was a single compound (2), more astute physicians realized that the diversity in clinical symptomatology ruled for chemical diversity (3,4), and that amyloid was a generic term signifying a disease complex (4). The early polarization studies of Congo red stained amyloid inherently implied a highly oriented ultrastructure which was proven by the earliest electron microscopic studies (5,6). X-ray diffraction studies revealing that all amyloid was composed of proteins in a β-pleated sheet configuration (7), and the chemical purification of the first AL proteins (8,9) suggested that "tissue depositon of anti-parallel, β-pleated sheet fibrils [may result] from portions of immunoglobulins other than light chains or of proteins other than immunoglobulins" (9). These suspicions were confirmed with the discovery of clinically distinct amyloid fibril proteins e.g. AL, AA, AF, AE, etc. (10). With the realization that all amyloid deposits are composed of β-pleated fibrils came the awareness that the polarization color after Congo red staining was due to the unusual predilection of Congo red for the β-structure (11,12) and was not the result, as was suggested, of the staining of glycoprotein deposits (2) even though a rare amyloid protein has been found to have a polysaccharide moiety (13). Furthermore, structures without polysaccharide such as the Congo red-polarized intracellular paired helical filaments found in the neurofibrillary tangles in e.g. Alzheimer's disease now appear to have a β-structure (14) despite the fact that the filaments are 120 Å in width (15) and do not correspond to the so-called "classic dimensions" (16) of amyloid fibrils. Thus there are no classic dimensions for amyloid fibrils (12) anymore than there is chemical uniformity. The finding of diverse protein compositions for amyloid fibrils and the evidence that proteolytic cleavage of a precursor was one mechanism for amyloid fibril formation (17) led to the concept of the "amyloidogenic" protein i.e. there are certain sequences in proteins which on proteolysis lead to formation of amyloid fibrils (18). We now know that the lambda VI light chain is amyloidogenic (19) and that prealbumin when substituted in position 30 with a Gly for a Thr predisposes to the formation of an amyloid fibril (20). This concept was testable with the SAA protein. Attempts to relate amyloid formation to high levels of this protein were unconfirmable (21) nor could the 11% of rheumatoid arthritis complicated by amyloidosis (22) be thus explained. It could, however, be explained by assuming SAA is not a single protein, but a variety of subspecies, one or more of which is amyloidogenic (10). Subspecies of SAA have been detected in mice (23) and humans (24) and recently an isotypic variant has been shown to be amyloidogenic (25). In passing it is important to mention that all compounds associated with amyloid fibrils are not necessary a part of the fibril protein or even related to its formation. A case in point is the so-called plasma "P-component" (AP) which was initially thought to be a component of the fibril (26) or causative in its formation (27). Neither concept has stood the test of either confirmation or time (28,29). To this day, the physiologic function of SAP has not been determined. A warning, therefore, arises when whole undenatured paired helical filaments from Alzheimer's disease neurofibrillary tangles are used as immunogen and the antibodies obtained are ascribed to a filament origin (30,31).

With these lessons from the past an attempt to look into the future of amyloid research presents its warnings of pitfalls within pitfalls. There are, however, certain possibilities that are apparent and logical. To these we will focus our attention.

2.Pathogenesis

In the AL series of amyloid fibril proteins there is a marked diversity of tissue localization from case to case, while AA protein distribution is relatively uniform. This can best be explained by the chemical diversity of SAL precursor proteins as compared to that of SAA. Assuming two amyloidogenic chemically different light chain proteins in an individual, if one is hydrolyzed in sites A, B, C and D and the second in sites A and B one could assume that because of the chemical composition of the second SAL protein only sites A and B contain proteolytic enzymes capable of cleaving both substrates, while sites C and D have an inadequate enzyme complement to cleave the second. However, if the first substrate is formed into fibrils in sites A, B, C and D and the second in sites E, F and G then we must assume lysosomal enzyme diversity i.e. the "lysosomal" proteolytic enzyme complement must vary in some tissues (Fig. 1). The fact that this is the case has been shown by the presence of the "lysosomal" enzyme, lysozyme in the macrophage of the lung and in monocytes (32) and relative absence from other tissue sites. For those amyloidogenic substrates for which proteolytic cleavage is considered a mechanism in the formation of amyloid fibrils, e.g. SAL and SAA species, "lysosomal" enzyme diversity must be considered in amyloid fibril pathogenesis.

Glenner

LYSOSOMAL ENZYME/PROTEIN DIVERSITY

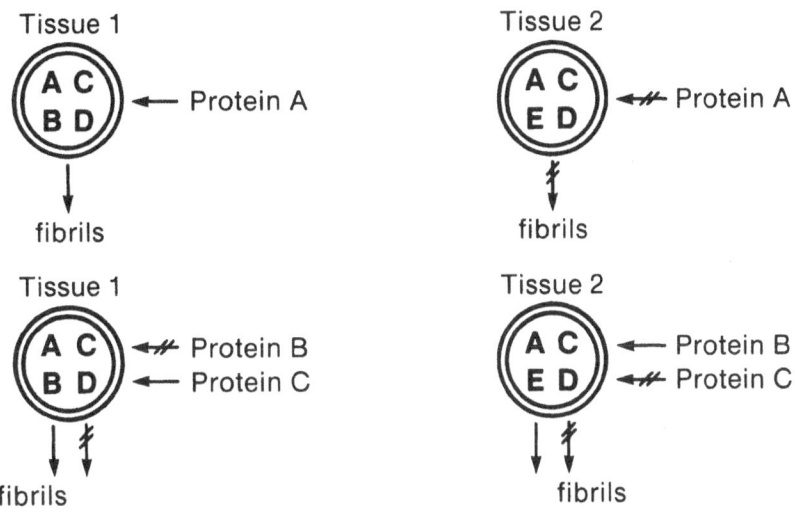

<u>Figure 1</u>: Proteolytic enzymes A, B, C, D, and E act on amyloidogenic proteins A, B and C of different amino acid sequence. When the enzyme B in tissue 1 is replaced by E in tissue 2, protein A is not formed into fibrils. When proteins B and C are exposed to proteolysis by enzymes A, B, C and D, only protein B is formed into fibrils. This illustrates the potential of different amyloidogenic proteins to afford different amyloid tissue patterns of localization in the presence of proteolytic enzyme diversity.

3.Other Amyloid Fibril Proteins

There is little question that the discovery of new, novel amyloid fibril proteins will be found based on the unique clinical condition in which they occur, e.g. Finnish familial amyloidotic polyneuropathy, or their unique site of deposition e.g. corneal lattice dystrophy and pancreatic insular amyloidosis. Although the chemical nature of the neurofibrillary tangles of Alzheimer's disease has resisted attempts at definition for over 15 years (31,33), its nature and composition should fall shortly to innovative and creative approaches. Thus far three isotypic amyloidogenic variants of prealbumin have been reported (34). It is a possibility that there is more than one human SAA amyloidogenic isotype with different ones perhaps being found in different individuals. We should define if the different SAA subspecies are the result of the stimulus or are individual genetic variants, (10) for how does one explain the high incidence of amyloidosis found associated with tuberculosis: 50% (35), as compared to that in cystic fibrosis: 0.1% (36)?

4. Diagnosis

Some utility in non-invasively detecting amyloid deposits has been claimed for ^{99m}Tc-diphosphonate (37) presumably based on its capacity to react with calcium liganded to amyloid deposits, much as AP/SAP chelate amyloid bound calcium (27). However, biopsy is still the method of choice, (perhaps following ^{99m}Tc-diphosphonate localization) to define not only the presence of amyloid but also its chemical nature. Antibodies can be obtained for immunohistochemistry (38) to AA and pre-albumin proteins and many to AL type subgroups are available. Amyloid in metastatic medullary carcinoma can be detected with calcitonin antibodies. When specific antibodies become available to the various pre-albumin isotypes these conditions should also be sub-classifiable. Needless to say these immunohistochemical methods can be misinterpreted with mistaken identification of the amyloid protein being made (39) unless stringent techniques and controls are performed.

An ingenious method for the detection of prealbumin-30 in serum has been developed (40) which, because of its selectivity to the amino acid sequence of prealbumin-30, may not be applicable to other amyloidogenic serum proteins.

A whole new technology now makes an alternative method of diagnosis of amyloid diseases possible. Using recombinant DNA methodology, the gene for prealbumin-30 synthesis has been identified (41) and this can be used for _in vivo_ diagnosis. There is a likelihood that this approach may yield diagnostic methods for other amyloidoses once the amyloidogenic sequences of proteins in addition to that of the $AL_\lambda VI$ and the prealbumin isotypes are defined.

5. Treatment

The results of the prophylactic therapy (42) of the amyloidosis of familial Mediterranean fever (FMF) lends an optimistic note to the potentiality of therapy for other amyloidoses. If an animal model for each type of amyloidosis were available, the therapeutic search, as it was in FMF, might be easier. We still do not know how colchicine produces its prophylactic effect in FMF, unless by reducing the inflammatory component of the processes that induces the synthesis of an amyloidogenic SAA subgroup, perhaps genetically predetermined.

With a genetic predispositon assumed for the familial diseases, we still are not completely cognizant of the pathogenesis in all types of amyloidosis. Thus, approaches to potential treatment tend to be empiric at the least (Fig. 2).

One approach is to denature or remove the amyloid deposit. Although DMSO has been advocated and attempted for the acquired systemic amyloidoses (43), its efficacy is not yet clear (44) and its major drawback appears to be its pungent odor as it is excreted via the lungs. Perhaps other protein denaturants to which the body has high tolerance

THERAPY

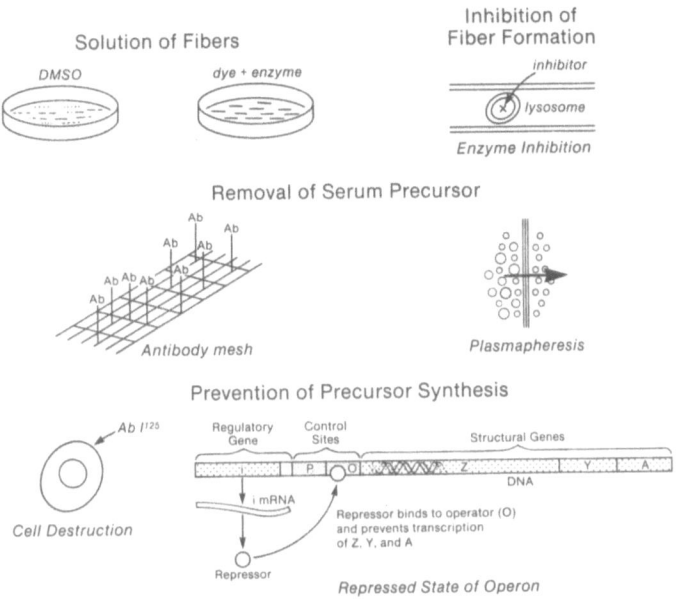

Figure 2: Approaches to the treatment of amyloidosis.

might be efficacious. The potential exists of attaching a covalently-
-linked, broad spectrum proteolytic enzyme, e.g. pronase, to a
relatively selective amyloid dye such as Congo red to produce proteolytic cleavage with time (45) of the fibers. This concept could be
modified by the use of an amyloid dye to a covalently-linked denatur-
ant.

Once the enzymes active in fiber formation in the AL type of
amyloidosis (and perhaps others) are known it may be possible to em-
ploy specific non-competitive or competitive inhibitors to prevent
proteolysis of the amyloidogenic precursor protein. This would appear
to be a highly viable approach to inhibit fiber formation.

To remove the serum precursor plasmapheresis has been employed
(46) with few satisfactory results (perhaps since it represents only a
partial serum depletion). Akin to this approach is the potential use of
specific antibodies to amyloid serum protein precursors attached covalently to synthetic meshes (47). In theory the bound amyloidogenic
protein could be eluted and removed and the antibody activity, regen-
erated.

Prevention of the synthesis of the amyloidogenic precursor could be approached in at least two ways. Both are current approaches being used in cancer chemotherapy. The first is to produce monoclonal antibodies to the plasma membrane of the cell of origin of the protein and destroy the cell using specific radiolabelled cytotoxic monoclonal antibodies (48). A cell-specific cytotoxic drug also is feasible and has been used, e.g. Melphalan with prednisone, and has had significant results with some subgroups of AL patients (49,50). Obviously these are feasible only if the cell in question is not essential to the body's economy.

Another approach to prevent protein synthesis is the use of specific gene repressors which by binding to the operator site prevent transcription. We are unaware of this approach to therapy having thus far been studied extensively.

Perhaps the focus on therapy in amyloidosis will increase sharply as the staggeringly large number of victims (3 million in the USA) of Alzheimer's disease acts as an impetus. The rewards of successful treatment would be enormous in terms not only of lives, but also in terms of entire families saved (51).

References

1. Virchow, R. Cellular Pathology (F. Chance, transl.) Lippincott, Philadelphia, 511, 1863.
2. Cohen, A.S. International Review of Experimental Pathology, Richter, C.W., Epstein, M.A., Eds. Academic Press, New York, 4, 159-243, 1965.
3. Snapper, I. & Kahn, A. Myelomatosis Fundamentals and Clinical Features, University Park Press, Baltimore, 380, 1971.
4. Heller, H., Gafni, J. & Sohar, E. In The Metabolic Basis of Inherited Disease, 2nd Edition. Stanbury, J.G., Wyngaarden, J.B., Fredrickson, D.S., Eds. McGraw-Hill, New York, 995-1014, 1966.
5. Spiro, D. Am. J. Pathol. 35, 47-73, 1959.
6. Cohen, A.S. & Calkins, F. Nature 183, 202-1203, 1959.
7. Eanes, E.D. & Glenner, G.G. J. Histochem. Cytochem. 16, 673-677, 1968.
8. Glenner, G.G., Harbaugh, J., Ohms, J.I., et al. Biochem. Biophys. Res. Commun. 41, 1287-1289, 1970.
9. Glenner, G.G., Terry, W., Harada, M., et al. Science 172, 115--1151, 1971.
10. Glenner, G.G. New Engl. J. Med. 302, 1283-1292, 1980.
11. Glenner, G.G., Eanes, E.D. & Page, D.L. J. Histochem. Cytochem. 20, 821-826, 1972.
12. Glenner, G.G., Eanes, E.D., Bladen, H.A., et al. J. Histochem. Cytochem. 22, 1141-1158, 1974.
13. Harada, M., Isersky, C., Cuatrecasas, P., et al. J. Histochem. Cytochem. 19, 1-15, 1971.
14. Kirschner, D.A., Abraham, C.A. & Selkoe, D.J. Proc. Natl. Acad. Sci. USA 82, 1-5, 1985.
15. Kidd, M. Nature 197, 192-193, 1963.
16. Shirahama, T. & Cohen, A.S. J. Cell. Biol. 33, 679-708, 1967.
17. Glenner, G.G., Ein, D., Eanes, E.D., et al. Science 174, 712-714, 1971.
18. Glenner, G.G., Ignaczak, T.F. & Page, D.L. In Metabolic Basis of Inherited Diseases, 4th Edition. Stanbury, J.G., Wyngaarden, J.B., Fredrickson, D.S., Eds. McGraw-Hill, New York, 1308-1339, 1978.
19. Dwulet, F.E., Strako, K. & Benson, M.D. In Amyloidosis. Glenner, G.G., Osserman, E.F., Benditt, E.P., Calkins, E., Cohen, A.S., Zucker-Franklin, D., Eds. Plenum Press, New York, 497-502, 1986.
20. Dwulet, F.E. & Benson, M.D. Proc. Natl. Acad. Sci. USA 81, 694-698, 1984.
21. Rosenthal, C.J. & Franklin, E.C. J. Clin. Invest. 55, 746-753, 1975.
22. Arapakis, G. & Tribe, C.R. Ann. Rheum. Dis. 22, 256-262, 1963.
23. Anders, R.F., Natvig, J.B., Sletten, K., et al. J. Immunol. 118, 229-234, 1977.
24. Bausserman, L.L., Saritelli, A.L., Herbert, P.N., et al. Biochim. Biophys. Acta 704, 556-559, 1982.
25. Hoffman, J.S., Ericsson, L.H., Eriksen, N., et al. J. Exp. Med. 159, 641-646, 1984.
26. Cathcart, E.S., Skinner, M. & Cohen, A.S. Immunology 20, 945-954, 1971.

27. Pepys, M.B., Baltz, M.L., Dyck, R.F., et al. In Amyloid and Amyloidosis. Glenner, G.G., Costa, P.P., Freitas A.F., Eds. Excerpta Medica, Amsterdam, 373-383, 1980.
28. Ram, J.S., DeLellis, R.A. & Glenner, G.G. Int. Arch. Allergy Appl. Immunol. 34, 269-282, 1968.
29. Hind, C.R.K., Collins, P.M., Caspi, D., et al. In Amyloidosis. Glenner, G.G., Osserman, E.F., Benditt, E.P., Calkins, E., Cohen, A.S., Zucker-Franklin, D., Eds. Plenum Press, New York, 233-238, 1986.
30. Yen, S.H., Crowe, A. & Dickson, D.W. Am. J. Pathol. 120, 282-291, 1985.
31. Selkoe, D.J. & Abraham, C. In Amyloidosis. Glenner, G.G., Osserman, E.F., Benditt, E.P., Calkins, E., Cohen, A.S., Zucker-Franklin, D., Eds. Plenum Press, New York, 709-715, 1986.
32. Osserman, E.F., Carrfield, R.E. & Beychak, S. Lysozyme Conference. Academic Press, New York, 641, 1974.
33. Shelanski, M.L., Albert, S., De Vries, G.H., et al. Science 174, 1242-1244, 1971.
34. Castro, C.W., Ball, R.D., Smith, E.M., et al. Clin. Res. 34, 704A, 1986.
35. Pirani, C. In Amyloidosis. Wegelius, O., Pasternack, A., Eds. Academic Press, New York, 33-49, 1976.
36. Canciani, M., Pederzini, F., Mastella, G., et al. Acta Paediat. Scand. 74, 613-614, 1985.
37. Janssen, S., Van Rijswijk, M.H., Piers, D.A., et al. Eur. J. Nucl. Med. 9: 538-541, 1985.
38. Fujihara, S., Balow, J.E., Costa, J.C. et al. Lab. Invest. 43, 358-365, 1980.
39. Shirahama, T., Skinner, M. & Westermark, P. Am. J. Pathol. 107, 41-50, 1982.
40. Nakazato, M., Kangawa, K., Ninamino, N., et al. Biochem. Biophys. Res. Commun. 122, 712-718, 1984.
41. Sasaki, H., Sakaki, Y., Matsuo, H., et al. Biochem. Biophys. Res. Commun. 125, 636-642, 1984.
42. Ravid, M., Robson, M. & Kedar(Keizman), I. Ann. Intern. Med. 87, 568-570, 1977.
43. Osserman, E.F., Sherman, W.H. & Kyle, R.A. In Amyloid and Amyloidosis. Glenner, G.G., Costa, P.P., Freitas, A.F., Eds. Excerpta Medica, Amsterdam, 563-569, 1980.
44. Van Rijswijk, M.H., Ruinen, L., Donker, A.J.M., et al. In Amyloid and Amyloidosis. Glenner, G.G., Costa, P.P., Freitas, A.F., Eds. Excerpta Medica, Amsterdam, 570-577, 1980.
45. Kim, I.C., Franzblau, C., Shirahama, T., et al. Biochim. Biophys. Acta 181, 465-467, 1969.
46. Nicholls, A.J., Platts, M.M. & Triger, D.R. Br. Med. J. 287, 726, 1983.
47. Trevan, M.D. Immobilized Enzymes: An Introduction and Applications in Biotechnology, J. Wiley, New York, 138, 1980.
48. Accolla, R.S., Carrel, S. & Mach, J.P. Proc. Natl. Acad. Sci. USA 77, 563-566, 1980.
49. Buxbaum, N.J., Hurley, M.E. & Chuba, J. Am. J. Med. 67, 868-878, 1979.
50. Kyle, R.A, Wagoner, R.D. & Holley, K.E. Arch. Intern. Med. 142, 1445-1447, 1982.
51 Glenner, G.G. In Senile Dementia of the Alzheimer's Type. Hutton, T.J., Kenny, A.D., Eds. Alan R. Liss, New York (In press).

CONTRIBUTORS

CONTRIBUTORS

ALLSOP, D.A.   VI.2
Dept of Pathology,
Univ of California, School of Medicine,
La Jolla, California 92093, U.S.A.

ANDEL, A.C.J. van   IV.9, 1V.10
Dept of Vet Pathology, University of Utrecht,
P.O. Box 80.158, 3508 TD Utrecht, The Netherlands.

ARAKI, S.   V.2
Kumamoto University Medical School,
First Dept of Internal Medicine,
1-1-1, Honjo, Kumamoto 860, Japan.

BAUSSERMAN, L.L.   VII.6
The Miriam Hospital,
164 Summit Avenue, Providence, Rhode Island 02906, U.S.A.

BEER, F.C. de   IV.3
Dept of Internal Medicine, University of Stellenbosch,
Posbus 63, Tygerberg, 7505 South Africa.

BENDITT, E.P.   IV.1
Dept of Pathology,
University of Washington,
Seattle, Washington 98195, U.S.A.

BEYREUTHER, K.   IV.7
Institute of Genetics, University of Cologne,
Fed Republic of Germany.

BOUDREAU, L.   VII.2
Dept of Pathology, Queen's University,
Kingston General Hospital,
Kingston, Ontario, Canada K7L 3N6.

CATHCART, E.S.   VII.9
E.N. Rodgers Memorial Veterans Hospital,
200 Springs Road, Bedford, MA 01730, U.S.A.

COE, J.E.   VII.7
National Institutes of Health, Lab of Persistent Viral Diseases,
Rocky Mountain Laboratories,
Hamilton, Montana 59840, U.S.A.

COETZEE, G.A.   IV.3
UCT/MRC Muscle Research Unit,
Dept of Medical Biochemistry University of Cape Town,
Cape Town, South Africa.

COHEN, A.S.   I.1, II.5, III.3
Arthritis Center, K-5,   III.4, VII.1
Boston University School of Medicine,
71 East Concord Street, Boston, MA 02118, U.S.A.

COLTEN, H.R.   IV.2
Washington University School of Medicine,
Children's Hospital,
400 S. Kingshighway Blvd., St. Louis, Missouri 63110, U.S.A.

CROWTHER, R.A.   IV.8
Medical Research Council, Lab of Molecular Biology,
Hills Road, Cambridge CB2 2QH, England.

DOWTON, S.B.   IV.2
Washington University School of Medicine,
Children's Hospital,
400 S Kingshighway Blvd., St. Louis, Missouri 63110, U.S.A.

Contributors

FALK, R.   III.2
Arthritis Center K-5,
Boston University School of Medicine,
71 East Concord Street, Boston, MA 02118, U.S.A.

FUKS, A.   VII.5
Dept of Medicine, N.Y. University Medical Center,
550 First Avenue, New York, NY 10016, U.S.A.

FURUYA, H.   V.3
Lab for Genetic Information, Kyushu University,
Fukuoka 812, Japan.

GLENNER, G.G.   VI.1, VIII.1
University of California, School of Medicine,
Dept of Pathology (M-012),
La Jolla, California 92093, U.S.A.

GRUYS, E.   IV.9, IV.10
Dept of Vet Pathology, University of Utrecht,
Postbus 80.158, 3508 TD Utrecht, The Netherlands.

HAYES, K.C.   VII.9
Geriatric Research Center,
E.N. Rogers Memorial Vet Adm Hospital,
200 Springs Road, Bedford, MA 01730, U.S.A.

HEM, G.K. van der   III.1
Dept of Internal Medicine, Div of Nephrology,
University Hospital,
Oostersingel 59, 9713 EZ Groningen, The Netherlands.

HIGUCHI, K.   VI.7, VII.3
National Institutes of Health,
NHLBI, MBD Bldg 10, Room 7N117,
Bethesda, Maryland 20892, U.S.A.

HOL, P.R.   IV.10
Dept of Vet Pathology, University of Utrecht,
Postbus 80.158, 3508 TD Utrecht, The Netherlands.

HUSBY, G.   II.1
Institute of Clinical Medicine, University of Tromsø
P.O.Box 977, N-9001 Tromsø, Norway.

JANSSEN, S.   III.1
Dept of Internal Medicine, University Hospital,
Oostersingel 59, 9713 EZ Groningen, The Netherlands.

KANGAWA, K.   V.3
Dept of Biochemistry, Miyazaki Medical College,
Kiyotake, Miyazaki 889-168, Japan.

KISILEVSKY, R.   VII.2
Queen's University, Dept of Pathology,
Kingston, Ontario, Canada K7L 3N6.

KURIHARA, T.   V.3
Third Dept of Medicine,
Miyazaki Medical College,
Kiyotake, Miyazaki 889-168, Japan.

LAHTI, D.   VII.9
Geriatric Research Center,
E.N. Rogers Memorial Vet Adm Hospital,
200 Springs Road, Bedford, MA 01730, U.S.A.

LESLIE, C.A.   VII.9
Geriatric Research Center,
E.N. Rogers Memorial Vet Adm Hospital,
200 Springs Road, Bedford, MA 01730, U.S.A.

Contributors

LUTZ, B.T.G.   IV.9
Dept of Vet Pathology, University of Utrecht,
Postbus 80.158, 3508 TD Utrecht, The Netherlands.

MARRINK, J.
Dept of Internal Medicine, Div of Immunochemistry,
University Hospital,
59 Oostersingel, 9713 EZ Groningen, The Netherlands.

MASTERS, C.L.   IV.7
Royal Perth Hospital, Dept of Neuropathology,
Box X2213, G.P.O.Perth, Western-Australia 6001.

MATSUKURA, S.   V.3
Third Dept of Medicine, Miyazaki Medical College,
Kiyotake, Miyazaki 889-168, Japan.

MATSUO, H.   V.3
Dept of Biochemistry, Miyazaki Medical College,
Kiyotake, Miyazaki 889-168, Japan.

McADAM, K.P.W.J.   VII
London School of Hygiene & Tropical Medicine,
University of London,
Keppel Street, London WC1E 7HT, England.

MEIJER, S.   III.1
Dept of Internal Medicine, Div of Nephrology,
University Hospital,
Oostersingel 59, 9713 EZ Groningen, The Netherlands.

MESSING, M.W.J.   IV.9
Dept of Vet Pathology, University of Utrecht,
Postbus 80.158, 3508 TD Utrecht, The Netherlands.

MEYDANI, S.M.   VII.9
Geriatric Research Center,
E.N. Rogers Memorial Vet Adm Hospital,
200 Springs Road, Bedford, MA 01730, U.S.A.

MUCKLE, T.J.   VI.6
Laboratories Chedoke McMaster Hospitals
P.O. Box 2000, Station A, Hamilton, Ont. L8N 3Z5, Canada.

NAKAZATO, M.   V.3
Miyazaki Medical College, The Third Dept of Medicine,
5200 Kihara, Kiyotake Miyazaki 009 16, Japan.

NIEWOLD, Th.A.   IV.9, IV.10
Dept of Vet Pathology, University of Utrecht,
Postbus 80.158, 3508 TD Utrecht, The Netherlands.

PEPYS, M.B.   II.4, IV.4
Royal Postgraduate Medical School,
Hammarsmith Hospital,
Immunological Medicine Unit,
Ducane Road, London W12 OHS, England.

PRAS, M.   V.1
Department of Medicine,
Tel-Hashomer Hospital,
52 621 Tel-Aviv, Israel.

RAMADORI, G.   VII.4
First Dept of Internal Medicine,
Mainz, Fed Rep of Germany.

RIJSWIJK, M.H. van   III.1
Dept of Internal Medicine, Div of Rheumatology,
University Hospital,
Oostersingel 59, 9713 EZ Groningen, The Netherlands.

369

Contributors

RUINEN, L. III.1
Dept of Internal Medicine,
University Hospital,
Oostersingel 59, 9713 EZ Groningen, The Netherlands.

RYAN, L.M. VI.5
Rheumatology Section, Dept of Medicine,
Medical College of Wisconsin,
MCMC Box 118,
8700 West Wisconsin Avenue, Milwaukee, WI 53226 U.S.A.

SAKAKI, Y. V.3
Lab for Genetic Information,
Kyushu University,
Fukuoka 812, Japan.

SASAKI, H. V.3
Lab for Genetic Information,
Kyushu University,
Fukuoka, 812 Japan.

SHIRAHAMA, T. II.5, III.3
Boston University School of Medicine, III.4, VII.1
Arthritis Center K-5,
71 East Concord Street, Boston, MA 02118, U.S.A.

SIPE, J.D. VII.4
Boston University School of Medicine,
Arthritis Center K-5,
71 East Concord Street, Boston, MA 02118, U.S.A.

SKINNER, M. III.3, III.4
Boston University School of Medicine,
Arthritis Center K-5,
71 East Concord Street, Boston, MA 02118, U.S.A.

SLETTEN, K. II.1, II.2
Biokjemisk Institutt, Universitetet i Oslo, VI.4
Postboks 1041, Blindern 0316, Oslo 3, Norway.

SNOW, A.D. VII.2
Dept of Pathology, Queen's University,
Kingston General Hospital,
Kingston, Ontario, Canada K7L 3N6.

SUBRAHMANYAN, L. VII.2
Dept of Pathology, Queen's University,
Kingston General Hospital,
Kingston, Ontario, Canada K7L 3N6.

TAKEDA, T. VI.7, VII.3
Kyoto University, Chest Disease Research Institute,
Sakyo-Ku (606), Kyoto, Japan.

TAN, R. VII.2
Dept of Pathology, Queen's University,
Kingston General Hospital,
Kingston, Ontario, Canada K7L 3N6.

TURNELL, W. IV.4
Royal Postgraduate Medical School,
Hammersmith Hospital,
Immunological Medicine Unit,
Ducane Road, London W12 OHS, England.

WESTERMARK, P. II.3, VI.3
University Hospital, Dept of Pathology, VI.4, VII.8
S-75185 Uppsala, Sweden.

Contributors

WESTHUYZEN, D.R. van der   IV.3
UCT/MRC Muscle Research Unit,
Dept of Medical Biochemistry, University of Cape Town,
Cape Town, South Africa.

WISCHIK, C.M.   IV.8
Cambridge Brain Bank Laboratory,
Addenbrooke's Hospital,
Hills Road, Cambridge CB2 2QQ, England.

WONG, C.W.   VI.1
University of California School of Medicine,
Dept of Pathology (M-012),
La Jolla, CA 92093, U.S.A.

WOO, P.   IV.5
Clinical Research Centre,
Division of Rheumatology,
Watford Road, Harrow, Middlesex HA1 3UJ, England.

YAMAMOTO, K.   IV.6
Kanazawa University,
Cancer Research Institute 13-1,
Takara-Machi, Kanazawa, Ishikawa 920, Japan.

ZUCKER-FRANKLIN, D.   VII.5
New York University Medical Center,
550 First Avenue, New York, NY 10016, U.S.A.

SUBJECT INDEX

Subject Index